FORGOTTEN

Forgotten

Narratives of Age-Related Dementia and Alzheimer's Disease in Canada

MARLENE GOLDMAN

McGill-Queen's University Press

Montreal & Kingston · London · Chicago

© McGill-Queen's University Press 2017

ISBN 978-0-7735-5092-6 (cloth)
ISBN 978-0-7735-5093-3 (paper)
ISBN 978-0-7735-5227-2 (ePDF)
ISBN 978-0-7735-5228-9 (ePUB)

Legal deposit fourth quarter 2017
Bibliothèque nationale du Québec

Printed in Canada on acid-free paper that is 100% ancient forest free
(100% post-consumer recycled), processed chlorine free

This book has been published with the help of a grant from the Canadian
Federation for the Humanities and Social Sciences, through the Awards
to Scholarly Publications Program, using funds provided by the Social
Sciences and Humanities Research Council of Canada.

McGill-Queen's University Press acknowledges the support of the
Canada Council for the Arts for our publishing program. We also
acknowledge the financial support of the Government of Canada
through the Canada Book Fund for our publishing activities.

Library and Archives Canada Cataloguing in Publication

Goldman, Marlene, 1963–, author
    Forgotten: narratives of age-related dementia and Alzheimer's disease
in Canada / Marlene Goldman.

Includes bibliographical references and index.
Issued in print and electronic formats.
ISBN 978-0-7735-5092-6 (hardcover). – ISBN 978-0-7735-5093-3
(softcover). – ISBN 978-0-7735-5227-2 (ePDF). –
ISBN 978-0-7735-5228-9 (ePUB)

    1. Dementia – Social aspects. 2. Alzheimer's disease – Social aspects.
3. Diseases in literature. 4. Old age in literature. 5. Mental illness
in literature. I. Title.

RC521.G64 2017   306.4'61   C2017-904248-3
                                                  C2017-904249-1

This book was typeset by Marquis Interscript in 10.5 / 13 Sabon.

Contents

Acknowledgments

I began to research in the area of mental illness and Alzheimer's disease in 2008, and I owe a tremendous debt of gratitude to my husband, Bob, and my children, Luke and Emma, for giving me the time and support to see this project to its fruition.

My friends and colleagues at the University of Toronto at Scarborough and the graduate English Department – Andrew DuBois, Michael Lambek, Lora Carney, Russell Brown, Donna Bennett, Linda Hutcheon, Jill Matus, Malcolm Woodland, Neil ten Kortenaar, Naomi Morgenstern, Lawrence Switzky, Eleanor Cook, and Alice Maurice – provided excellent advice and ongoing support. Michael Lambek kindly invited me to participate in his PhD thesis seminar on medical anthropology and he also introduced me to fellow anthropologists Paul Antze, Zoe Wool, and Margaret Lock, who offered helpful resources and guidance. When I hit on the idea of researching and writing on pathological memory loss, I was extremely fortunate to meet and work with Andrea Charise. Together with Linda and Michael Hutcheon, Andrea and I hosted an international conference, "Aging, Old Age, Memory, and Aesthetics," at the University of Toronto in 2011. We also co-edited a special issue of Stanford's online journal *Occasion* in 2012. The ongoing working groups on aging sponsored by the Jackman Humanities Institute (JHI) at the University of Toronto since 2010 have also been wonderfully inspiring, and I am very grateful to the JHI and to the members of these groups. Particular thanks go to Larry Switzky who shares my passion for age studies and aesthetics. Together, in 2015, we co-hosted the international conference, "Playing Age" and we also co-edited a special issue of *Modern Drama* on age studies and theatre, published in 2016.

I also want to thank my graduate students at the University of Toronto. From 2012 to 2014, students who took my class "Pathological Forgetting in Canadian Literature" joined me in exploring representations of dementia in a host of literary and filmic narratives. It was a delight to co-write an article with Sarah Powell on Alice Munro's and Sarah Polley's treatment of dementia. I consider myself very fortunate to be able to share my ideas with Katherine Shwetz, Katie Mullins, Michael Collins, Gillian Bright, and Angelo Murreda. I have also greatly benefitted from the help of Russell Bent, Aynsely Moorhouse, Max Karpinski, Norah Franklin, and Sarah de Jong Carson, who researched and edited chapters of my book.

As one might expect, the research for this book took me beyond the University of Toronto. I am grateful to the specialists in nineteenth-century Canadian writing – Ceilidh Hart, Jody Mason, Carole Gerson, Jennifer Henderson, Misao Dean, Janice Fiamengo, and Andrea Cabajsky – who enthusiastically responded to my email queries and directed me to fascinating examples of pathological forgetting in early Canadian literature. I am also thankful to Heather Gardiner and Nancy MacArthur, who graciously provided me with an introduction to the Alzheimer's Society of Ontario and supported my research into the early days of the organization at the local and national levels. I also want to thank Andrew Ignatieff and Lori Dessau, who agreed to be interviewed about their experience with the Alzheimer's Society. Medical historians David Wright and Edward Shorter also generously provided insight and support along the way. I was lucky to be able to work closely with Renee Saucier, a medical historian and highly accomplished editor. I also benefitted greatly from the encouragement and advice of scientists and clinicians, many of whom work in the areas of geriatric medicine and dementia, including Gary Naglie, Michael Gordon, Ruth Goldman, Carol Loffelmann, Rosemary Fitzgerald, Peter Whitehouse, Tiffany Chow, David Conn, Jason Karlawish, and Sandra Black.

Many of the ideas in this book were first presented as conference papers and brief articles. I want to express my gratitude to my colleagues and friends who invited me to speak and to publish articles on my research. I owe a huge debt to my age studies colleagues and friends – Stephen Katz, Amelia DeFalco, Kim Sawchuk, Josie Dolan, Sally Chivers, Barbara Marshall, Michelle Massé, Erin Lamb, Leni Marshall, Cynthia Port, Kate de Madeiros, Pia Kontos, Julia Gray, Elinor Fuchs, Margaret Morganroth Gullette, Roberta Maierhofer,

Ulla Kriebernegg, and Aagje Swinnen – who have welcomed me with open arms into the vibrant and supportive community of scholars and activists associated with the North American Network of Age Studies (NANAS), the European Network of Age Studies (ENAS) and Aging, Communication and Technology (ACT). My research on Munro, dementia, and surrealism – which formed the basis for chapter nine – was inspired by marathon conversations with Paul Higgs at the inaugural ACT meeting in Montreal in 2014; an essay based on this research was later carefully edited by Paul Higgs and Chris Gilleard for publication both as an article and in the Sociology of Health and Illness's monograph on *Ageing, Dementia and the Social Mind.* I am also thankful to Stephen Katz for giving me the opportunity to air the early results of my research on Munro and surrealism at his interdisciplinary conference on mild cognitive impairment at Trent University in 2015 – one of the most inspiring conferences I have ever attended. I remain in debt to the age-wise scholars and staff at Trent, particularly Sally Chivers, Jeannine Crow, Suzanne England, May Chazan, and Mark Skinner for their ongoing support and enthusiasm for my interdisciplinary research.

I also want to thank the editors of journals and book chapters as well as the anonymous reviewers who helped me to sharpen my ideas and my prose. In my conclusion, the analysis of the apocalyptic narrative elements in David Chariandy's and Sheila Watson's novels benefitted from Aagje Swinnen's and Mark Shweda's very helpful suggestions. My examination of John Mighton's *Half Life*, also in the conclusion, was likewise sharpened by the editorial expertise of Eleanor Ty and Cynthia Sugars. The exploration of Munro's "The Bear Came over the Mountain" in chapter nine was greatly aided by the anonymous reviewers and by Laura Moss, editor of *Canadian Literature*.

I also want to thank early readers of discrete chapters in my book – friends and colleagues who took time from their work and busy lives to help me clarify my arguments – Lora Carney, Russell Brown, Danielle Torbay, Eleanor Cook, Mark Abley, and Cielidh Hart. I would also like to thank the anonymous readers who vetted the book for McGill-Queen's University Press; their enthusiasm for the project and their detailed and inspired suggestions improved the book tremendously. I am particularly grateful to Kathryn Simpson for her skill as a copy editor. My intellectual and emotional lifeline through this book is, as always, my dear friend and steadfast editor,

Kristina Kyser. I continue to cherish and rely on her patience, courage, and intellectual rigour.

Excerpts from earlier versions of chapter nine and the conclusion appeared in journals issued by *Canadian Literature* and in books published by Oxford University Press, Wiley Press, and Bielefeld. I am grateful for permission to publish revisions of the following essays: "Gothic and Apocalyptic Portrayals of Dementia in Canadian Fiction," in *Popularizing Dementia: Public Expressions and Representations of Forgetfulness*, Aging Studies series, eds A. Swinnen and M. Schweda, Bielefeld, 69–88; "'Their Dark Cells': Transference, Memory, and Postmemory in John Mighton's *Half Life*" in *Canadian Literature and Cultural Memory*, eds Eleanor Ty and Cynthia Sugars, Oxford University Press, 118–33; "Reimagining Dementia in the Fourth Age: The Ironic Fictions of Alice Munro," in *Ageing, Dementia and the Social Mind*, Sociology of Health and Illness monograph series, eds C. Gilleard and P. Higgs, Wiley, 285–302; "Alzheimer's, Ambiguity, and Irony: Alice Munro's 'The Bear Came over the Mountain' and Sarah Polley's *Away from Her*," co-written with Sarah Powell, in *Canadian Literature* 225 (Summer 2015): 82–99.

FORGOTTEN

INTRODUCTION

Why Apocalypse Now?

Novelists, poets, and dramatists play a profound role in any period's understandings of illness and disease. The idea that fiction, more than medicine, is responsible for shaping our concepts of disease[1] is central to the analysis of Canadian biomedical, media, and literary depictions of age-related dementia and Alzheimer's disease in this book. My engagement with Alzheimer's began when I was writing *DisPossession: Haunting in Canadian Fiction* (2012). As I learned from my historical research on the relationships among haunting, trauma, and hysteria in early modern Europe, accusations of witchcraft and demonic possession gradually gave way to medical explanations and diagnoses of "dotage" or "hysteria" (Cohen, *No Aging* 72–4). In the nineteenth century, during the "great age of confinement" (see Katz, *Cultural* 37–52), clinicians simultaneously classified two seminal forms of pathological memory loss – hysteria and Alzheimer's disease.[2] Hysteria emerged as the emblematic ailment of the nineteenth century. When fears of hysteria waned, society became preoccupied by the threat of tuberculosis, then cancer, and in the 1980s, AIDS. But now, according to the medical anthropologist Lawrence Cohen, we have entered an "Age of Alzheimer's" (*No Aging* 7). In 2000, Alzheimer's was hailed as the "disease of the century" (Thomas in Post 249).[3]

In *AIDS and Its Metaphors* (1989), Susan Sontag reflects on how in the 1980s AIDS eclipsed prior fears of cancer. As she explains, society has a tendency to identify a particular disease and align it with evil: "In recent years some of the onus on cancer has been lifted by the emergence of a disease whose charge of stigmatization, whose capacity to create spoiled identity, is far greater. It seems that societies need to have one illness which becomes identified with evil, and attaches blame to its 'victim,' but it is hard to be obsessed with more than one" (*AIDS* 16). Just as AIDS eclipsed "the popular misidentification of cancer as an epidemic," I would argue that Alzheimer's has, following Sontag, "banalized" AIDS (*AIDS* 44).[4] Americans now fear Alzheimer's more than any other disease, even cancer, according to a survey from *MetLife*.[5] Equally critical, according to Sontag, the language of "epidemics" and "plagues" are the principal metaphors by which these "evil" diseases, most recently Alzheimer's, are understood (*AIDS* 44). The current "Age of Alzheimer's" is likewise characterized predominantly by fears of an epidemic of terrifying proportions.[6]

In his book *The Longevity Revolution* (2008), gerontologist Robert Butler explicitly warns that "unless we find ways to prevent or cure Alzheimer's and other severe dementing diseases, the world will shortly be confronted with epidemic proportions of these diseases" (121). The media also relies heavily on Gothic and apocalyptic metaphors to describe Alzheimer's. As Sontag explains, what she terms "master illnesses," including TB, cancer, AIDS – and, I would add, Alzheimer's – are invariably perceived as the "germ of death itself" (19). It is these types of fatal disease, Sontag argues, "thought to be multi-determined (that is, mysterious) that have the widest possibilities as metaphors for what is felt to be socially or morally wrong" (61). In other words, these mysterious illnesses inspire dread and, as Sontag reminds us, they are also categorized as "evil" (*AIDS* 16). Once categorized as morally wrong and horrifying, these illnesses are, in effect, transported into the territory of the Gothic – a literary mode that typically features monsters and monstrous transformations. At bottom, the meanings attributed to the suffering and loss instigated by "master illnesses" such as Alzheimer's disease – as well as the delegation of blame, culpability, and agency – are mediated through narrative and, more precisely, through literary modes such as the Gothic, which articulate the desires for the revelation of secrets and for mastery. Apocalyptic narratives, which prophesy the end of the world, feature terrifying plagues, and install divisions between the elect and the non-elect that are also popular ways in which to master fear and uncertainty.

The media frequently adopts a Gothic and apocalyptic perspective on Alzheimer's disease. An NBC report, entitled "Alzheimer's: The Silent Killer" (5 March 2014), for example, calls Alzheimer's "one of the deadliest diseases of our time," and warns that "the number of people affected by Alzheimer's – one of the most common forms of dementia – is growing rapidly." It then goes on to list a series of alarming facts:

1 An estimated 5.4 million Americans have the disease, according to the Alzheimer's Association;
2 Experts anticipate that number will grow to over 13 million by 2050;
3 Alzheimer's disease is the sixth leading cause of death in the U.S.,
4 It is the only cause of death that can't be prevented, cured, or slowed;
5 Every 68 seconds, another person contracts the crippling [sic] illness;
6 Exactly what causes Alzheimer's still has experts baffled.

Such facts and statistics, which are controversial and at times exaggerated, are repeatedly cited to convey the horrors associated with the Alzheimer's "epidemic."[7] This approach remains popular in spite of the fact that "in some countries and with certain patient groups," the epidemic may be slowing (Ingram 155).[8] Research has shown, in fact, that Alzheimer's rates are dropping in Britain, the US, Germany, Norway, and Sweden, but they are rising in poor nations.[9]

The question I want to ask is: why have narratives featuring epidemics and apocalyptic disasters enveloped discussions of what was once termed "senility"? Put differently, why would North Americans want to figure age-related cognitive impairment as a Gothic horror story? Brain injury and Parkinson's disease, both of which result in cognitive decline, are less feared than Alzheimer's. We do not treat people with mobility differences in this way.[10] Is there something about contemporary culture – what sociologists such as Stephen Katz term "neuro culture" (a term that reflects the role neuroimaging and brain sciences play in contemporary society) – that makes us obsessed with the brain and, more precisely, cognitive function and memory? Why, as many people with autism wonder, are we obsessed with the "neurotypical" rather than embracing "neurodiversity"?[11] What concerns a number of scholars, myself included, who have traced the increasing Gothic emphasis in society on memory, cognition, and attention, is that this focus on the brain reduces personhood to cognitive ability. We have stigmatized pathological memory loss to the extent that people feel as if a decline in cognitive function effaces their humanity.

Adding to the shame, Alzheimer's also supposedly threatens the security and prosperity of the nation. Picard notes the claim, by a London-based consumer group called Alzheimer's Disease International, that "35.6 million people worldwide are living with dementia and that the annual global cost of dementia has been pegged at $604 billion (US) – the equivalent of the revenues of the mega-corporations of Walmart and Exxon Mobil combined. If dementia were a country, it would be the 18th largest economy, ranking between Turkey and Indonesia" (A1). In the film adaptation of *The Forgetting*, based on David Shenk's best-selling book about Alzheimer's disease, Shenk likewise describes Alzheimer's as an epidemic: "We absolutely have to stop this disease," he says. "There's just no choice. As a nation, as an economy, as a civilization, we have to end it now" (in Basting, *Forget* 36). I cite these dire pronouncements not because they are accurate, but because they demonstrate that the public meaning of Alzheimer's is inextricably connected to notions of cost and value – ranging from the socio-economic to moral values and, at times, the very survival of the nation-state.

Rather than embrace a particular approach, this study analyzes a broad range of biomedical, media, and literary narratives associated with age-related dementia and Alzheimer's disease. My aim is to analyze both the use and the impact of the various narrative approaches to "express" – both in the sense of telling *and* expelling – the ambivalence and uncertainty that attends this mysterious illness (Jackson 4–5). Although my book analyzes the inflated rhetoric frequently used in discussions of Alzheimer's disease, I do acknowledge that the experience of dementia can be very hard. I know firsthand, as Anne Davis Basting insists, that Alzheimer's can "take a heavy emotional, physical, and financial toll on families" (*Forget* 39). My mother recently received a diagnosis of mild cognitive impairment. Although she was treated with remarkable kindness and respect by her geriatric psychiatrist, I witnessed how the label transformed her in the eyes of family members.

Like other dementia scholars such as Anne Davis Basting, Margaret Gullette, and Peter Whitehouse, I worry that our current fixation on pathological memory loss makes us forget that people diagnosed with Alzheimer's disease remain resilient and have enduring attributes. In *Agewise*, Gullette relates her experience of caring for her mother after the latter suffered cognitive decline due to a stroke. She tells the story of her repeated encounters with the director in the nursing home, who started to use the word "dementia" in relation to her mother (189). Rather than accept the director's insistent narrative of decline, Gullette focused instead on her mother's recent stellar Scrabble score and on her equally admirable qualities. As Gullette observes, "intelligence, logic, creativity, warmth, humor, empathy, imagination, and moral judgement, survive for a long time in people living along the whole spectrum of impairments" (179). One day, utterly exasperated, the director turned to Gullette and said furiously, "Your mother is *failing*!" As Gullette explains, "To her, my mother's strengths were irrelevant. Once embarked on the decline story, the reality instructors notice nothing else" (189). Sadly, this is a story many of us know too well. But what of the other stories? What narratives about dementia and Alzheimer's have been forgotten?

SECTION I: AN AGE STUDIES APPROACH TO ALZHEIMER'S DISEASE

The history of old age and its diseases is a fairly new field in Canada. Until the 1990s, Canadian scholars writing on old age typically presented top-down bureaucratic histories or focused on the present rather than the past (Dillon, *Shady* 9). Moreover as historian Thomas Cole notes, in the last fifteen years, scholars who have pioneered the new history of old age "have taken their basic orientation from the social and biomedical sciences, which generally view old age as an engineering problem to be solved or at least ameliorated" (xxi). In contrast to the social scientific and biomedical approaches, and in keeping with the work of contemporary social historians and age critics, my book offers an age studies approach to illness and relies on close readings of fictional and non-fictional narratives to bring an alternative perspective to bear on the experiences of aging and age-related dementia. As Elinor Fuchs explains: "Age Studies ... has emerged, since the 1990s, out of a resistance and an inspiration – resistance to accepting decline as the primary fact of advancing age, from early middle age on, and inspiration from the 'materialist' identity theories, especially the body-based theories of race and gender that have pierced the screen on biological determinism to expose cultural constructions of the self" ("Estragement" 69). I think Cole puts it best when he says, "growing up and old is not only a *process,* rooted in our biological existence, structured by social and historical circumstances. It is also an *experience*, an incalculable series of events, moments, and acts lived by an individual person" (xxxii). Whereas the process remains the purview of scientists and clinicians, the experience and its often elided and repressed features are the domain of writers. Literature is especially critical to age studies because biomedical narratives often ignore the texture of people's lives. As sociologist Stephen Katz asserts: "If we are to deal with aging, we have to imagine it first."[12] My decision to address the past and to consider narrative accounts thus aligns with a relatively recent phenomenon – part of a growing trend influenced by narrative theory "to render visible the previously invisible" (Dillon, *Shady* 15; see also Katz, *Cultural* 39).

British historian Pat Thane writes that old age – and, I would add, age-related dementia – "cannot simply be a social construct, an artifice of perception, or fashioned through discourse – unquestionably bodies age, change, decay – but the images, expectations, and experience of older men and women have been constructed in different ways at different times and for differing people at any one time" (5). Narratives are crucial to my study precisely because they offer insight into the "images, expectations, and experience" that have changed and, in many cases, been forgotten over time. To broaden the view of Alzheimer's disease and dementia beyond theoretical or biomedical terms, I explore the stories literary authors and journalists have told over the years about age-related dementia – stories that enable us to recognize it as not only a biological process but also a malleable, socially mediated experience.

In the spirit of prior studies that call into question the tightly woven threads that bind illness and metaphor, the aim of my book on Alzheimer's disease is "to calm the imagination, not to incite it" (Sontag, *AIDS* 14).[13] One way to do this is to look at how dementia (or "senility" as it was once termed) was viewed in the past. As a Canadian, I wanted to understand the history of dementia and Alzheimer's within Canada – a nation with its own unique history and healthcare system. Virtually all of the major critical analyses of aging, dementia, and Alzheimer's address the history and culture of the US and Britain. Even Canadian age critics frequently adopt an international approach.[14] By choosing to examine conceptions of age and age-related illnesses now and in the past in Canada, and by relying on an interdisciplinary methodology, my book uses what Gullette calls "the leverage of history – the whisper that 'everything can change'" (*Agewise* 17) – to question current narratives about

Alzheimer's and dementia in the Canadian nation-state. I see my book as complementing the excellent work of other age critics including Kathleen Woodward, Margaret Gullette, Stephen Katz, Elinor Fuchs, and Sally Chivers, who are likewise questioning what Gullette calls "decline narratives" – the name she gives to "the entire system that worsens the experience of aging past youth" (5).[15]

My work dovetails, in particular, with that of scholars who address narrative. Amelia DeFalco's *Uncanny Subjects* (2010), for example, analyzes uncanny narratives about old age. Basting's *Forget Memory* (2009) addresses the mass media's obsession with "tragic tales of dementia" (33), in the popular sense of "a sad story." As Basting explains, dementia is associated with two types of tragic stories – the first portrays dementia as "a calamity that can only be eliminated if scientists are given enough time and money to find the cure" (ibid.). The second tells the story of "the loss of an accomplished, inspiring person ... slowly emptied out by a devastating illness" (ibid.). Basting supplants these decline narratives with more positive accounts featuring innovative programs that offer more ethical and person-centred care for people with dementia. In *The Silvering Screen* (2011), Sally Chivers explores the plots of recent mainstream films to show how they maintain the decline narrative while trying "to reduce old age to a manageable and controllable set of representations" (xviii).

While I share this focus on language and stories, my book investigates how narratives of dementia have shifted over time from the elegy to the Gothic. The elegy – a classical genre that long preceded the Gothic – traditionally attempts "to lament, contextualize and possibly grant larger and lasting meaning to a person (and occasionally a group) who has passed away" (Hogle, "Elegy" 565).[16] By contrast, Gothic fiction, which emerged in the mid-eighteenth century with the publication of Horace Walpole's *The Castle of Otranto* (1764), treats death as both a crime and a mystery that a "subsequent narrative works to explain, thus providing another avenue for contextualizing and finding meaning in primal loss" (ibid. 565–6). As I argue below, when applied to the medical framework, the Gothic promotes the identification of illness as unequivocally evil, and treats disease as a mystery and a crime to be solved. Ultimately, the purpose of this book is to help readers regard Alzheimer's and other forms of age-related dementia as if they were merely illnesses – serious ones, but "not a curse, not a punishment, not an embarrassment" (Sontag, *AIDS* 14).

To counter the alarmist and apocalyptic language associated with Alzheimer's disease as well as the prevailing stigma attached to people with Alzheimer's, my book investigates these narrative patterns. My book also turns to history to illuminate the great differences in stories that have been told about late-onset dementia and Alzheimer's disease in Canadian culture and fiction since the late nineteenth century. I am particularly fascinated by the emergence and ramifications of an ironic tension between what is normal and what is pathological, and an increasing reliance on Gothic and apocalyptic rhetoric in the vast range of stories that have circulated about Alzheimer's disease. Rather than offer an encyclopedic account of dementia narratives in Canada, I have selected a group of illustrative and innovative literary examples to explore how and why approaches to aging, old age, and dementia are implicitly and explicitly predicated on elegiac and, later, Gothic and apocalyptic narrative patterns and elements. My aim is to examine the types of narrative features used to describe Alzheimer's disease and to clarify their impact on our understandings of aging, old age, and dementia.

Why an Age Studies or Cultural (or Critical) Gerontology Approach?

In considering the role of literary studies and literature to the field of gerontology, Katz observes that gerontologists have always recognized the need to account for the reciprocal relationship between medicine and culture. He cites the introduction to Edmund Vincent Cowdry's edited volume of the foundational text in gerontology, *Problems of Ageing* (1939), in which John Dewey says: "We need to know the ways in which social contexts react back into biological processes as well as to know the ways in which the biological processes condition social life. This is the problem to which attention is invited" (in Katz, "What" n.p.). I would argue further that language – specifically, clusters of familiar metaphors and literary genres such as tragedy and the Gothic – constitutes the central medium for the ongoing interplay between biology and culture.

As a literary scholar who has joined the growing ranks of critical or cultural gerontologists – also known as age studies critics or age critics – focusing on Alzheimer's disease and dementia, I pay particular attention to language and genre. As the modifier "critical" in the title "critical gerontology" also suggests, I adopt a set of practices that as Katz reminds us "are associated with the Frankfurt School of critical theory, whose thinkers such as Max Horkheimer and Theodor Adorno emphasized theoretical reflexivity, not taking for granted the assumptions, principles and practices that any field of political agenda claims as its canonical heritage" (ibid.). In probing the history of Alzheimer's, my study also relies on what the philosopher Michel Foucault described as "the genealogical method," "a multidisciplinary technique for discovering the contingent historical trends that underpin contemporary society's structures, discourses, and practices" (Katz, *Cultural* 72). This method enables me to ask why "certain vocabularies, disciplinary approaches, and informed opinions took on the status of truth at specific historical junctures, while others were marginalized or disparaged" (ibid. 73). A genealogical analysis of Alzheimer's disease (AD) is useful because, currently, experts are questioning and reframing the category of Alzheimer's: "possible category fragmentation or reshuffling [is] ... in the air, making for a plethora of unknowns" (Lock 2).

Although age analysis is popular in the social sciences, currently there are fewer age critics in the humanities.[17] And yet the perspective afforded by humanities on questions of aging and age-related illnesses is particularly valuable because, as Katz points out, humanities-based age critics "are liberated from some of gerontology's disciplinary and scientific commitments" ("What" n.p.). My training in literary studies enables me to step back from authoritative and popular narratives about aging and age-related diseases to consider how they are narratively constructed, whose interests they serve, and, in some instances, to challenge their Gothic and apocalyptic pronouncements. Rather than simply accept stories that appear in medical journals or the media as the truth, I explore how their "truthiness" is generated by a familiar set of metaphors, rhetorical techniques, and generic conventions that shape popular and scientific models of aging and disease alike.

I began this work at a time when, as medical anthropologist Margaret Lock observes, technological innovations "had recently resulted in research findings that, together with remarkable epidemiological insights, were forcing researchers to confront head-on the ontological question of what exactly constitutes AD" (2). As a result, "acknowledgement that the AD phenomenon is deeply entangled with the very process of aging could no longer be conveniently set to one side, as had usually been the case to date, raising difficulties about what counts as normal and what as pathological" (3). The timing of my research also coincides with the fact that the first members of the baby boomer generation (the large cohort of persons born between 1946 and 1963) turned sixty-five – the standard definition of old age – in 2011.

To date, Alzheimer's disease has been the focus of research by bench scientists, clinicians, voluntary associations, and social scientists. An age studies approach – and, more precisely, a literary one – is called for to explain why, since the late 1970s, Gothic and apocalyptic metaphors have increasingly constellated around this "dread disease." A literary and historical approach can also shed light on controversies among researchers and on approaches to senile dementia that have been eclipsed by the dominant biomedical perspective. In the nineteenth and early twentieth centuries, for examples, doctors focused on diet, exercise, and education. Ultimately my study cautions against privileging one model over another. Instead I advocate using the one to illuminate the other; ultimately, my aim lies in transforming our experience of both.

Although literature plays a central role in my analysis, my project is interdisciplinary and also constitutes, in part, a medical history.[18] The chapters that follow trace Canadian society's shifting understanding of Alzheimer's disease from the 1860s to the present. To aid readers who might not be familiar with key medical terms, in section two below, I offer working definitions for Alzheimer's disease, dementia, age-related dementia, mild cognitive impairment, and related neurodegenerative diseases associated with Alzheimer's and dementia including Down syndrome and Parkinson's disease. By broadening the scope of my book to include stories featuring the latter, I am following the lead of other age studies critics such as Sally Chivers and Leni Marshal who argue for the need to bring age studies and disability studies into conversation. My ultimate goal in drawing connections between discrete forms of disability associated with Alzheimer's disease lies in showing how slippages between the search for a cure, euthanasia, and eugenics hover over Alzheimer's as they did over other forms of difference during and prior to the Second World War.

I refer to the information cited below as "working definitions" because despite the authoritative aura that hovers over biomedical labels, they remain cultural constructs and are fiercely contested. Like prior disease entities legitimized by biomedicine such as drapetomania,[19] the meanings attributed to Alzheimer's and related terms including dementia and mild cognitive impairment (MCI) remain in flux.

SECTION II: WORKING DEFINITIONS
AGE-ASSOCIATED MEMORY IMPAIRMENT

As the Alzheimer Society of Canada explains on its website: "Almost 40 per cent of people over the age of 65 experience some form of memory loss. When there is no underlying medical condition causing this memory loss, it is known as 'age-associated memory impairment,' which is considered a part of the normal aging process."[20] Despite their claim that there is a difference between pathological and normal or age-associated memory loss, several authoritative and famous studies have demonstrated that "there is, at best, a blurred line between normal cognition, mild impairment and full-on dementia – a declining straight line" (Ingram 123). Simply put, there is no clear distinction "between normal mental functioning and Alzheimer's" (122).

Dementia

The oldest known appearance of the term "dementia" – which is primarily a group of symptoms, rather than a disease – was in Roman texts, where it meant "being out of one's mind."[21] "Dementia" emerged as a legal concept in the seventeenth century and as a medical concept in the eighteenth century, when it was regarded as an end stage for various mental disorders and as "a synonym of madness."[22] At this time, dementia was not considered irreversible, linked to an age group, or used exclusively to refer to cognitive impairment;[23] rather, it broadly "referred to states of psychosocial incompetence of varied origin."[24]

During the nineteenth and early twentieth centuries, the concept of dementia was narrowed to "'the cognitive paradigm,' i.e. the view that the essential feature of dementia was intellectual impairment."[25] Dementias associated with insanity were reclassified, as were symptoms such as "hallucinations, delusions, and mood and behavioural disorders," while memory loss assumed conceptual importance.[26] A more "syndromatic" view of dementia, which entailed interpreting a group of symptoms as if they collectively indicated or characterized a disease, emerged as "states of cognitive impairment mostly affecting the elderly, and almost always irreversible."[27] "By 1900 'senile dementia'" – aging-related intellectual decline due to degeneration of the brain – "became the prototype of the dementias; by 1970, AD had become the flagship of the new approach."[28]

In contemporary usage, dementia is understood as "acquired cognitive impairment," that is, a range of symptoms including memory loss and impaired thought, sensory and language processes.[29] Causes include "more than 50 medical, psychiatric, and neurological conditions" that interfere with or damage the brain, of which Alzheimer's is reported as the leading cause among the elderly.[30] As Margaret Gullette argues, however, there are "many reasons to stop using the term 'dementia'"; for one, "it is useless as a differential diagnosis" (*Agewise* 195). Gullette cites Dr Vladimir Hachinski, who writes in the *Journal of the American Medical Association* that "the concept of dementia is obsolete. It combines categorical misclassification with etiological imprecision."[31]

Alzheimer's Disease

As Margaret Lock explains, there have been "repeated efforts to standardize an Alzheimer diagnosis – a task that continues to be extraordinarily difficult to achieve" (50). Contemporary scientists maintain that Alzheimer's disease is characterized by a fairly predictable pattern of tangle and plaque formation (within the hippocampus, the amygdala, and the deeper layers of the neocortex), whereas other forms of dementia may be more non-specific or have different distribution patterns; additionally, the disease is accompanied by extensive synaptic loss – loss of connections between nerve cells – whereas other dementias are not (see Perl). Alzheimer's disease is now recognized as the most common cause of dementia. The initial symptoms are often "impairment of recent memory and disorientation in time and space," progressing to impairment of overall cognitive function, impacting language, judgment, comprehension and abstract reasoning."[32] Progressive neurological degeneration ultimately leads to death over a course of years.[33]

The disease's etiology is uncertain, but early onset – before age sixty-five – has been attributed to mutations in three genes.[34] Early onset Alzheimer's accounts for up to 5 per cent of cases. With respect to age-related Alzheimer's, the risk of developing the disease increases steadily after age sixty-five, particularly for women, who "are affected twice as often as men."[35] Pharmaceutical treatments have been developed in an attempt to slow the disease's progression, but these have not proven effective. Treatment is mainly in the form of "nursing and social care" as the disease interferes with day-to-day life.

As Gullette observes, however, in addition to "the four subtypes of possible Alzheimer's, there are dementias of the Lewy body type, vascular cognitive impairments, frontotemporal [dementia], traumatic brain injury ... and 'cognitive impairment without dementia'" (*Agewise* 195). Moreover, many of these dementias appear in patients as mixed. Creating a singular disease does not do justice to the clinical complexity, and explains why neurologist and Alzheimer's researcher Peter Whitehouse refers to Alzheimer's disease as a "myth" (see *Myth*). Equally problematic, observations of caregivers in several settings have found that the disease carries with it a powerful stigma: "once the label Alzheimer's is applied, even normal behavior is interpreted in terms of disease 'stages' ... and few opportunities are provided to continue meaningful activity."[36]

Mild Cognitive Impairment (MCI)

MCI is a concept applied to individuals affected by "a measurable degree of cognitive impairment that does not meet the diagnostic criteria for dementia."[37] The concept has attracted increasing attention since the mid-1990s with continuous "uncertainty and lack of consensus about what it actually means."[38] The liminal term, used as a descriptor and set of symptoms, has existed alongside "more than a dozen terms referring to mild changes in elderly people's cognition."[39] In some cases, it "can refer to the early stages of other dementing disorders or conditions," including Alzheimer's disease, while in other cases it is ultimately a stable or even reversible condition, with various underlying causes.[40]

As in the case of the Alzheimer's diagnosis, there are also problems associated with using MCI as a label – problems that recall Sontag's insights about the ethical minefield surrounding testing people with AIDS to determine who harbours the virus:

The obvious consequence of believing that all those who "harbor" the virus will eventually come down with the illness is that those who test positive for it are regarded as people-with-AIDS, who just don't have it ... yet. It is only a matter of time, like any death sentence. Less obviously such people are often regarded as if they do have it ... Infected means ill, from that point forward. "Infected but not ill," that invaluable notion of clinical medicine (the body "harbors" many infections) is being superseded by

biomedical concepts which, whatever their scientific justification, amount to reviving the antiscientific logic of defilement, and
make infected-but-healthy a contradiction in terms. (AIDS 32)

In the case of MCI, unlike AIDS, there is no test for a discrete pathogen
and, as noted above, the condition can disappear – there is dementia
and there is also "amentia" (cognitive improvement) associated with
MCI. For this reason, Canadians are increasingly concerned with
the MCI diagnosis. Recently, an article cautioned that accepting the
new label "MCI" would allow "doctors to investigate and medicate
potentially healthy people and create needless fears"; the Canadian
medical system has also been urged to think carefully before adopting the US guidelines with respect to MCI because the latter advocate
treating potentially healthy people as if they have Alzheimer's and
using them as test subjects for drugs.[41]

Down Syndrome

Down syndrome is a "relatively common" genetic condition that in
nearly all cases results from a chromosomal anomaly: the presence of
three chromosomes in pair number 21 ("trisomy 21").[42] Individuals
with the syndrome experience typical physical and neurological symptoms including marked facial characteristics, hyperflexibility, organ
anomalies such as congenital heart defects, developmental delays,
and intellectual disability to varying degrees. There has long been
an observed association between Down syndrome and "advanced
maternal age."[43] Standard definitions of Alzheimer's disease note that
it is almost always associated with individuals with Down syndrome,
who "tend to demonstrate neuropathological findings consistent with
Alzheimer-type senile dementia."[44] Individuals with Down syndrome
have a far greater risk of developing Alzheimer's-like dementia, and
typically experience cognitive decline at an earlier age – in their forties and fifties.[45]

Parkinson's Disease

Parkinson's disease is "a slowly progressive degenerative neurological disorder generally occurring in later life involving tremor, rigid
muscles, slow movement, difficulties with balance, a distinctive walk,
and a 'masklike' face."[46] It is more common among men than women.

According to the Alzheimer's Association website, individuals with Parkinson's have a risk of developing dementia, typically later in the progression of the disease; as many as 80 per cent of people with Parkinson's will develop dementia. As the website states: "As Parkinson's brain changes gradually spread, they often begin to affect mental functions, including memory and the ability to pay attention, make sound judgments and plan the steps needed to complete a task."[47] Individuals with "Parkinson's disease dementia" also develop plaques and tangles – changes linked to Alzheimer's disease.[48]

Although I critique the inflammatory rhetoric Alzheimer's researchers, clinicians, and physicians sometimes use, my study has been greatly enriched by the insights and compassion of a group of clinicians and researchers who have helped guide this project and generously offered their expertise.[49] Fundamentally, my view of Alzheimer's does not contradict that of leading researchers. I understand that changes in the brain commonly glossed as dementia are undeniably real (see Lock 11). And I concur with researchers and clinicians that dementia has many causes, "some of which are well understood" (ibid.). Yet I would also suggest that, to a great extent, the threat posed by Alzheimer's to people's quality of life and to their sense of well-being (and that of their family) springs from the fact that the condition, first formally named as a disease in 1908, remains an enigma. As Lock observes, efforts have been repeatedly made to map the clinical and neuropathological features of Alzheimer's with the goal of finding a cure (1). Despite governments having poured billions of dollars into research over the past few decades, "scientists have not found a cure and, at present, only four drugs are available on prescription that variably alleviate symptoms for a period of some months, often with side effects, and by no means in all patients" (1). To date, there is neither a clear understanding of the cause of, nor a cure for, the disease. In fact, there is growing controversy – a controversy as old as the disease concept itself – as to whether Alzheimer's is even a disease or rather part of the process of aging. As prominent and well-respected Alzheimer's researcher Martin Samuel puts it: "If we lived long enough, would we all become demented, with plaques and tangles? Is Alzheimer's just another name for aging?" (in Groopman 42–3).

One of the most paradoxical elements that both early and more recent research into Alzheimer's disease has shown irrefutably is that large numbers of people with so-called Alzheimer's neuropathology in their brains never become demented in old age (see Groopman;

see also Ingram 99–126). This finding, which has been known for many decades, is now undeniable due to neuroimaging. Yet, as Jerome Groopman observes, it is ignored in the Alzheimer's research world, and no one can explain what it is that protects some people from dementia.

Due, in part, to its status as an enigma, Alzheimer's has become a screen for the projection of society's worst fears about aging and death. It has also served as an anxious site for exploring the fundamental difficulties inherent in distinguishing between what constitutes "normal" as opposed to "pathological" changes during later life. Equally relevant, the fact that the disease can be present but have few or no significant clinical symptoms undermines science's attempt to create a definitive map of the relationship between mind and body. This indeterminacy introduces complexities into biomedical discussions concerning old age and dementia that are often unacknowledged. It is precisely this link between mind and body, or between ideas and disease, that shapes my interest in the relationship among models of dementia and Alzheimer's, in particular.

SECTION III: THE PARAMETERS OF THE STUDY
THE TEMPORAL AND GEOGRAPHIC SCOPE

As medical historians observe, diseases such as Alzheimer's "demand an outsider's vantage point, and, oddly enough, our ancestors can furnish this perspective" (Ingram 10). For this reason, as noted above, my book is in part a medical history. In keeping with the practice of medical historians, for the most part, my project focuses on a specific geographic site and maintains a linear temporal arc. I begin in Europe during the nineteenth century and, more precisely, in Germany because this was where the disease concept was created. Chapter two shifts to Upper Canada – the predecessor of modern Ontario – in the 1850s because this was a key period and locus for asylum construction in Canada. I examine the rise of asylums because it is crucial for people to understand how older adults with dementia were initially transformed into patients within the newly built asylums – institutions that served as a foundation for later models of biomedical, state-supported care.[50]

To address the roots and the enduring legacy of the Gothic view of dementia, I consider connections between the writings of the English philosopher John Locke (1632–1704), the rise of asylums, and the

Canadian anti-asylum movement during the late 1960s. As I argue below, Locke's *Essay Concerning Human Understanding* (1689) laid the foundation for the Gothic view of dementia by creating a new class of beings, which Locke termed "idiots" and distinguished it from the category of "Man." By segregating people with mental illness from the rest of society, the asylum movement represents an extension of Locke's philosophy, which condemned "idiots" to a social death under British law. Although the anti-asylum movement in the late 1960s and 1970s liberated people from institutions and increased society's sympathy for individuals with cognitive and physical disabilities,[51] it failed to transform society's stigmatized, Gothic view of elderly people with dementia.

In keeping with my book's initial focus on Upper Canada, the popular and literary narratives under consideration, particularly in the early chapters, are restricted to eastern Canada. This selection is both pragmatic and advantageous because the region is central to Canada's cultural identity, medical advances, and economic force. As I explain in chapter five, owing to the intricate connections between researchers at the University of Toronto and grassroots activists, the story of the Alzheimer Society of Canada could only have happened in Toronto. In chapters eight and nine, I venture beyond Ontario to explore fiction written in Vancouver in the 1980s, which addresses crucial connections among the stigma associated with homosexuality, AIDS, and late-onset dementia.

The Literary Context – English Canadian Fiction

Since the publication of Margaret Laurence's *The Stone Angel* in 1964, Canadian writers have continued to produce some of the most compassionate and compelling accounts from any country of mental illness, age-related dementia, and Alzheimer's, including Mordecai Richler's *Barney's Version* (1997) and Alice Munro's story "The Bear Came over the Mountain" (*New Yorker*, 27 Dec 1999).[52] With the exception of chapter three, which analyzes fiction written from the early twentieth century to the 1960s, my book concentrates on texts from the 1980s to the present. Although Canadians wrote about mental illness during the 1960s and 1970s, in this youth-oriented period, they typically approached the topic from the perspective of people in the first half of the life course rather than the last. With the exception of Alice Munro, Canadian authors also tended to explore psychosis and schizophrenia rather than late-onset dementia.[53] Munro's work features prominently in my book because her short story collections, which immortalized the lives of the inhabitants of southwestern Ontario, portray a range of people with illnesses and disabilities throughout the life course. Characters in her early collections including *Dance of the Happy Shades* (1968), *Lives of Girls and Women* (1971), and *Who Do You Think You Are?* (1978) have cognitive and physical disabilities such as Parkinson's disease, Down syndrome, and Alzheimer's.[54]

In representing age-related dementia and Alzheimer's, Canadian literature powerfully engages with the historical and contemporary controversies surrounding dementia. Whereas biomedical and cultural discourses typically write about and not from within dementia, the works considered in this study – Caroline Adderson's *The History of Forgetting* (1999), Michael Ignatieff's *Scar Tissue* (1993), Stephen Leacock's *Sunshine Sketches of a Little Town* (1912), Alice Munro's short stories, Mordecai Richler's "The Summer My Grandmother Was Supposed to Die" (1969), and Jane Rule's *Memory Board* (1987) – convey what fiction portrays so well, namely, "res cogitans," the space of the mind, which cannot easily be illustrated in other discourses (Hutcheon, *Theory* 3). In essence, both biomedicine and literature offer models of pathological forgetting, but they must be taken together if the various representations these discourses produce are to help us understand and critique Western culture's evolving response to age-related dementia.

Since my goal lies in tracing the transformations in representations of dementia and Alzheimer's from the elegy to the Gothic in biomedical, popular, and literary narratives, I have selected texts in each category that best highlight these shifts over time. Rather than offer a comprehensive exploration of Canadian dementia narratives, I have chosen the most representative and, in some cases, the most innovative works I came across in the course of my research. All of the works I have selected highlight the tension between religious and scientific approaches to dementia. I focus primarily on fiction rather than poetry, drama, or film because, with a few exceptions, fiction best illustrates the metamorphosis from the elegy to the Gothic. Readers interested in learning more about imaginative treatments of dementia in Canadian culture are invited to consult the appendix, which provides as complete as possible a list of English-Canadian texts – films, plays, fiction, graphic novels, and poetry – that focus or touch on dementia.

As Kathleen Woodward observes in the preface to her important essay collection *Figuring Age* (1999), as early as 1976 the American historian Andrew Achenbaum was concerned with the lack of "heterogeneity of aging" in his research (xxiii). Woodward concedes that diversity is likewise lacking in her collection. This remains true in the case of this book. With the exception of David Chariandy's novel *Soucouyant*, the texts under consideration approach the experience of Alzheimer's and dementia from a predominantly white perspective. Although sociologists and anthropologists such as Lawrence Cohen, Kristin Jacklin, and Karen Kobayashi are increasingly addressing the culturally diverse experiences of dementia,[55] mainstream media and fictional treatments of Alzheimer's in the global north continue to reflect the erroneous belief that Alzheimer's victims are white. This has resulted in the equally problematic emphasis on white people's experience of the illness.

SECTION IV: ALZHEIMER'S AND THE PROBLEM OF EVIL

In his book *Caring for Mentally Ill People* (1982), Alexander Leighton writes: "One could argue that all diseases seen as chronic and life threatening or incurable make people uneasy … But I think that our response to insanity has additional dimensions of intensity and irrationality. There is something particular in these disorders that evokes in human beings existential apprehension that is akin to the fear of the dead and of ghosts, demons, trolls and other apparitions" (8). In contemporary Western society, what society deems dreadful or, to use an even more morally loaded term, "evil," is increasingly aligned with contemporary forms of age-related "mental disintegration" – "cognitive decline" and, more recently, MCI. In using the term "evil," I am drawing on the fact that evil once had a far broader meaning than it does nowadays, encompassing forms of suffering that accrued simply by virtue of being mortal as well as the forms associated with errors in human judgement (Corey 2). During the Enlightenment, as drama scholar Paul Corey observes, "the event that prompted the most discussion about evil was not a political or moral atrocity but rather a natural catastrophe: the Lisbon earthquake of 1755" (ibid.).

After the Enlightenment, the notion of evil began to narrow to the point that the term now merely connotes the antithesis of rationality and morality – nothing more than "just extreme human wickedness" (ibid.). The shifting definitions of evil and their relationship to the Gothic are relevant to my study because disease in general, and Alzheimer's disease in particular, typically arouses profound dread and is frequently personified as a monstrous evil. In keeping with earlier understandings of the term, the evils that constellate around Alzheimer's include both individual and familial suffering as well as moral transgression, since current victims of Alzheimer's are implicitly subjected to blame for supposedly not taking the appropriate measures to ensure brain health and neuroreserve in old age (see Katz et al.). As I argue in chapter two, in the late nineteenth century, later-life dementia likewise became a lightning rod for moral arguments concerning "good" and "bad" forms of aging.

In many respects, the mainstream media's treatment of Alzheimer's and its victims also recalls prior Gothic and apocalyptic representations of cancer and, later, AIDS, as a menace. As Sontag asserts, "simplified terrors are raised by crude statistics brandished for the general public" (*Illness* 70). Nowadays, as the statistics concerning Alzheimer's cited above demonstrate, alarmist and apocalyptic discussions about demography pervade biomedical and media narratives about age-related dementia – discussions that instigate new forms of fear and terror or what age studies scholar Kathleen Woodward terms "statistical panic" (*Statistical*). When it comes to the media's treatment of Alzheimer's, the overriding message is that we are being stalked by a disease that steals our minds and instigates a monstrous Jekyll-and-Hyde transformation – one which affects both individual bodies and the body politic (see Khatchaturian). Even the supposedly neutral language of science used to describe the neuropathology draws on the Gothic: in the course of the dread disease, healthy neurons are replaced by what neurologists term "fossilized skeletons" of neurons, also known as "ghost" or "tombstone" tangles (Braak and Braak, *Concepts* 55).

The reliance on Gothic and apocalyptic metaphors in the diverse accounts of Alzheimer's serves as my point of entry for two reasons. First, as a literary scholar, I have researched and written extensively on the literary and socio-political dynamics of this mode and its related concern with resolving who or what is accountable for moral crimes, in essence, the cause of human suffering or "evil." Second, Canadian writers and critics have learned to adopt a self-conscious and skeptical approach to the Gothic due to the close historical connections between the Gothic and the cultural construction of the Canadian nation-state. An understanding of the origins of this form in the Canadian nation-state helps to underscore some Canadians' long-standing negotiation with a Gothic, divided self that arises "from a settler-invader identity that *constitutes* and *encounters* a 'foreign element'" (Sugars, "Canadian" 418). As a result, Canadian critics may be particularly well positioned to interrogate the Gothic.

In her introduction to her essay "Canadian Gothic" (2012), Cynthia Sugars explains that the extensive colonization of North America in the eighteenth and nineteenth centuries "coincided with the rise of the Gothic as a genre in Europe," a historical fact that explains why so many early Canadian writers applied this mode to their "experiences in the New World" (410). Simply put, Canada "learned to read itself through a Gothic lens" (411). During the nationalist revival period in the 1960s and 1970s, Canadian Gothic fictions became so popular that scholars coined the term "Southern Ontario Gothic" to describe the predominant mode in the works of Alice Munro, Margaret Atwood, Robertson Davies, Timothy Findley, and others (418). This phase of the Canadian Gothic was largely responsible for putting Canada on the global Gothic map. Canada's ongoing, reflexive negotiations with both the Gothic and apocalyptic discourses make the Canadian context a critically productive site for the analysis of the governing metaphors and assumptions that constellate around age-related dementia and Alzheimer's disease. A historical analysis highlights the tensions between elegiac, Gothic, ironic, and surrealist approaches to old age and dementia. In light of my study's aim to analyze a range of narratives in terms of literary tropes and genres, it is helpful to review the key conventions of these modes and to comment on critical views of their socio-political valences.

SECTION V: FROM ELEGIAC CONSOLATION TO IRONIC DOUBT

The common denominator that makes elegy and the Gothic appealing genres for the depiction of Alzheimer's disease – a terminal illness primarily affecting older people – is that they both invoke the spectre of death. Although they have undergone profound changes throughout the centuries, "in their most frequent and imitated forms" both genres are nearly always concerned "with one or more deaths" (Hogle, "Elegy" 565). In essence both the elegy and, later and more urgently, the Gothic address how one can face and potentially transcend mortality by adopting and adapting references to theologies and belief systems that are no longer entirely compelling. Whereas the Gothic stages terror, the traditional elegiac three-part response involves "lamentation for an individual's death, confrontation with the fact of human mortality, and consolation for the inescapability of death" (Vickery 1).

In keeping with psychoanalytic and literary theorist Julia Kristeva's view of literature as a "staging of affects" ("On the Melancholic" 1), John Hollander advises that elegy is "a mood rather than a formal mode" (200). Although elegy began as a poetic form, modern prose writers such as Virginia Woolf and James Joyce adopted and adapted the traditional elegy's basic triad in their fiction, making it what Dennis Kay has called "a form without frontiers" (7). In her diary entry for 27 June 1925, for example, Woolf writes: "I have an idea that I will invent a new name for my books to supplant 'novel.' A new — by Virginia Woolf. But what? Elegy?" (34). In accordance with Woolf's proposition, her novels ushered in what critics now refer to as the "prose elegy."

Due to the waning power of traditional ideologies and religious modes of consolation, the trope of irony emerges instead as central to both modern and contemporary literary confrontations with death and with the spectre of death in conditions like age-related dementia. "The modern elegiac temper's confrontation with loss," Vickery writes, "is that of doubt. A dominant attitude emerges of ironic, sceptical uncertainty as to whether a viable resolution of the trauma of loss is possible" (6).

SECTION VI: IRONY AND ILLNESS

The modern elegist's expression of "ironic, sceptical uncertainty" is particularly relevant to my study of Alzheimer's disease. As medical anthropologist Michael Lambek observes, "there is often something in situations of illness that resembles irony or that brings the recognition of irony to the fore" (*Irony* 1). He goes on to assert that therapeutic practices and discourses "can be described and distinguished according to the degree to which they recognize or refuse irony" (ibid.). In using the term irony, Lambek, following contemporary Greek philosopher Alexander Nehamas, refers to its most famous classical Greek expressions: Sophoclean tragic irony, in which spectators know what is happening but characters are unable or refuse to acknowledge or accept it; and Socratic irony, a rhetorical stance characterized by turning questions back on the questioner to demonstrate the gaps in the latter's ostensibly rational thinking (5). Ultimately, both the tragic and the philosophical ironic forms underscore "the limitations and ambiguity of praxis" (ibid.).

Fundamentally, irony relies on the possibility of arriving at more than one meaning. For Roman rhetoricians, including Cicero and Quintilian, "*ironia* denoted a rhetorical figure and a manner of discourse, in which, for the most part, the meaning was contrary to the words"; indeed, this "double-edged nature" appears to be an enduring feature of irony (Cuddon 458, 460). Verbal irony oscillates between the simultaneous "perception of the said and the unsaid" (Hutcheon, *Irony's* 39) – between literal and inferred meanings. In general, "most forms of irony involve the perception or awareness of a discrepancy or incongruity between words and their meaning, or between actions and their results, or between appearance and reality. In all cases there may be an element of the absurd and the paradoxical" (Cuddon 460). Visual irony likewise depends on the possibility of two or more interpretations of what at first glance appears to be a single image (see fig. 1). In narratives about Alzheimer's disease, irony is particularly relevant because it remains virtually impossible to distinguish between normal and pathological brain aging.

For the most part, contemporary discourses from the biomedical field, volunteer organizations, and the media represent and categorize Alzheimer's non-ironically as a medical problem, and stress the socio-economic costs to society that attend the diseased individual's loss of personhood – costs that are graphically outlined in the articles cited above. These discourses also typically adopt an apocalyptic tone and, as American author Jonathan Franzen observes, portray the illness as a terrifying scourge that "refracts death into a spectrum of its otherwise tightly conjoined parts – death of autonomy, death of memory, death of self-consciousness, death of personality, death of body" (89). Equally important, the current biomedical discourse subscribes to the "most common trope of Alzheimer's: that its particular sadness and horror stem from the sufferer's loss of his or her [cognitive] 'self' long before the body dies" (ibid). In other words, the non-ironic discourses portray Alzheimer's primarily as a disease that destroys the individual's memory and, hence, personal identity.

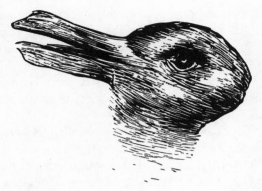

Figure 1.

As noted above, in his *Essay Concerning Human Understanding* Locke famously distinguishes between personal identity and human identity. The latter corresponds to substance and is dependent on bodily or physical continuity. In contrast, personal identity, the identity of the self, is a function of the continuity of consciousness. For Locke, personal identity equates to the ability to remember one's own actions and to narrate past experiences in the present (see Whitehead 53–8). As Canadian philosopher Ian Hacking puts it, for Locke "the person is constituted not by a biography but by a remembered biography" ("Memory Sciences" 81). According to Locke, only our memory – rather than, say, our embodied experience – holds these evanescent perceptions together and grants them, and us by virtue of them, a sense of our ongoing existence. Simply put, Locke's theory maintains that both experience and perceptions of experience are fleeting and, hence, intrinsically elegiac. Equally relevant, those who lack the capacity for abstracting from experience and for formulating memories are, according to Locke, not classifiable under the category of "Man." In formulating the category of "Man" in this way, Locke "contributed to contemporary views of idiocy as a mental state that lies 'beyond what is human' and aligned it with monstrosity" (Goodey 227). As Locke puts it: "Shall a defect in the Body make a Monster; a defect in the Mind (the far more Noble, and, in the common phrase, the far more Essential Part) not?" (in ibid. 232). The view of idiocy as monstrous thus constitutes a Gothic legacy from the Enlightenment. In hindsight, the irony of Locke's contribution is striking. During the Age of Reason, Locke argued for the elevation of humankind by creating a new and debased category composed of individuals formerly considered human, which he called "monsters."

In her discussion of diseases that arouse the greatest dread, Sontag argues that "the most terrifying illnesses are those perceived not just as lethal but as dehumanizing, literally so" (*AIDS* 38). Locke's link between defects in the mind and monstrosity presages the prevailing fear that Alzheimer's disease – a neuro*degenerative* disease – is a malevolent form of degeneration, the most dreaded disease precisely because it seemingly instigates "mutations into animality" (ibid. 41). "What counts," Sontag maintains, in the case of master illnesses, is that they supposedly reflect "underlying, ongoing changes, the dissolution of the person" (ibid.). This type of dissolution is portrayed by writers on Alzheimer's in both biological and mechanistic terms. Basting, for example, cites an article in *Time* that opens by inviting readers to "imagine your brain is a house filled with lights. Now imagine someone turning off the lights one by one ... and you succumb to the spreading darkness."[56]

In his account of his father's struggle with Alzheimer's disease, Franzen questions the validity of mechanistic models – models that substitute the artifact for the individual – and insists that his father's brain is not "simply a computation device running gradually and inexorably amok." He thus challenges both Locke's emphasis on cognitive memory and the biomedical conception of self (89–90). Equally important, Franzen wonders whether the various deaths cited earlier – of autonomy, of memory, of self-consciousness, of personality, of body – "can ever really be so separated, and whether memory and consciousness have such secure title, after all, to the seat of selfhood" (89). In contrast to the stories that insist that selfhood is erased in the late stages of Alzheimer's disease, Franzen states: "I can't stop looking for meaning in the two years that followed his loss of his supposed 'self,' and I can't stop finding it" (ibid.). Skeptics may be tempted to assert that Franzen is merely fooling himself – understandably consoling himself with fantasies of his father's continued presence in the face of the latter's inexorable decline. Yet this view overlooks the fact that from birth to death, our entire experience of selfhood is predicated on intersubjective relations. It also overlooks how multiple, contradictory, and non-continuous so-called ordinary consciousness is. Hence, what constitutes our "self" may well be elided or effaced when others cease to perceive us. At bottom, Franzen's essay underscores the role played by narrative in asserting agency or mastery and in offering consolation in the face of illness. His comments also highlight the difficulty of parsing whether the consolations and resolutions proffered by narrative are ever plainly false. Irony pervades Franzen's conflict with the medical establishment's view of his father. Whereas the medical framework sees only a machine winding down – the equivalent of the image of the duck in fig. 1 above – Franzen sees his father and qualities that endure in the latter despite illness – the hidden figure of the rabbit.

Having been repeatedly struck by the Gothic and apocalyptic rhetoric in widely diverse discussions of Alzheimer's, I began to wonder about the practical and ethical stakes involved in the materialist, biomedical presentations of Alzheimer's as a quantifiable "disease" as compared to representations of Alzheimer's as an illness. Calling it a disease entails adopting a positivistic approach and calibrating its values and costs. It also offers people coping with dementia a name for their condition and something to war against. To treat Alzheimer's as an illness requires the recognition that it is shaped by culture and, hence, is open to interpretation and change (see Lambek, *Irony* 2 and Kleinman). Whereas the disease model offers an opponent to conquer, the illness model also entails acknowledging profound uncertainty with respect to both the ontology of the disease and the physician's, sufferer's, and caregiver's agency, reason, and control. Acknowledging the status of Alzheimer's disease as an enigma implicitly or explicitly underscores the uncertain and therefore ironic possibilities associated with late-onset dementia.

For many authors, reframing age-related memory loss and Alzheimer's disease entails adopting a critical approach that allows for skepticism, humility, irony, and ambiguity – an approach that has affinities with contemporary, feminist elegiac responses to loss and death.[57] In the majority of the literary works under consideration, this alternative approach entails challenging the genre of Gothic, which pits supposedly "healthy," most often young, individuals against aged, "abnormal" people who have succumbed to a monstrous "brain-killing disease."

As noted above, physicians know that labels such as Alzheimer's and, more recently, MCI can be stigmatizing or what sociologist Erving Goffman calls "identity spoiling" and iatrogenic. In other words, the label itself makes people ill because individuals, who are much more than their cognitive abilities, are led to believe that their cognitive capacity is everything. If their memory fails, they feel they are nothing but a useless burden to their families and society. Citing Peter Whitehouse, Jay Ingram acknowledges that "there is likely more harm than good in diagnosing Alzheimer's when the diagnosis, at least when compared to that of other illnesses, is very slippery … If you compare the blow delivered by the diagnosis to the inadequate options for treatment, it's hard to argue with that point of view" (165). The stigma associated with Alzheimer's has become increasingly pressing in light of the Supreme Court of Canada's decision to revise the laws concerning assisted suicide.[58] In prompting individuals to read against the grain, the ironic approach does not deny that people face profound challenges that usually increase as they age; nor does it minimize the real suffering that attends age-related cognitive impairment. Instead, ironic narratives associated with Alzheimer's may offer us a view of the person coping with dementia as an individual deserving of compassion and respect. As well, ironic narratives enable us to see vulnerability and dependency as part of the entire life course and, therefore, as something that need not strike terror into our hearts.

SECTION VII: ALZHEIMER'S DISEASE AND THE GOTHIC

In the nineteenth century, elements of the Gothic derived from Walpole's *The Castle of Otranto* were disseminated into various modes, including more realistic Victorian novels. At the end of the nineteenth century, as in the *fin de siècle* of the previous century, there was another surge in Gothic fiction that culminated in the production of classic examples featuring monstrous transformations, degeneration, and mental illness, including Oscar Wilde's *The Picture of Dorian Gray*, Bram Stoker's *Dracula*, Charlotte Perkins Gilman's "The Yellow Wallpaper," and Henry James's *The Turn of the Screw* (see Hogle, *Cambridge* 1–2). Many scholars conceive of the Gothic as the flipside of eighteenth-century rationality and morality – the reverse of Enlightenment values (Botting 2). More precisely, the Gothic condenses threats to Enlightenment values since it is associated with supernatural and natural forces, imaginative excesses and delusions, religious and human evil, social transgressions, mental disintegration, and spiritual corruption (ibid.).

As I explain in my book *DisPossession*, scholars find it increasingly difficult to define the Gothic, a complex poetics that "mutates across historical, national, and generic boundaries as it reworks images drawn from different ages and places" (Smith 4). Drawing on the story of Frankenstein's monster, Maggie Kilgour likens the Gothic to a literary patchwork, "assembled out of bits and pieces" (4). Unlike the British Gothic, which developed during a definable time period and has a recognized coterie of authors, the American Gothic is even less easily specified (Goddu 3). Critics have noted, however, the presentist focus of the American Gothic, which is largely shared by Canadian writers. In this regard, Lloyd-Smith's view that "the distinctive theme and deepest insight of American Gothic, the sense that there is something behind, which may not be, as in European Gothic, the Past, but some perpetual and present Otherness hidden within, behind, somehow below the apparently benign 'natural surface'" also holds true for the Canadian Gothic (86). His views are echoed by Eric Savoy's sense that "the entire tradition of the American Gothic can be conceptualized as the attempt to invoke 'the face of the tenant'" within (14). In Canadian writing, the Gothic is typically mobilized to identify and resolve what a particular society deems dreadful or evil. As I argue in *DisPossession*, in the case of early Canadian literature, the landlord is typically the belated arrival, the settler-invader, and the tenant is the Native North American. Since the publication of Sheila Watson's *The Double Hook* in 1959, however, behaviours associated with dementia such as transgressive wandering have also played a profound role in the Gothic characterization of the monstrous Otherness hidden within.

    In an effort to recapture the classical awareness, which has been forgotten, that evil is not solely something that we do but also something that we suffer, psychoanalyst C. Fred Alford offers new insight into the workings of the Gothic, and in the process helps us to understand its pervasive deployment in portrayals of Alzheimer's disease. Alford explains evil as "an experience of dread," which is "the uncanny experience of discomfort we have of being human, vulnerable, alone in the universe, and doomed to die" (in Corey 7). Affirming Alford's hypothesis, Corey argues further: "In dread, we are terrified by the reality of violation, pollution, infection, confusion and destruction. We fear that the limits that secure our physical well-being, mental health, and societal order will be crossed, afflicting us with suffering and chaos. This fear is aggravated by the ever-present reality of death, which reminds us that ultimately we cannot escape being victims, no matter how secure we are in our daily lives" (7). In

Gothic narratives, these internal states are projected onto the setting, characters, and plot of the story in an effort to symbolize and master the dreadful feelings aroused by disease and death.

It is well established that Alzheimer's disease is strongly correlated with age. The closer one gets to death, the more likely it is that one will experience dementia. According to the most recent statistics, one of every two people over the age of eighty-five is demented (Ingram 21, 201). The recent construction of the disease concept in the 1970s may represent an attempt to contain society's dread of illness and death. Jesse Ballenger argues that representing a person with dementia as a victim of a dread disease theoretically preserved old age as a stage of life relatively free of deterioration and dependency. Attempts to preserve old age as a utopian stage also include differentiating between what sociologists in Europe term the "third and fourth ages" (the former is associated with healthy old age; the latter, with illness and death). By establishing the terms such as Alzheimer's disease and the third and fourth ages, the threat of illness and death could be contained within the sharper, more restricted boundaries of a particular disease category and a stage in the life course. Citing Alford, Corey explains that the motivation for committing an evil deed can be traced to a desire to evacuate the experience of dread "by inflicting it on others, making them feel dreadful by hurting them" (in Cory 7). The evildoer attempts "to transform the terrible passivity and helplessness of suffering into an activity" (ibid.). As Corey warns, in adopting this course of action "we fool ourselves into thinking that by causing dread we can escape dread" (7). Corey's insights prompt me to wonder to what extent contemporary biomedical narratives about Alzheimer's have aided in transforming society's sense of passivity and helplessness into the related activities of naming and fighting diseases. In the case of MCI and Alzheimer's, given that there is no cure for age-related dementia and that those so labelled suffer from stigma, we may have fallen into the trap of thinking that "by causing dread" – separating the normal from the pathological and labelling the latter as "diseased" – we can "escape dread."

Kristeva likewise considers the experience of dread and the role of narrative in asserting agency in the face of loss – literally expressing what society deems dreadful. As noted earlier, she argues that literary representation is a "staging of affects," which "possesses a real and imaginary efficacy that, cathartic more than of the order of elaboration, is a therapeutic method utilized in all societies through the ages"

("On the Melancholic" 1). Kristeva specifically aligns the mood of dread and the ghosts and grotesques that populate the Gothic with what she terms "the abject" and products of "abjection" – terms that she derives from the literal meaning of ab-ject: "throwing off" and being "thrown under" (see Hogle, *Cambridge* 7). According to Kristeva, the dead body is "the most sickening of wastes ... the utmost of abjection ... death infecting life ... [that] beckons to us and ends up engulfing us" (Kristeva, *Powers* 3–4). In the case of the Gothic, however, whatever is expelled or hastily buried insistently returns to haunt the living.

As a terminal condition that leads to death, age-related dementia, and, more precisely, Alzheimer's disease – which can only be accurately diagnosed post-mortem – is inextricably connected to the abject and to society's fear of death and the corpse. Taken together, Corey's, Alford's, and Kristeva's theoretical observations shed light on both the motivations for and the potentially harmful ramifications of unselfconsciously deploying apocalyptic and Gothic discourses to represent Alzheimer's disease. "Through ... an inappropriate pursuit of the good," Corey writes, "we lash out at our doom and cause harm" (7). His statement recalls the recent announcement by the Canadian Broadcasting Corporation (CBC) that attempts on the part of scientists to treat mild cognitive disorder (found to progress to Alzheimer's in 17 per cent of cases) have failed; worse, the drugs used to treat patients have, in many cases, rendered otherwise healthy individuals severely ill ("Alzheimer's Drugs"). These theoretical considerations and the practical outcomes associated with Gothic attempts at mastering Alzheimer's disease emphasize the need to remain open-minded and avoid clinging to a singular model in the face of a host of potential triggers.

Given that new factors including anxiety and loneliness are understood to affect dementia, it is equally important to explore the imaginative and political ramifications of alternative rhetorical tropes and genres. Such alternative approaches include irony, the feminine elegy – which, as Melissa Zeiger argues and as I discuss in detail below, is a form of elegy that does not promote psychologically detaching from and replacing the deceased – and surrealism – an aesthetic movement based on the work of a coterie of writers, painters, and poets living in Paris after the First World War. Following the Dadaists, the Surrealists famously rejected order and logic – which, in their view, had given rise to the war – in favour of chaos. Their primary goal lay in liberating the imagination. André Breton, one of the founders of the Surrealist movement who studied medicine and psychiatry, promoted an extremely compassionate view of mental illness. Taken together, irony, the feminine elegy, and surrealism allow for ambiguity, the process of mourning, and, in the case of surrealism, an acceptance of alternative states of consciousness.

Nowadays we are accustomed to thinking of the Gothic and the elegy in predominantly aesthetic terms. I would suggest, however, that these modes also inform biomedical and media accounts of dementia. As David Kennedy observes, both the elegy – and, I would add, the Gothic – and anatomy rely "on the actualities of death in order to model life" (107). As a result, it is not surprising that historically, elegy in its canonical sense "starts to be writeable at the same time as early modern anatomical scientists begin to map the body" (ibid.). He argues further and more fancifully that "if we consider that elegy, like medicine, derives from dead bodies, then elegy itself, in its consolatory turn, starts to look like a species of medicine and one that is particularly concerned with hygiene and healing" (ibid. 51). Following Kennedy, I maintain that both biomedical and literary discourses play a seminal role in society's efforts to heal individuals, communities, and nations.

Whereas Kennedy limits his exploration to the relationship between biomedical discourse – particularly anatomy and pathology – and the elegy, my study complicates matters by distinguishing between masculine and feminine elegiac approaches to dementia. I also argue that, most recently, the Gothic has played an equally profound role in biomedicine's ongoing attempt to tell the story of Alzheimer's disease – an attempt that entails prising apart the natural from the unnatural to elucidate the secret workings of what is now widely understood as a terminal "disease," in the hopes of forestalling death.

In contrast to traditional masculine elegy's reluctant acceptance of death, the Gothic text takes "a series of narrative or dramatic steps toward revelations of the 'primal crimes' behind deaths and burials, as in the detective fiction that the Gothic later helped to spawn" (Hogle, "Elegy" 567). The Gothic thus expresses society's struggle to view illness and death within a modern scientific framework that refuses to accept the latter as "natural." Viewed in this light, Gothic narratives serve as defence mechanisms that offset the experience of helplessness by offering a sense of agency in the face of illness and death. As Hogle writes: "The Gothic enacts a passage out of a decaying, but still beckoning past ... toward an emerging, if not completely modern world, albeit haunted by vestiges of the past, now driven by the ideologies of middle-class and Protestant 'inner determination' that have grown in power with the expansion of post-1750 'free enterprise' 'Enlightenment' science, and pre-industrial, industrial or post-industrial capitalism" ("Elegy" 567). The legacy of these modern ideologies continues to fuel the contemporary biomedical battle against Alzheimer's disease.

In light of the connections I am positing between biomedical approaches to Alzheimer's disease, the elegy, and the Gothic, it is helpful to consider Mary Shelley's famous Gothic novel, *Frankenstein* (1818). In keeping with the Gothic's haunting and uncanny approach to death, in the wake of his extreme grief at the death of his mother – a trauma that leaves Shelley's protagonist "feeling so 'rent by the most irreparable evil'" – the quasi-scientific Victor attempts "to defy death by creating a haunting creature from the pieces of the dead in 'charnel houses' as well as fragments of medieval alchemy and modern biochemistry" (Hogle, "Elegy" 566). Rather than accept his mother's death as natural and mourn in an elegiac fashion, Victor deems her death an unjust crime – an "evil" – and he takes it upon himself to defy death. Ironically, Victor's quest results in the deaths of virtually everyone he holds dear. In this regard, Victor can be viewed as "an elegist manqué," a "failed mourner" (Sacks 64, 65).[59]

Victor Frankenstein's defiant response to his mother's death, and determination to use scientific training to undo and seek revenge for it, suggest that the Gothic is motivated by similar impulses. I would argue further that in its account of Alzheimer's disease, contemporary biomedicine views death as a mystery and crime to resolve, rather than as a natural facet of the life course, and this reliance on the Gothic and its twin, the genre of Gothic detection,[60] likewise forestalls – or at the very least defers – the difficult yet crucial work of mourning.[61] Put somewhat differently, the prevailing biomedical Gothic approach to Alzheimer's disease – which conceives of age-related cognitive impairment as an "evil" wholly distinct from the normal process of aging – urges people, in the words of Dylan Thomas, not to "go gentle into that good night," but, instead, to "rage, rage against the dying of the light,"[62] thereby legitimating the costly, apocalyptic "war" on dementia.[63] Although it is tempting to rank the efficacy of narrative strategies, including those Freud termed "mourning" and "melancholia," virtually all of the imaginative treatments of

Alzheimer's disease considered in my study demonstrate the limited ability of any tactic to wholly resolve the powerful anxieties and grief aroused by dementia.

SECTION VIII: ALZHEIMER'S DISEASE AND APOCALYPSE

As I observe in my book *Rewriting Apocalypse* (2005), the apocalyptic paradigm pervaded Canadian literature from its beginnings. In the hands of Canadian writers, the paradigm has also been used to figure intranational struggles between different generations, genders, and races. In contrast to the traditional biblical apocalypse, which includes a transformative catastrophe and a subsequent revelation of ultimate truth, Canadian fiction often balks at celebrating the destruction of evil and the creation of a new world. Instead, these works highlight the devastation wrought by apocalyptic thinking on those deemed the non-elect (5).

As I suggest in *Rewriting Apocalypse*, one of the easiest ways to become acquainted with the distinctive political, structural, and thematic features of the apocalypse is to consider Revelation, the biblical text on which many Canadian fictions rely. In essence, the narrative of Revelation relies on binary oppositions between "the totally good and the absolutely evil" (Abrams 11). Equally important, "the consummation of history ... occurs not by mediation between these polar opposites, but only after the extirpation of the forces of evil by the forces of good" (ibid.). Ultimately, by exposing the pervasiveness of the apocalyptic paradigm and analyzing its ruthless exclusion of difference, Canadian fiction typically invites readers to reconsider apocalypse from the perspective of what Canadian poet Leonard Cohen called "the beautiful losers" (1966). In the fictions under consideration, older adults suffering from dementia fall into this category of exclusion.

I argue further that among sociologists, primarily in Europe, the distinction between the "third and fourth ages" likewise serves to separate the supposed elect from the non-elect. Invoking the well-known model of the four ages of man, Peter Laslett was one of the first to identify the third age as "an era of personal fulfilment" in contrast to a fourth age as "an era of final dependence, decrepitude and death" (4; see also Hazan 11). To date, there have been many useful elaborations and critiques of both the theory and the concepts of the third and fourth age (see, for example, Neuberger; Holstein; Scharf; Calasanti and King). Although Canadians do not typically refer to the third and fourth ages, the media braids apocalyptic motifs together with elements of the Gothic to drive home the uncanny horror of dementia. As Sontag emphasizes, binary divisions between third and fourth ages and apocalyptic narratives forcibly emerge when people feel the need "to master" their fears of what seems "uncontrollable" by installing a largely imaginary binary between heaven and hell (*AIDS* 87). While literary treatments of Alzheimer's install elements of Gothic and apocalyptic rhetoric to express these heightened fears, they frequently include facets of the elegy, thereby opening a space for grief and mourning in everyday life.

SECTION IX: MASCULINE VERSUS FEMININE ELEGY

In referring to the elegy, it is important to distinguish between masculine and feminine forms. Feminist critics such as Melissa Zeiger argue that both the traditional forms of the Gothic and the masculine elegy are shaped by patriarchal gender politics that position the male as the hero/quester and the female as the passive object. In the traditional elegiac model of Orpheus and Eurydice, for example, the hero seeks his beloved in the underworld, but inevitably relinquishes her and returns to the world of the living, where he is celebrated as a culture-hero. For Zeiger, such narrative frameworks doom women to death and silence. Zeiger aligns the masculine elegy with Freud's conception of mourning, which, she argues, likewise promotes detachment and substitution. Simply put, for the bereaved hero, a skill, a work of art, or an artifact (knowledge, religious consolation, etc.) ultimately serves to replace the beloved. The tendency to accept the substitution of the "artifact for the living being" in masculine elegiac texts is part of this dissociative trend. Yet, as my summary of Mary Shelley's *Frankenstein* cited above suggests, attempts at substitution are prevalent in Gothic narratives as well.

In contrast to this masculine movement of detachment and mastery, Zeiger argues that some women's elegies promote "an alliance and continuity with the dead" (64). She also maintains that issues of "presence, voice, and embodiment become central in the self-position of modern and contemporary women elegists" (ibid.). In keeping with the concerns of women elegists, a key facet of my study involves questioning the tendency to substitute scientific knowledge about

Alzheimer's disease for the loss of individual sufferers. My study likewise resists the elegiac and Gothic association of women "with death, silence, darkness, and, above all, loss of the body" (ibid.). For example, chapter one's historical account of Alois Alzheimer – the "culture-hero" who reputedly discovered the disease that bears his name – relies on medical records to trace the elided experience of his infamous patient, Auguste D.

Following her death in an asylum, Auguste D.'s brain was removed, dissected, and stained using a newly invented technique to reveal the disease's supposed characteristic features – the notorious plaques and tangles.[64] In his book *The Forgetting* (2001), David Shenk goes so far as to offer a detailed account of how the brain was prepared for its journey from the asylum to Alzheimer's Munich clinic. The ongoing fascination with the treatment of Auguste D.'s brain serves as a concrete and graphic example of the tendency to substitute "the artifact for the living being" (ibid.). Currently, in the Canadian media's narratives of contemporary Gothic detection, scientists are "detectives" and "sleuths" who "chase clues hidden in protein" and follow "the trail of the mind killer."[65]

In keeping with chapter one's counter-reading of elegiac and biomedical strategies of detachment and substitution, my book focuses on both the theories of the principal psychiatrists and researchers who developed the disease concept *and* the frequently elided experiences of people with dementia and their caregivers, who, today as in the past, are predominantly women. Analyzing the metaphors surrounding the disease and taking a step back from the hyperbolic rhetoric also helps us to see how traditional Gothic and apocalyptic language implicitly supports the intensive and "heroic" drive for a pharmaceutical cure, which due to the complexity of the illness has proved highly elusive.

In contrast to the search for a cure, a growing number of experts including Carol Brayne[66] and Peter Whitehouse are circling back to prior historical perspectives on senile dementia adopted in the nineteenth century that addressed people's lifestyles.[67] Some Canadian physicians are also questioning the dominant biomedical and pharmaceutical approach and strongly suggesting forms of prevention that take a public health approach. The latter entails assessing the need for lifestyle changes, reduced exposure to toxins, and reduction in poverty; evaluating the level of community support; and considering other factors that are, as Lock insists, likely to reduce the global prevalence of dementia "to a much greater extent than will an approach confined to expensive molecular micro-medical management of privileged populations deemed to be at risk" (4). Citing the most recent findings associated with protections against dementia, Ingram explains that education is the one that stands out the most (143). Both Ingram and Peter Whitehouse observe that people who are bilingual have a built-in buffer against dementia – a neuroreserve – that no drug has thus far been able to match (see ibid. 145). Recently, the Ontario Brain Institute identified exercise as the single most beneficial preventative strategy (in ibid. 241). Researchers are exploring links between glucose intake and toxins (nitrosamines) that also negatively impact brain health (ibid. 248–9). Factors associated with the decline of dementia in certain groups include better blood vessel health, avoiding concussions and brain injury, not smoking, better fitness, and better care of high blood pressure and cholesterol (ibid. 161). Education, exercise, and diet are factors that society can actively address.

Viewed in light of the controversies associated with the nature of late-onset dementia and its elusive cure, it is not surprising that alternative psychological and sociological perspectives on Alzheimer's, which have always shadowed the biomedical disease model, have become increasingly important in social science and in aesthetic representations of Alzheimer's. Within these discourses, age-related dementia is not always labelled as a disease; nor is it unequivocally equated with the quantifiable and absolute erasure of agency, reason, meaning, and personhood. Instead it serves as a more potent, albeit ironic source of meaning. Rather than maintain a restricted focus on the constituent parts – the molecules and DNA of the "diseased" individual suffering from dysfunctional cognition – the non-biological approaches typically offer a broader sociological context that helps to explain why particular types of stories about aging and dementia are told at specific historical moments. Non-biomedical approaches also shed light on who is best served by particular stories and, equally important, how the different stories we tell influence families and, in some cases, the nation-state's attempts to cope with dementia.

SECTION X: AN OVERVIEW OF THE CHAPTERS

In my study of the development of the disease concept and the shift from the elegy to the Gothic, the focus of the first half of my book,

I adopt an age studies approach to the biomedical records to re-orient our focus from the heroic exploits of well-known scientists and the brains of infamous Alzheimer's patients – most notably, Auguste D. – to the experience of people with dementia in asylums for the mentally ill at the turn of the nineteenth century. To highlight the generative tensions among different approaches to Alzheimer's, I analyze a wide variety of narratives – by researchers, clinicians, journalists, and members of Alzheimer's associations – that have circulated among the public. In chapters one through six, I trace the construction of the concepts of senile dementia and Alzheimer's disease from their beginnings in the mid- to late nineteenth century to their contemporary, twenty-first century biomedical and cultural representations.

The first six chapters address a set of related questions: how and why did Alois Alzheimer's research on the brain in the late-nineteenth century contribute to the formation of the disease that bears his name? Is there a relationship between the two most prominent diseases of forgetting – namely, hysteria and Alzheimer's disease? How has our understanding of the latter disease evolved and, in some cases, been contested in biomedical discourses? Finally, what stories have institutions in Canada – most notably, the Alzheimer Society of Canada – helped to fashion and disseminate concerning age-related dementia and Alzheimer's disease?

Whereas, as noted earlier, the majority of scholars have traced the shifting understanding of Alzheimer's disease in Europe and the US, I analyze when, how, and why the changing story of age-related dementia was narrated north of the 49th parallel from the turn of the nineteenth century to the present. My study draws on a variety of sources including asylum records, historical accounts of medicine and psychiatry, articles in the national newspapers, and literary works. Taken together these materials provide a foundation for my argument that the meaning of aging and senile dementia in Canada was shaped by a range of cultural narratives that altered radically over time.

For most of the nineteenth and twentieth centuries, the fate of aged individuals, including those suffering from dementia, was not a widespread social concern. Equally significant, dementia or "senility," as it was known, was considered part and parcel of aging.[68] Our contemporary interest in historical attitudes toward and the treatment of the dependent elderly is thus driven largely by the current concerns of the baby boomer generation. Whereas contemporary Western society is preoccupied with concerns about old age and dementia, the fate of children was the paramount concern during the Victorian period and into the twentieth century; the Commonwealth was riveted by the issues of childbirth, child mortality, child-rearing practices, child labour, and, more broadly, enhancing Canada's growing population through increased fertility and immigration (see Dillon, *Shady*). This was, as historian Sharon Anne Cook explains, "an era in which the child was glorified and the aged merely maintained" (35).

Chapter one traces the twin birth of hysteria and Alzheimer's disease in late-nineteenth century European asylums to illustrate that the changing meanings accorded to Alzheimer's disease, whether in biomedical or literary accounts, cannot be prised apart from their discrete historical contexts. In the process of illuminating the controversies surrounding the hasty baptism of Alzheimer's disease and in keeping with the female elegiac approach, chapter one offers a detailed account of the often-elided experience of Alzheimer's famous patient, Auguste D. My aim lies in showing how the biomedical preoccupation with the features of her illness in conjunction with her doctor's desire to retain her brain for post-mortem analysis contributed to what might best be described as her Gothic erasure.

Chapter two shifts from late-nineteenth century Europe to the New World, specifically Ontario at the *fin de siècle,* to consider several fundamental and interrelated factors that contributed to the change from a more elegiac acceptance of senility to the contemporary, Gothic pathologizing of senility. These factors include (1) the gradual shift from a more elegiac, religious acceptance of the illnesses associated with old age to an increasingly scientific approach that distinguished between a healthy and a diseased old age; (2) the creation of purpose-built asylums to house the new class of "patients" with mental illnesses; and, finally, (3) the disputes among asylum superintendents, politicians, and concerned families about who should look after the elderly in their "dotage." Owing to the mounting costs accrued by the newly built asylums, debates raged as to whether people with dementia should be admitted or cared for at home by their families. Although these debates were not unique to Canada, they had a profound impact on Canadians caring for elderly people with dementia – an impact that was vividly represented by a host of Canadian writers.

To complement chapter two's analysis of the controversies associated with the rise of the asylum at the end of the nineteenth century, chapter three relies on close readings to analyze the treatment of dementia in the popular media – specifically *The Globe*, *The Daily Mail*, *The Toronto Telegram*, and *The Guardian* – and in literature from, and reflecting on, the late 1800s to the 1960s. In comparing media, biomedical, and fictional accounts over that century, I trace the workings of two competing and enduring Victorian theories that were applied to dementia and that relied on the opposing concepts of "waste" and "repair." As I argue, the theory of "waste" was tied to the Gothic view of dementia. As I explain in chapter three, there are very few late-nineteenth and early twentieth century fictions that portray dementia.[69] The Victorian concern with waste and repair surfaces in Leacock's short stories (1912) and again, more forcibly, in literary works written in the 1960s and 1970s by Richler, Munro, and Laurence. The latter authors used the images of waste to reflect on both the experience of dementia and the related, broader theme of the wastefulness associated with modern life.

Chapter three's comparative analysis of media and literary discourses from the 1860s to the 1960s also reveals a wide variety of approaches toward dementia, including a subset of views that supported the asylum superintendents' rhetoric of the "menace" of the feeble-minded, aging population. Although not tied exclusively to aging bodies, the early twentieth century's creation of the concept of the "feeble-minded" and its panicked response to this newly fabricated demographic category bear a striking similarity to our current anxieties about the economic "burden" posed by sufferers of Alzheimer's disease. At the dawn of the twentieth century, eugenicists invoked apocalyptic images of "a rising tide"[70] of "feeble-minded" people – images now applied to elderly people suffering from dementia – that would supposedly instigate the degeneration of the nation-state. These largely forgotten historical and philosophical underpinnings of our understanding of dementia are crucial because they led to some of the darkest chapters in modern history: the massive sterilization campaigns in both Canada and the United States in the 1930s and the Nazi death camps during the Second World War.[71]

The literary portrayals of dementia I analyze in chapter three by Stephen Leacock, Alice Munro, Mordecai Richler, and Margaret Laurence that reflect on the late nineteenth and early twentieth centuries do not engage with the dark chapter in the history of mental disability that culminated during the Second World War. They nevertheless adopt the negative view that dementia is both inevitable and dreadful. Their work upholds this perspective not because of Alzheimer's disease, which was only understood to play a role in dementia in the late 1970s and early 80s, but because of the prevailing medical beliefs concerning the relationships between dementia, arteriosclerosis, and the effects of stress or "shattered nerves." During the late nineteenth century, when dementia was found not to be the result of alcoholism or syphilis, it was attributed to the effects of a stroke, a nervous breakdown, or some other dementing illness such as Parkinson's disease. These precipitating causes are explicitly cited in the texts under consideration: Leacock's *Sunshine Sketches of a Little Town*, Munro's "The Peace of Utrecht," Richler's "The Summer My Grandmother Was Supposed to Die," and Laurence's *The Stone Angel*. Unlike our current view of Alzheimer's disease, these fictions accept an array of biological origins of dementia, and they promote a compassionate, elegiac response to those suffering from its effects. Equally important, and in keeping with the historically specific meanings of age-related dementia, the fictional portrayals link dementia to the accelerated decline and waste associated with the effects in Canada of industrialization and modernity.

Chapter four continues to trace the rise of the contemporary Gothic understanding of the disease concept by exploring the views of age-related dementia that prevailed from the 1930s to the 1950s, a period when psychological stress was viewed as a prime instigator of age-related dementia. Given the prevailing dominance of the biological or somatic approach to dementia today, it is notable that in North America during this period, an emphasis on stress – and more generally a psychological rather than somatic approach to cognitive decline – remained dominant, and profoundly influenced clinicians and researchers studying aging and old age. The "sociopsychiatric" approach, as it was termed, found one of its greatest champions in David Rothschild, a Canadian-American researcher trained in pathology and psychoanalysis in Germany. His insights into the role of stress, particularly the effects of anxiety and loneliness, are now being cited as factors affecting the development of dementia (Ingram 125).

In chapter four, I show how the increasing popularity of the biological approach to geriatric psychiatry in Canada in the 1950s traces its roots to the research of Dr Vojtech Adalbert Kral in Montreal, Quebec. Like David Rothschild, Kral worked in an environment heavily influenced by the research findings of Hungarian-born endocrinologist Hans Selye, who served as the director of the Institute of

Experimental Medicine and Surgery at the University of Montreal. In the era after the Second World War, however, Kral's research tempered the prevailing emphasis on psychological factors and ultimately led to the collapse of German psychiatrist Emil Kraepelin's initial distinction between Alzheimer's and senile dementia. The 1950s also saw the introduction of newly discovered medications that controlled psychosis and severe mood disorders (most notably chlorpromazine, introduced in Canada by Dr Heinz Lehmann), as well as the discovery of antidepressants. These biologically oriented treatments increasingly eclipsed psychological approaches and played a key role in the de-institutionalization movement in the 1960s.

In keeping with my study's emphasis on exploring and, where appropriate, calling into question the masculine elegiac and Gothic habit of substituting the artifact for the individual, chapter four juxtaposes Rothschild's and Kral's theories to accounts of clinical experience that shed light on the actual experiences of individuals suffering from dementia in the 1950s – which, in Canadian asylums after the Second World War, were horrific. In the early 1960s, the Canadian government's ongoing desire to cut healthcare costs and the increasingly negative view of state-run mental institutions led to the "massive disgorgement of disabled asylum patients to the rough care of the streets" (Shorter, *A History* 238).

To analyze literary responses to the influence of the anti-asylum movement on individuals – particularly lower-income, elderly women suffering from dementia – in chapter five, I offer a close reading of Alice Munro's short story "Powers" (2004). In addition to providing insight into the challenges posed by de-institutionalization, Munro's story offers a useful corrective to the view that only biological and Gothic models of dementia rely on a process of reductive substitution whereby the person is replaced by ever smaller artifacts – a diseased brain, pathological brain cells, and aberrant protein molecules. "Powers" demonstrates that in an attempt to offer consolation in the face of illness and loss, literary genres such as the masculine elegy also engage in the analogous and equally distorting processes of substitution.

Chapters six and seven are paired. They focus on the experience of two Canadian brothers, Michael and Andrew Ignatieff, who coped in very different ways with their mother Alison's dementia, which took her life in 1992. Alison Ignatieff was diagnosed at a watershed moment in the history of Alzheimer's disease, when researchers, most notably Robert Katzman, recast early onset and senile dementia as a single entity and pronounced it "the fourth or fifth most common cause of death in the United States" (in Ballenger, *Self* 104) As a result of this paradigm shift in the 1980s, old people and old age itself were cast as major contributors to an ongoing, global healthcare crisis. Faced with this crisis, Andrew joined the newly established Alzheimer Society, a worldwide organization that was originally founded in Toronto. In contrast to Andrew's approach – which I cite as an example of an elegiac approach, a turn toward "ordinary ethics," and an instance of the growing shift from cure to care – Michael opted for a literary and philosophical response that culminated in his Gothic and melancholy novel *Scar Tissue*. Taken together, their responses, viewed in the context of prevailing media and biomedical accounts, highlight the social repercussions from the late 1980s to the present when Alzheimer's was reconfigured as the disease of the century.

Chapters eight and nine deepen my book's literary focus on Alzheimer's and widen the geographic scope by offering a close reading of two novels set in Vancouver. Caroline Adderson's novel *A History of Forgetting* (the focus of chapter eight) and Jane Rule's *Memory Board* (analyzed in chapter nine) depict long-term, homosexual relationships in which one partner suffers from Alzheimer's. In essence, both texts align late-onset dementia with queer forms of aging. Both novels also allude to the traumatic effects of the Second World War. By drawing a connection between the discrimination against queers, Jews, and elderly people with dementia, Rule's and Adderson's narratives forge an analogy between elderly individuals with dementia and marginalized groups that were persecuted during the Second World War. Equally important, rather than locating the Gothic monster solely within the "queer" body of the person suffering from Alzheimer's and within the boundaries established by a disease category, *Memory Board* and *A History of Forgetting* cast Gothic shadows over Western society's heteronormative fantasies of interminable youth and sexual allure.

Whereas Adderson's and Rule's novels offer counter-arguments to the Gothic representation of the diseased individual and the related calls for a war against Alzheimer's disease, Munro's short stories, the central focus of chapter nine, offer a distinctly ironic, trickster-inspired response to age-related dementia. Unlike *Memory Board*, which engages in a utopian rewriting of the past and portrays individuals coping with dementia welcomed into the larger community, Munro's stories maintain a bleak view of society's response to people suffering from cognitive decline. Nevertheless, her fiction insists on a fundamentally ironic view of dementia as having unknowable meanings beneath the surface of things.

Moreover, by drawing on surrealist elements, her stories recall alternative ethical and political perspectives on disability and dementia associated with the Surrealist movement that, as noted above, originated in France after the First World War. Rather than fear mental illness and dementia and valorize the powers of reason and memory, the French founders of surrealism drew inspiration from the insights provided by the imagination and the irrational thought processes afforded by altered states of consciousness and dreams. As André Breton proclaims in his *Second Manifesto of Surrealism* (1930), "We want nothing whatever to do with those ... who use their minds as they would a savings bank" (*Manifestoes* 129). Later, Breton boldly writes: "And let it be clearly understood that we are not talking about a simple regrouping of words or a capricious redistribution of visual images, but of the re-creation of a state which can only be fairly compared to that of madness" (175). In contrast to the Lockean view of personhood predicated on intelligence and cognitive fitness, Breton and, more forcibly, avant-garde artist Antonin Artaud recognized that intelligence is "the purest contingency" (Sontag, "An Essay" xxi). Recalling the experience of dementia, Artaud used metaphors to portray the mind "either as a property to which one never holds clear title (or whose title one has lost) or as a physical substance that is intransigent, fugitive, unstable, and obscenely mutable" (ibid. xx). In the final chapter, I argue that Munro's short stories can be usefully read in light of surrealism, a movement that opposed all hierarchical theories of the mind that "[make] one part of consciousness superior to another part" (ibid. xxiii). By figuring the dreams and surreal effects of the imagination of people coping with dementia, Munro's stories, like that of Artaud, promote neurodiversity by upholding "the democracy of mental claims, the right of every level, tendency, and quality of mind to be heard" (ibid.).

For the most part, the fictions analyzed in chapters seven through nine respectfully acknowledge biomedicine's efforts to name and find a cure for Alzheimer's disease – efforts outlined in detail in the first six chapters of the book. However, the literary works under consideration repeatedly highlight the limitations of Gothic tropes and the biblical narrative of apocalypse, with its promise of revelation and the destruction of absolute evil. Rather than re-install Gothic and apocalyptic narratives, the literary portrayals of age-related dementia offer an alternative form of revelation – one that, in keeping with the female elegy and surrealism, entails exposing the humanity of individuals with a dementing illness. Equally important, they also reveal the importance of the geographic and historical contexts in which the illness occurs in constructing the meanings associated with the illness. Rather than join the war against Alzheimer's disease, Canadian fiction explores the fate of the combatants and their families, fleshing out the broader, historical interpersonal and intergenerational relationships often obscured by reified portrayals of this "master illness" as a Gothic monster that supposedly can be located and vanquished on the molecular level.

Cultural theorist Ian Baucom observed recently that over the past decade or so the biological natural sciences have posited "a new theory *of* the human being; one which describes human personhood as reducible to a series of molecular, neuronal, or genetic determinations; one that provides a profound challenge to the notion of the human being long advanced by the humanities; one which for *that very reason* ... it is the responsibility of the humanities to engage" (23). In keeping with Baucom's insight, my study traces the ongoing construction of age-related dementia and Alzheimer's to determine how, in the face of a terminal illness, literary and biomedical narratives alike deploy familiar genres and rhetorical tropes in an effort to establish the meaning of this ailment, allocate agency and blame, and console us for our losses.

I

A Forgotten History:
The Late-Nineteenth- and Early
Twentieth-Century Construction
of the Disease Concept

In the introduction, I referred to two classical forms of irony that often attend discussions of illness: Sophoclean tragic irony, in which spectators know what is happening but characters are unable or refuse to acknowledge or accept it; and Socratic irony, a rhetorical stance characterized by turning questions back on the questioner to demonstrate the latter's gaps in ostensibly rational thinking (Lambek, *Irony* 5). As historian Jesse Ballenger observes, one of the most notable examples of irony in our relationship to Alzheimer's is that public discussion of a disease that robs people of their memory "proceeds with so little appreciation of its past" (*Self* 3).[1] Contingencies and ironies abound when one probes the history of Alzheimer's. For example, as an illness category, Alzheimer's was effectively born in the 1970s (Gubrium 181). Before this time, Alzheimer's disease referred to a disease that affected individuals in their forties and fifties and occasionally even younger, and was considered to be quite rare. Older people with comparable symptoms and pathologies were diagnosed with senile dementia. In 1976, Robert Katzman convincingly argued that these two forms of dementia were, in fact, a single disease. Now the dominant biomedical discourse "holds that dementia of the Alzheimer type (DAT) is a disease without age boundaries that is qualitatively and quantitatively different from 'normal aging' – except that age represents the single most important risk factor for its onset" (Holstein 159). Since "the basic pathological features, identified almost a century ago, remain mysterious enough to be open to differing interpretations," several scholars wonder how we have come to talk about a disease at all (Whitehouse et al. 2).

In this chapter, I trace the rise of the disease concept in Germany in the late nineteenth century – when modern medicine "reconstructed the body in terms of pathological anatomy, displacing degenerative processes to micro-levels of tissues and cells" (Katz, *Cultural* 29; see also Jewson).[2] I aim to identify the distinct and sometimes contradictory paradigms by which the disease has been understood: the Alzheimer/Kraepelin concept of the late nineteenth and early twentieth century, the psychodynamic approach that peaked in the 1950s, the molecular and, more specifically, cholinergic hypothesis of the 1970s, and the current genetic model. My specific interest lies with examining the set of issues that have consistently been at play in the development of Alzheimer's disease as a clinico-pathologic entity from Alois Alzheimer's time to the present. These issues include the related problems of differentiating the normal from the pathological (particularly in women's bodies), distinguishing aging from disease, and exploring the various roles that psychosocial, environmental, and genetic factors have been reputed to play in producing dementia (Whitehouse et al. 48). As noted in the introduction, these issues and the protracted confusions they raise lend Alzheimer's disease its "dreadful" and morally "evil" connotations. Moreover, all of these issues remain contested – Alzheimer's is a disease for which there is presently no cure and no effective treatment.

As neuroscientist Peter Whitehouse argues, thinking historically is crucial since part of the challenge in grappling with Alzheimer's entails recognizing "that disease entities are as much linguistic labels and social constructions as they are the business of science and medicine" ("History" 259). In his account of the history of Alzheimer's disease, professor of psychiatry G.E. Berrios contrasts the two prevailing metaphors for the formation of disease concepts. The first envisions the clinician as "cataloguing" pre-existent "species of disease in an exotic garden" ("Alzheimer's" 356). By contrast, the "creationist" or constructivist view envisions diseases as cultural constructs: "At its basis is the assumption that there is no such thing as the final description for a disease, that clinical boundaries, symptom content, and even anatomical description constitute temporary scripts cribbed from the ongoing medical discourse. In other words, a disease is defined not only by the power of resolution of the ongoing science, but also by periodic backroom decisions taken by her self-appointed mandarins" (ibid.). In keeping with Whitehouse's view, Berrios maintains that the history of Alzheimer's disease offers strong support for "the creationist view" of historical nosology – the branch of science dedicated to the construction and classification of diseases. Nevertheless, many of those involved in the description and dissemination of information about Alzheimer's disease take the non-ironic (cataloguing) stance.

An awareness of historical and cultural contexts associated with the conflict-ridden development of the disease concept is critical since "they bring some observations, interpretive possibilities and options into focus while obscuring others" (Holstein 160). Familiarity with the historical development of Alzheimer's reveals a host of elided features and ironies that help us to appreciate why the unanswered questions associated with age-related dementia continue to haunt contemporary biomedical and aesthetic accounts. In what follows, I adopt a humanistic approach to dementia by exploring the twin birth of hysteria and Alzheimer's disease within late-nineteenth-century European asylums. Focusing initially on the Salpêtrière – the public women's hospital in Paris whose inmates were largely insane, poor, and aged women (Katz, *Cultural* 41) – allows me to illustrate how gender profoundly inflected both the theories and treatments of hysteria and Alzheimer's disease.

This chapter's detailed analysis of the early papers concerning Alzheimer's disease also reveals important, related connections among gender, disease, and aging in nineteenth-century theories of dementia. As the patient population in institutions such as Salpêtrière suggests, Alzheimer and his colleagues were working in a scientific context that legitimated the view that aging was closely aligned with disease and the female body and its physiological processes. Their approach contrasts with contemporary views that rigorously divide so-called "healthy aging" from disease. More precisely, late-nineteenth-century clinicians shared the widely held belief that "involution" – the life changes associated with menopause in women and what was known as "the climacteric" in both women and men – were closely connected with disease processes including dementia. These views help to explain some of the most significant and hidden aspects of the conventional story of Alzheimer's disease, namely, that when early researchers, including Alois Alzheimer himself, found evidence of dementia in an individual who was comparatively young – in her fifties – they did not believe that they had discovered a distinct and novel disease process. Instead, Alzheimer and his colleague Gaetano

Perusini repeatedly insisted that they had merely stumbled on an odd case of atypical senile dementia. Hindsight allows us to recognize that Alzheimer's employer, Emil Kraepelin,[3] who bestowed the name "Alzheimer's disease" on what were considered to be rare cases of early onset dementia, was for a host of reasons deeply enmeshed in a constructivist endeavour. Yet, to the end, Alzheimer and Perusini opposed Kraepelin's view because they remained unconvinced that they had discovered a new disease at all. Instead, in their eyes, what they were dealing with was merely senile dementia – an unfortunate, but common feature of aging – manifesting earlier in the life course.

SECTION I: THE EARLY STORY
OF ALZHEIMER'S DISEASE

In *Cultural Aging* (2005), Stephen Katz poses an intriguing question: "Why have scholars paid such little attention to the senilizing of women's bodies in light of their sophisticated analysis of hysteria?" (42). As Katz astutely observes, Jean-Martin Charcot, the infamous "Napoleon of Neurosis" (Ellenberger 95) and doyen of the Salpêtrière – who was responsible for entrenching the (now obsolete) disease category known as hysteria[4] – was equally famous for penning the seminal work entitled *Clinical Lectures on Diseases of Old Age*. Originally published in France in 1867, Charcot's *Clinical Lectures* laid the foundations for the discipline later known as geriatrics. Yet, as Katz observes, "while most histories on gerontology, aging, and old age accent the canonical power of Charcot's text, few of them comment on the bodies and identities of these women who formed gerontology's first institutionalized population of aged subjects" (40). My exploration of the fraught history of Alzheimer's disease responds to Katz's invitation to scholars to consider the lived experience of the women whose minds and bodies gave rise to both hysteria and Alzheimer's disease – the "master illnesses" of the nineteenth and twentieth centuries, respectively.

By the mid-1600s, the Salpêtrière had become a public hospital for destitute women and prostitutes; later it also became a women's prison (Katz, *Cultural* 40). In the seventeenth and eighteenth centuries the Salpêtrière was the largest asylum in Europe, holding between 5,000 and 8,000 persons at a time when the entire population of Paris was only 500,000 (Goertz in ibid. 41). Like many Old and New World asylums in the nineteenth century, the Salpêtrière was also a popular tourist attraction: "Its reputation as a terrible and terrifying place of confinement on the edge of the city, what Yannick Ripa refers to as the 'capital of female suffering' (1990, 9) in mid-nineteenth-century Paris, did not prevent it from becoming a popular and frequently visited site where its unfortunate inmates were subjected to the humiliation of public display and exhibition" (*Cultural* 41). Axel Munthe, a Swedish doctor practicing in Paris at the time, gave a vivid description of Charcot's Tuesday lectures when "the huge amphitheatre was filled to the last place with a multicoloured audience drawn from tout Paris, authors, journalists, leading actors and actresses, fashionable demimondaines" (in Showalter, "Hysteria" 311). According to Elaine Showalter, Charcot's female hysterics "put on a spectacular show before this crowd of curiosity seekers" ("Hysteria" 311). Some of Charcot's working-class women patients, Showalter writes, "became stars of his public lectures and supermodels in his photography albums" (*Hystories* 34).

Charcot was also the first European psychiatrist or alienist (doctor at a state-run asylum), as they were known at the time, to install a full-time photographer, Albert Londe, in his clinic (Gilman et al. 352).[5] Familiarity with this historical context allows us to appreciate why disease concepts such as hysteria and Alzheimer's could not have evolved without these types of institutions, which sanctioned the confinement of individuals, many of them women, for the purposes of medical, moral, and aesthetic scrutiny. Both the construction of the hysteria diagnosis – indeed, the term (*hystera*, uterus, Gr.) signals the pathologization of the reproductive organs of the female body – and the creation of Alzheimer's disease reveal the prevailing nineteenth-century view that the female body and the physiological processes of puberty, menstruation, pregnancy, birth, and menopause trigger or underlie various psychiatric disorders.[6] Enlightenment definitions of "man" privileged the capacity for abstract reasoning and the faculty of memory. Both hysteria and Alzheimer's disease were viewed as threatening illnesses precisely because they compromised the ability to reason and instigated pathological memory loss.[7] It is well established that Alzheimer's disease is associated with the destruction of memory and, more specifically, of recall – the ability to access events or information from the past. Yet Freud viewed precisely this symptom as characteristic of hysteria. As he explains, hysterics are unable to tell a complete, "smooth and exact" story about themselves: "their communications run dry, leaving gaps unfilled, and riddles

unanswered … The connections – even the ostensible ones – are for
the most part incoherent, and the sequence of different events is
uncertain" (Freud, *Dora* 45–6).

The bodies of women were thus at the site of the birth of hysteria,
geriatrics, and Alzheimer's disease (see Katz, *Cultural* 42). The profound relationship between geriatrics and asylum culture populated by
female inmates prompts Katz to question further whether the discipline of geriatrics as a whole, "like hysteria," is similarly "a prolifera-
tive, positivist and performative science" (ibid. 3). I would suggest that
it is also important to consider the ways in which Alzheimer's disease
is likewise the product of late-nineteenth-century and early twentieth-
century German asylum culture, with its own globally celebrated,
middle-aged "supermodel," Auguste D. (Showalter, *Hysteries* 34).[8]

SECTION II: THE ACTORS: AUGUSTE D. AND ALOIS ALZHEIMER

In considering the fate of Auguste D., it is crucial to recognize that
her photographic image and accounts of her experience, both prior
to and following her incarceration in the asylum, are entirely limited by and mediated through Alzheimer's and Perusini's case reports.
These documents are fascinating for several reasons: first, they offer a
sense of the fundamental preoccupations of some of the leading male
neurologists and psychiatrists in the early twentieth century. Second,
they allow readers intermittent access to Auguste D.'s voice – a crucial feature missing from virtually all accounts in which she has been
transformed almost entirely into a clinical object. Her humanity and
her experience in the asylum – what Ann Goldberg has called "the
social characteristics of madness (6) – have been all but forgotten in
light of contemporary society's obsession with her brain and its telltale stigmata of plaques and tangles.[9] From Alzheimer's careful notes,
however, we can read against the grain of this erasure of her subjectivity and gain a much clearer sense of Auguste's experience in the
Municipal Asylum for the Insane and Epileptic in Frankfurt am Main.

As luck would have it, Auguste D.'s original file was discovered in
the basement of the University Clinic in Frankfurt on 4 June 1977.
The documents "comprised 32 well-preserved pages in a dark blue
folder tied up in string. The cover shows the patient's personal data:
Auguste D., wife of a railway worker, born on 16 May 1850, of the
Reformed faith" (Lage 17). The file records the onset, symptoms,

and course of the disease, the cause of death, and the autopsy findings. There are six pages written by Alzheimer. Four of them, dated between 26 and 30 November 1901, describe conversations between the doctor and his patient, and include samples of Auguste's writing. Four photographs of Auguste taken by Rudolphe, the hospital photographer, were also found (ibid.).

In the late nineteenth century, psychiatric care in Germany was divided between large state-run asylums – including the Frankfurt asylum where Alzheimer worked initially under the director, Professor Emil Sioli – and the new University hospital clinics that emerged after the 1860s, where Alzheimer later worked under Emil Kraepelin. As Eric Engstrom explains, the state-run asylums "charged mainly with caring for indigent patients," were conceived "on a model patriarchal family; the director (or alienist) lived with the patients as an ambiguous blend of father, physician, and judge who oversaw a moral regime of therapeutic intervention" (406). It was within this type of "model patriarchal family" that Auguste D. lived out the end of her life and died.

The assistant physician, Dr Nitsche, examined Auguste on the day she was admitted and informed Alzheimer that the patient showed unusual clinical symptoms. With respect to her male doctors' overarching concerns, it is significant that after entering her name and marital status, Alzheimer focuses on Auguste D.'s mother's health following menopause. Alzheimer notes, for example, that the latter "suffered convulsive attacks" after menopause, but she did not "lose consciousness and did not drop objects that she was holding in her hands" (in Maurer et al. 12). After duly inscribing the causes of death of Auguste D.'s parents, Alzheimer observes further that Auguste had "three healthy brothers. No alcoholism or mental illness in the family history" (ibid.). The report notes that "she lived quite happily, married in 1873, had a healthy daughter and no miscarriages. She was a polite, hard-working, shy and slightly anxious woman. There is no data that leads us to believe that either she or her husband have a syphilitic infection" (in Lage 17). This information emphasizes the extent to which alcoholism and syphilis were viewed as potential causes of dementia.[10] In addition to enquiring whether certain forms of disease and degeneracy were apparent in Auguste D.'s family, the physician's initial focus on Auguste's mother's experience of menopause further underscores the prevailing belief that "involution" in women can trigger mental illness, and that such illnesses were hereditary.

Admitted on 25 November 1901, Auguste was interviewed extensively by Alzheimer the following day. As the translators of the case
report observe, the questioning goes on for many pages. For the purposes of my analysis, I have chosen specific passages that highlight:
her doctors' concerns, Auguste's own often anguished and puzzled
response to her sudden confinement, and facets of Auguste's experience in the asylum that have been eclipsed by late-twentieth- and early
twenty-first-century scientists' preoccupation with her pathological
brain. The contemporary and relentless focus on her brain is, as Katz
observes, driven by trends in science that continue to displace "degenerative processes to micro-levels of tissues and cells" (*Cultural* 29).[11]

The first entry for 26 November 1901 reads: "ALZHEIMER'S
NOTE: She sat on her bed with helpless expression" (in Maurer et
al. 13).[12] Alzheimer's report then records how he began to quiz her
repeatedly; within this initial interview, Alzheimer poses over fifty
questions. He begins by asking her to state her name and that of her
husband. Midway through the interview, when he asks her to say her
husband's name again, she replies, "I do not know how I came to this.
I cannot go on this way." Alzheimer repeats his question five times,
until, according to Alzheimer, she "suddenly and quickly answered,
'August Wilhelm Carl'" (ibid. 15).

Later, in response to her inability to remember objects he has shown
her, Alzheimer states, "It is difficult, isn't it." Auguste replies that she
is "anxious, so anxious." Without commenting on her response, he
holds up three fingers and asks her to count them. She answers correctly and easily. He enquires if she is "still anxious" and she replies
"Yes." Following this, Alzheimer notes, "When she has to write, 'Mrs.
Auguste D.,' she writes 'Mrs.,' and we must repeat the other words
because she forgets them. The patient is not able to progress in writing, and repeats, 'I have lost myself'" (ibid. 15).

I cite these aspects of Alzheimer's report because, in addition to
emphasizing the implicitly patriarchal concern with Auguste D.'s
marital status, this initial entry also offers a poignant glimpse of her
understandable grief, anxiety, and helplessness in the face of both her
confinement and her illness. Ironically, contemporary research cites
anxiety and loneliness as factors affecting the development of dementia (Ingram 125). Although Auguste D. did indeed lose her home,
her husband, her daughter, and all of her social connections, roles,
and responsibilities, there is little indication that Alzheimer or anyone else – the orderlies, domestics, and other patients – responded

compassionately to her repeated confessions of anxiety or her insightful plaint that she had lost herself.

Given her inability to produce the desired, accurate responses to the volley of questions Alzheimer directed at her in his initial clinical assessment, it is not surprising that the following day, as Alzheimer reports, Auguste D. says, "with a worried expression, when the doctor nears her bed, 'You don't seem to think well of me'" (Perusini, "Histology" 83). When Alzheimer asks her why he would be upset with her, she responds: "I don't know, we have not had debts, or something similar. I am only upset; you must not be angry with me" (83). In interpreting Auguste D.'s anxiety, it is helpful to know that she was, in fact, accused of many things, including of losing "all sense of the value of money" (Lage 17). Viewed in this light, Auguste may well have been attempting to assure her physician that she is still a responsible housewife (she has no debts) and has not, in fact, done anything to warrant ill treatment and confinement. She may have thus been asking for someone to attest to her innocence. She may also have been asking for Alzheimer's compassion because, as she explains, she is "only upset" – a reference perhaps to both her physical and psychological distress. Auguste D.'s plight recalls my earlier discussion in the introduction concerning the historical relationship between the Gothic mode and the transformation of illness and death into a crime. Viewed in this light, it is significant that Auguste D. feels as if she is unjustly being treated as a criminal; as a sufferer of dementia, she lived within a Gothic plot.

As the days pass, however, Auguste's anxiety increases. On her third day of confinement, 28 November, 1901, Alzheimer writes: "She is always frightened, anxious, continuously repeats 'I do not want to be cut [also translated as 'hurt']' even though no one has tried to do anything to her" (in Perusini, "Histology" 83). Despite Alzheimer's protests that no one has harmed her, people had done many things to Auguste D. First, she was removed from her home and confined to a hospital where she was "repeatedly given sedatives" (Lage 18). She was also given therapeutic baths, sometimes with cold water, sometimes with hot, nearly every day (ibid.). By Alzheimer's own admission, on several occasions she was placed in isolation. Her comments make even more sense when read in light of the fact that Alzheimer, "nicknamed the psychiatrist with the microscope" (16), was renowned among his colleagues (and presumably among his patients, as well) for dissecting his patients and studying their brains: "By day he examined his patients with painstaking care and tenderness, and by night he sat at his microscope to study the samples he had prepared" (ibid.). Her fellow patients may well have told Auguste D. what lay in store for her. Certainly, in hindsight, her fears of being cut were uncannily prescient. After her death her brain was indeed cut into pieces; precious samples were sent to Alzheimer, who had moved to Heidelberg and later to Munich. To this day, scientists still marvel over the perfectly preserved "specimens."

In offering this interpretive commentary on Alzheimer's accounts, I am in no way suggesting that Auguste was not suffering from dementia.[13] Instead, I am asserting that she was also likely suffering from the trauma of being interned in a mental hospital. Nowadays, it is widely recognized that patients can suffer psychosis due to the repeated boundary violations that occur in hospitals as well as the disruptions that attend basic processes such as eating and sleeping. Moreover, as a host of geriatric psychiatrists have observed, brain disease is frequently accompanied by affective (emotional) disorders such as depression and anxiety. It is thus quite possible that Auguste D. suffered from brain disease, depression, and anxiety. Even formulating the relationship between mind and body in this way is misleading since the relationship between them is blurry at the best of times. Despite her illness, Auguste made efforts to communicate her emotional state to her physicians. Only in retrospect, it seems, were her emotions – anxiety, desolation, and terror – taken into account. As noted, although Alzheimer is reputed to have been an extremely humane clinician who readily adopted Pinel's "moral treatment,"[14] the records do not indicate whether the team of doctors, nurses, and orderlies who continued to assess and care for Auguste acknowledged her experience or responded with compassion.

During his third interview with Auguste on 28 November 1901, Alzheimer reports that she "acts as if she were blind, touching the other patients on their faces and when asked what she is doing, replies: 'I must put myself in order'" (in Perusini, "Histology" 83). Although none of her doctors could find any physical basis for this peculiar symptom, Auguste's "psychic blindness" (Perusini, "Histology" 85) persisted throughout her illness. As Alzheimer's researchers observe, "functional blindness" (blindness in the absence of visible lesions) is sometimes associated with dementia since damage to specific parts of the brain can lead to problems identifying objects and people.[15]

Of course, it is impossible to know why Auguste D. felt compelled to touch other people's faces to put herself "in order." In addition to signaling the presence of neurodegeneration, her sense of her own blindness, and her repeated attempts to deal with the problem through touch, may also speak to an inability to make sense of her new surroundings and a desire not to witness her current circumstances. Read figuratively, her blindness and repeated attempts to put herself in order by touching another person also poignantly underscore the fact that, as noted in the introduction in my discussion of Jonathan Franzen's compassionate response to his father, human identity is predicated on intersubjective relations. In other words, we become and remain "ourselves" and sustain our identities – we are literally put together and afforded order and coherence as subjects – only insofar as we continue to see ourselves mirrored as subjects (rather than as clinical objects) by others. Without these reciprocal, daily acts of recognition individuals are indeed lost to themselves and others.

In the case of Auguste D., Alzheimer's records attest to the fact that he and his staff had difficulty communicating with her. As a result, her basic needs and desires went unrecognized. On 30 November 1901 Alzheimer stated tersely: "It is difficult to figure out what she wants. Therefore, she must be isolated" (in Maurer et al. 18). There is no indication that Auguste was able to communicate meaningfully with her doctors from that point on. After the 30 November entry, Alzheimer's records end abruptly and resume in February 1902 – the precise day is not stated. Alzheimer writes: "She is in a state of fright, anxious and completely disoriented, violent towards everything. She lies in bed in a strange way. She turns everything upside down and covers herself with a pillow. When you go to her she often asks, 'What do you want? My husband will come soon'" (in Perusini, "Histology" 84). Following this, the entries are few and far between, and Auguste's mental and physical health swiftly declined. The statement for June 1902 is terse, and again conveys the sense that, to her physician's dismay, Auguste railed against her confinement: "Completely rebellious, screams and stamps her feet when someone goes near her. She refuses to be examined, screams spontaneously and often for hours" (84). In discussing elderly people's rage, Robert Butler compassionately suggests that it would "be more realistically interpreted if one became sensitive to the degree of outrage older people feel, consciously or unconsciously, at viewing their situation," and he adds: "Much of the rage is an appropriate response to inhumane treatment" (Butler et al. 86). A full two years and eight months pass before the next brief entry: "Feb. 1904. No change."

By November 1904, Auguste D. is incontinent of "feces and urine" and Alzheimer observes that she screams "less than before" (in Perusini, "Histology" 84). A year later, another entry: "Oct. 1905. She lies in bed without moving" (84). In December of 1905, she "mainly lies with her legs pulled up to her chest. She again screams a lot. Refuses to be examined" (84). For two years, Auguste lay on her bed, curled up under the blankets in the midst of her urine and feces. The last fifteen lines describe her final days: at the beginning of 1906 she developed bedsores. Her physical deterioration was progressive. Throughout the month of March 1906, she had a fever of up to 40°C. She was diagnosed with pneumonia and continued to be very agitated, crying out loudly. In early April, her stupor increased and her fever rose to 41°C. Finally, at quarter past six on 8 April 1906, she died (Lage 18). As the report confirms, for five years and three months, Auguste D. was mentally and often physically isolated. Until her death, she suffered grievously both from her illness and her incarceration.

After he left Frankfurt and moved to the smaller, urban university clinic in Munich, Alzheimer never saw the patients in distant asylums; he and his coworkers often had only the patients' files to work with. Those files had been compiled by third-party observers using different kinds of record-keeping, and often contained gaps in the clinical picture that extended for years (Engstrom 410). In contrast, then, to the psychiatrists in the university clinics, some mid-nineteenth-century alienists spent "a lifetime living and working among patients" (410). As Engstrom observes, "without in any way wishing to romanticize asylum practice, those same alienists had acquired profound knowledge of the progression of their patients' lives and illnesses – knowledge that Alzheimer and other academic psychiatrists could never acquire" (410).

While working in Heidelberg and Munich with Kraepelin at their urban, university clinics, Alzheimer had to rely on the director of the Frankfurt asylum to supply him with data and specimens (ibid. 408). Indeed, it was so difficult for Alzheimer to procure data and specimens from patients suffering from dementia that he went to great lengths to ensure that patients such as Auguste D. remained accessible for his research. In fact, two attempts were made to transfer

Auguste D. from the Frankfurt asylum to a much less expensive asylum in Welmünster, some thirty miles north of Frankfurt. First, shortly after her admission in 1901, her husband applied for a transfer; later, in 1904, after she had apparently become a charge of the state, local courts again sought to have her transferred (ibid. 409). On both occasions, however, Alzheimer intervened "to prevent the transfer – presumably in anticipation of her demise and the prospect of obtaining valuable pathological specimens" (409).

The gaps and silences surrounding Auguste's experience in the Frankfurt asylum recall Lambek's comment cited earlier that, in the case of illness, irony entails "the recognition that some of the potentially participatory voices or meanings are silent, missing, unheard, or not fully articulate, and that voices or utterances appearing to speak for totality or truth offer only single perspectives" (*Irony* 6). Whereas numerous scholars, myself included, have explored the lives of female patients purportedly suffering from hysteria in institutions such as the Salpêtrière, comparatively little attention has been paid to the fates and perspectives of women like Auguste D. who were admitted to mental asylums due to dementia. Although in this instance I am tracing the political and, more specifically, feminist significance of seeking out elided voices, the irony associated with the early chapters in the history of Alzheimer's disease also reflects a far more pervasive epistemological and psychoanalytical predicament. Simply put, the act of knowing (including self-knowledge) involves repressing or forgetting the gaps and limits associated with our knowledge, which always remains partial. Even as I attempt to tell a more accurate story about the history of Alzheimer's disease, I recognize that every account remains partial; this is an irony that no one can escape.

SECTION III: ALOIS ALZHEIMER

According to historians, Alois Alzheimer was a humble, hard-working man, perhaps a better researcher than a clinician, who had "fame thrust upon him by those who loved him well or had their own reasons to do so" (Berrios, "Alzheimer's" 365). For the most part, the basic details of Alzheimer's life are well known. He was born on 14 June 1864 in the small German village of Marktbreit am Main. When he graduated from high school, his teachers certified that "he was excellent in the sciences" (Maurer et al. 6). He went on to study medicine at Berlin, Würzburg, and Tübingen. As noted earlier, in

1888 he became an intern at the Municipal Asylum for the Insane
and Epileptic in Frankfurt. Although still young, he was awarded
a place as a resident by Professor Emil Sioli, director of the asylum
(Lage 16).

At the asylum in Frankfurt, Alzheimer started his lifelong association and friendship with Franz Nissl, who developed new nerve staining techniques bearing his name that, for the first time, allowed early
neurologists to view microscopic features of the brain.[16] Together
with Sioli, Alzheimer and Nissl "transformed the asylum into a sound
psychiatric clinic where two primary concerns were foremost: firstly,
to avoid the use of physical restraint to reduce patient agitation;
and secondly, to promote research by doing as many autopsies and
neurological studies as possible" (Lage 16). Kraepelin called Nissl
to Heidelberg in 1895, and Alzheimer joined them in 1903. While
at Heidelberg, under Kraepelin's supervision, Alzheimer completed
his "Habilitationsschrift" – a postdoctoral research project required
of all German PhD students planning to work in the university system. In October of the same year, Alzheimer moved to Munich, following Kraepelin, who had accepted the chair of psychiatry at the
Nervenklinik of the Ludwig-Maximilians-Universität. In Munich
Alzheimer was appointed head of the neuroanatomic laboratory,
which became an important centre for brain research. He was joined
by a host of renowned psychiatrists and neuropathologists including Gaetano Perusini and Francesco Bonfiglio, who shared cases and
wrote the case reports on dementia that Kraepelin used to create
the new disease concept named after Alzheimer (Maurer et al. 6–9).
The Friedrich-Wilhelm University of Breslau in Silesia (formerly in
East Germany though today it is in Wrocław, Poland) appointed
Alzheimer as chair of the Department of Psychiatry and director
of the University of Psychiatric Clinic on 16 July 1912. He viewed
the post as the fulfillment of his scientific and academic aims. On his
way to Breslau, however, Alzheimer caught a severe and persistent
cold; the bacteria remained in his system and developed into bac-
terial endocarditis. He died at age fifty-one from kidney failure on
19 December 1915, outliving his celebrated patient, Auguste D., by
a mere nine years.

In traditional biographical accounts of Alzheimer's life such as the
one cited above, historians rarely include details that challenge the
stereotypical view of Alzheimer as a modest and dedicated clinician,

who relentlessly pursued the biological origins of dementia. Yet this is only a partial account of a much more complicated and open-minded individual, whose work as a psychiatrist was extremely wide-ranging.[17] Alzheimer's cases and interests were far more eclectic than historians determined to emphasize his biological focus admit. For example, while working under Sioli, Alzheimer actively researched the psychological roots of mental illness. At one point, Alzheimer treated a patient suffering from sexual perversion, a shoe fetishist. Determined to prove "that the illness was psychologically caused," Alzheimer set up an elaborate experiment, which involved "arranging to have a pair of women's shoes clandestinely placed in the wardrobe of the head warden and instructing him to monitor O's [the patient's] behavior" (46–7).

Despite his eclectic pursuits and his interest in the psychological roots of mental illness, historians typically promote the view that Kraepelin disseminated of Alzheimer as a sober and exclusively empirical scientist committed to tracing the roots of illness to biology. According to Kraepelin, Alzheimer "possessed a thoroughness in research which was stopped by no obstacles, by no difficulty, but above all, an almost cruel self-criticism which could not be corrupted and which controlled all his thinking and a boundless caution in regard to all conclusions" (in Berrios, "Alzheimer's" 356). His students, however, recall a less formidable man, who suffered from his own brand of forgetfulness: "An inveterate cigar smoker, he would put a half-smoked cigar down on the table before leaning into a student's microscope for a consultation. A few minutes later, while shuffling to the next microscope, he'd light a fresh cigar, having forgotten about the smoke already in progress. At the end of each day, twenty microscopes later, students recalled, twenty cigar stumps would be left smoldering throughout the room" (Shenk 22). My point in elaborating on these little known biographical details is to correct the erroneous and reified historical portrait by emphasizing that Alzheimer was, in fact, an open-minded and liberal psychiatrist. Alzheimer's own inclinations and, later, the wealth he received after his wife's death prompted him to pursue a variety of research interests, which included tracing the behavioural and psychological as well as the biological origins of mental illness. Critically, his wealth also allowed him the liberty of disagreeing with Emil Kraepelin, although the details and protracted nature of their disagreement have been forgotten.

SECTION IV: CONTROVERSIES CONCERNING
THE NAMING OF ALZHEIMER'S DISEASE

It is generally agreed that the illness that now bears Alzheimer's name
was mentioned for the first time at a meeting of psychiatrists and
neuropathologists in Tübingen, Germany, in November of 1906. Alzheimer briefly reported a case study of his fifty-one-year-old patient
Auguste D., who showed early clinical symptoms that deviated from
the common ones associated with syphilis and arteriosclerosis. In
contrast to patients suffering from dementia instigated by syphilis, Auguste D. presented with "progressive cognitive impairment,
focal symptoms relating to higher cortical functions, hallucinations, delusions, and marked psychosocial incompetence" (Berrios,
"Alzheimer's" 358).

In his more detailed account of the same case, Alzheimer's colleague, Gaetano Perusini, explains that Auguste D., "the wife of an
office clerk, aged 51-and-a-half years," led a normal life until March
1901 (Perusini, "Histology" 82). As his notes demonstrate, however,
Auguste was plunged into a paranoid, Gothic world:

> Around March 18, 1901, the patient suddenly asserted, without
> any reason, that her husband had gone for a walk with a neigh-
> bour. From then she remained very cool towards him and the
> lady. Soon after she started to have difficulty in remembering
> things. Two months later she started making mistakes in prepar-
> ing meals, paced nervously and without reason in the apartment,
> and was not careful with the household money. She progressively
> became worse. She asserted that a wagon driver who often came
> to her home might do something to her and she assumed that
> all conversations of the people around her were about her. She
> had no language disturbances and no paralysis. Later, she often
> had a fear of dying, nervous anxiety during which she started
> to tremble, and would go and ring all the bells of the neighbours,
> and knock on their doors. She could not find certain objects
> which she had put away. (ibid. 82–3)

As noted above, Auguste D. was admitted to the institution where
Alzheimer and Perusini worked on 25 November 1901 (ibid. 83).
In his summary of the case, Perusini writes: "Here we see a singular
clinical picture. In a woman of menopausal age a psychic disturbance

develops without fits and in which misunderstanding of situations plays a role and which culminates shortly in a completely frightened state with psychic blindness" (85). Perusini's summary is striking because in conventional accounts Alzheimer's disease is solely equated with memory loss. Yet as indicated by the passage cited above – which goes on to report on Auguste D.'s inability to prepare meals and handle money and on her fears and anxieties – memory loss and other cognitive deficits were, relative to today, interpreted within a broader context. As in many historical periods, they were seen as less interesting than emotional and behavioural disturbances as well as the patient's inability to play his or her social role (see Ballenger, *Self* 84).

Auguste D.'s memory loss was, of course, duly noted. Alzheimer's brief two-page report explains that shortly after being admitted, Auguste D. experienced disturbances in her ability to memorize and to recall events. During her stay in the mental institution, she became totally helpless and disoriented in time and place. After five years of illness, she died. Alzheimer carefully insists that in spite of "all the care and attention given to her she suffered from decubitus" (2) – acute blood poisoning due to infectious bedsores. On postmortem examination her brain was found to contain numerous senile plaques and newly observed pathological structures including neurofibrillary tangles, made visible to microscopic observation through the recent development of silver staining.

By and large, the details concerning Auguste D.'s memory loss related thus far constitute the entirety of the conventional account of her condition, which has become part of the lore associated with the early history of Alzheimer's disease. As my previous discussion of Auguste's experience and Perusini's treatment of the case suggest, however, there are other, elided aspects of the story concerning the formation of Alzheimer's disease. A basic feature that is omitted from the conventional account of the putative discovery of Alzheimer's disease is the humility and skepticism expressed by these early neurologists and neuropsychiatrists concerning the legitimacy of their findings. In their case reports, these early researchers repeatedly questioned the accuracy and acknowledged the limits of their hypotheses. Katherine Bick, the editor and translator of the historic papers of Alzheimer and his scientific colleagues, observes that "one is struck over and over again" as one reads the scientific essays of these early pioneers "by their skepticism about their own methods and their reluctance to speculate too broadly on what were clearly to them shaky grounds" (vii). In considering the researchers' skepticism, as well as the contradictions and complexities that attend the early story, it is useful to heed Berrios's warning that "the psychiatry of the late nineteenth century is a remote country" (355). To a great extent its remoteness springs from the fact that "crucial concepts such as dementia, neuron, neurofibril or plaque had not yet been fully crystallized and meant different things for different people" (ibid.).

Nowadays we associate dementia with senescence, but in the late nineteenth century the term was used far more broadly to designate "any state of psychological dilapidation associated with chronic brain disease" (ibid. 356). Included within this term were various "deficit states related to the functional psychoses" (ibid.) – in medical parlance, "functional" means that the symptom's origin is uncertain, and "psychosis" refers to conditions that result in a break with reality. This explains why Kraepelin used the term "dementia praecox" (precocious or premature dementia) to describe what was later termed "schizophrenia" – a disease that often manifests in late adolescence (ibid. 357).[18] When dementia states occurred in the elderly they were called "senile dementia," and "had been so since the beginning of the century" (ibid. 356). Furthermore, in the nineteenth century, irreversibility was not considered a criterion of dementia (ibid.). Simply put, in 1900 the term "dementia" did not necessarily denote an irreversible process; nor did it "evoke an association with old age, as it tends to do nowadays" (ibid. 357). I cite this information to demonstrate the extent to which the current connotations of the word "dementia" have changed since the nineteenth century. Nowadays, the term "dementia" has been Gothicized, in the sense that it solely evokes the "dreadful" image of an elderly individual suffering from irreversible brain disease.

Our understanding of Alzheimer's disease ironically entails a forgetting of its origins, specifically, the uncertainty that surrounded the illness and the humility of the researchers who probed its etiology. Francesco Bonfiglio, for instance, concludes his case study of dementia not with affirmations and promises of a forthcoming cure, but with a host of questions about the problems associated with attempts at categorizing dementia, asking: "Into which of the known nosographic groups can this case which I have presented fall?" "Or does it not belong to its own separate group which further studies will teach us to distinctly separate from those known up to now?" (30). Similarly, Perusini, who as noted earlier examined and wrote up the most detailed case report on Auguste D., humbly attests to the limits of his knowledge about dementia. At several points he states: "I can say very little about this" ("Histology" 117). Perusini likewise confesses that "our knowledge of senile psychoses is still full of uncertainties" ("The Nosographic" 143). Extremely circumspect with respect to the implications of the findings associated with the new staining techniques, Perusini repeatedly cautioned against coming to firm conclusions, insisting instead that as "Alzheimer underscores, we must be aware of the limitations of our methods" ("Histology" 118). He concludes his essay by explicitly warning against using anatomo-pathological datum in a reductive fashion; although lengthy, his comments on this topic are worth citing in full:

> Of course, as usually happens when anatomo-pathological datum offers easy enticement, there will be more than one person who, on the basis of these findings will make the most useless and fanciful anatomo-psychic guesses, and those who amuse themselves with anatomically localizing the location of conscience, the will and related matters, would find a good playground, in which the tangles, for instance, might offer the most clear-cut explanation for the disorientation observed in the senile, demented patient, and the gaps filled by Redlich-Fischer plaques might demonstrate *ad oculus*, [meaning "obvious on sight" or "obvious to anyone that sees it"] the cause of memory failure or similar events. ("The Nosographic" 144)

In hindsight, Perusini's warning is profoundly ironic given that nowadays, researchers recognize that plaques "are frustratingly absent when they should be present; they can exist in significant numbers without having any apparent effect on the brain; and they may not even be the entity that should be targeted in any Alzheimer's therapy" (Ingram 103). The same confusion obtains with respect to tangles, the other hallmark of Alzheimer's disease, leading scientists to admit that these days "it's beginning to look as if the ultimate target might be neither plaques nor tangles" (ibid. 107). Although contemporary brain scientists readily admit that we need to "know a lot more about the brain itself" (ibid. 12), the stylistic practices in Perusini's day seemingly allowed for a more self-consciously circumspect approach. Nowadays, although clinicians and bench scientists continue to grapple with the vexing nature of age-related dementia, circumstances prevent them from articulating the range of qualifications expressed by Perusini and his fellow researchers. For the most part, current research has assumed that plaques are the "bad guys"; yet a host of Alzheimer's researchers insist that vascular issues account for 30 per cent percent of all cases called Alzheimer's (see ibid. 163; see also Black). The theory that plaques are the primary culprit has an "enormous political and financial pressure behind it," but "in the eyes of some, [it] has prevented the exploration of other much less well attested ideas" (Ingram 166). In Alzheimer's day, scientists recognized that very little was known about the relationship between the material aspects of the body and brain, changes associated with the life course – specifically, aging and the transformations associated with menopause – and disease.

The confusions concerning these relationships are glaringly apparent in Kraepelin's eighth edition of his textbook on psychiatry, where he first named Alzheimer's disease (1910). Kraepelin published two revised volumes; the first appeared in February 1909, while the second "and the most important of the two," devoted to clinical psychiatry, appeared in July 1910 (Lage 19). Kraepelin coined the term Alzheimer's disease in chapter seven of the second volume, in a long essay entitled "Senile and Pre-senile Dementias." The chapter opens with a lengthy meditation on the seemingly inextricable relationship between dementia and old age – and, more precisely, "the involutional processes" (32). At first, Kraepelin argues that old age seemingly *predisposes* individuals to disease; his opening statements posit a correlation between aging and dementia: "That the involutional processes, known in man as old age, can also influence mental health seriously is most clearly demonstrated by the well-known fact of senile dementia which in certain circumstances can lead to a progressive transformation and, finally, to the destruction of the personality in the last decades of life" (32). Yet correlation seemingly transforms into causation when Kraepelin later asserts that "several disease processes are actually characteristic of the involutional years" (32). The ambiguity associated with his views on the relationship between aging and dementia recalls Charcot's much stronger conviction concerning the connection between women and hysteria. On the one hand, Charcot defined hysteria as "a physical illness caused by a hereditary defect or traumatic wound in the central nervous system that gives rise to epileptiform attacks" (Showalter, *Hystories* 30). On the other hand, Charcot's practices implied that such symptoms were associated with all women; as a contemporary of Charcot reports: "One felt that in all the talk of this terrifying man, he barely distinguished between society ladies and the 'hysterics' he was treating in his ward and that if it had been up to him he would have placed the whole of society behind the bars of his institution" (Martin du Gard in Harris 207). In keeping with Charcot's theories concerning the relationship between women and hysteria, Kraepelin likewise argued for a connection between women and dementia. Perhaps the kernel of accuracy in this distortion is that repression and incoherence are much more endemic to human experience than is widely accepted.

Drawing on the uterine theories of disease circulating in his day, Kraepelin argued that his studies on women from forty-five to fifty years old led him to postulate a connection between menopause and dementia. Referring to the latter, Kraepelin writes: "Its development in women of middle age without any recognizable external cause as well as the demonstration of a general severe cortical disease seemed initially to suggest auto-intoxication in connection with the process of involution" (40). The term "auto-intoxication" recalls the prevalent belief that structures in the body such as the intestines and other glands could become diseased or toxic and lead to self-poisoning (see Shorter, *A History* 303). But the view of "auto-intoxication" was also linked to theories concerning the ovaries and womb, and thus intersected with theories about hysteria. In the latter disease, the uterus was presumed to be the agent that instigated the disease process. In his essay, Kraepelin in fact triangulates the relationship between menopause and dementia by linking the two with a specific form of depression – "melancholia" of the age of involution (33) – that was supposedly "favoured very much by the upheaval of this very period of life" (34).

Given the pervasive belief in the late nineteenth and early twentieth centuries that women's bodies – particularly menopausal bodies – were prone to disease, if not inherently diseased, it is perhaps not surprising that Kraepelin's preferred methods for treating dementia of the Alzheimer's type was predicated in part on a glandular, or what might be best termed an ovarian, theory of disease:

As a treatment for patients, because of the suspected causal relationship to the menopause, we tested first the administration of an ovarian preparation, but unfortunately without any success. Further, sufficient nutrition has to be provided and occasionally

the use of a gastric tube is necessary. The agitation of the patients
is barely influenced by drugs; we carried out a programmed
opium treatment and tried also other kinds of sleeping pills
and sedatives ... When the patients would not stay in their beds,
water therapy, frequently also wet wrappings were well tolerated.
We attempted to improve the general state of health by administration of iron and arsenic. (42)

Although nowadays arsenic is understood solely as a poison, in the
nineteenth century, prior to the advent of penicillin, it was frequently
used in the treatment of syphilis. Ultimately, just as Charcot's views on
aging and hysteria reflect the beliefs of his time, Kraepelin's hypotheses concerning treatments for dementia must likewise be understood
in a broader historical context – a context that aligned aging with
disease and viewed women's bodies as particularly susceptible to the
latter. Although he promoted this hypothesis, Kraepelin nevertheless
maintained sufficient skepticism to admit that "since we do not know
the true causes of these diseases, it must still remain doubtful whether
they are closely related to the involutional processes, or whether
these are only particularly favourable conditions for the appearance
of independent disorders, *per se*" (45).[19]

Yet Kraepelin's skepticism paled in comparison to that of
Alzheimer himself concerning the nature and very existence of the
eponymous disease. By far the most fascinating aspect of Alzheimer's
story, which remains untold, is that, in contrast to Kraepelin – who
took it upon himself to name Alzheimer's disease for reasons that
remain mysterious – Alzheimer repeatedly insisted that he had not
discovered a distinct disease. This fact is perhaps one of the greatest ironies associated with our current understanding of the disease.
As noted earlier, it was, in fact, his wealth and independence that
enabled him to publicly disagree with his employer. After delivering
the short report on Auguste D. ("A Characteristic"), Alzheimer "left
the task of producing a more detailed publication on the disease later
named after him to Perusini" (1910) (Möller and Graeber 30). The
following year, however, Alzheimer turned his attention again to the
disease and published "a long paper of his own on the clinical picture
and neuropathological background of the disease" (30). In contrast
to his two-page report published in 1907, his later paper describes
fully "his conceptualization of the disease and contains numerous illustrations, mainly drawings, which include several examples

of the histopathology of the first case together with a second case report – that of Johann F." (30). In this latter report, which "seemed most important to Alzheimer" (30), Alzheimer forcibly disagreed with Kraepelin.

Alzheimer's 1911 case report traces the illness of Johann F., a fifty-six-year-old labourer who was admitted to the Psychiatric Hospital on 12 September, 1907. In his notes, Alzheimer states:

> Wife died two years ago. Quiet; since half year very forgetful, clumsy, could not find his way, was unable to perform simple tasks or carried these out with difficulty, stood around helplessly, did not provide himself with lunch, was content with everything, was not capable of buying anything by himself and did not wash himself. Very dull, slightly euphoric, slow in comprehension, unclear. Slowed speech, rare answers, frequent repetition of the question. PTR (patellar tendon reflex l. more pronounced than r.) Sticking when naming things, motor apraxia, imitates in a clumsy way. Paraphasia, ideational apraxia, paragraphia, able to copy writings and drawings. Does not realize contradictions in speech, can read. Blurred demarcation of the r. optic disk, veins very filled, wavy. Does not find the toilet. Heart rate 68. Blood pressure 98–168. Eats a lot. Is tugging at his sheets. Repeats sentences without problems. (in Möller and Graeber 31–2)

In contrast to Auguste D., Johann F. was reportedly "happy" and laughed "a lot." While he was at the hospital, he was taught to sing by the other patients (35). Even when he became incontinent and could no longer speak, he would still sing, "'We are sitting so happily together,' when others start[ed] him off" (35). In 1909, however, his health declined precipitously, and he died on 3 October 1910 of pneumonia after three years at the Psychiatric Hospital of the University of Munich. The autopsy book cites the findings of "Alzheimersche Krankheit" (Alzheimer disease); both the initial clinical diagnosis and the autopsy entry were most likely "written by Alois Alzheimer" (32). The results of the autopsy were peculiar, as Alzheimer explains: "Rather remarkably, numerous preparations produced from very many different areas of the brain did not show a single cell with the peculiar fibrillary degenerations I have previously described. This form of cell change, which occurred very frequently in the other case descriptions of this peculiar disease and which is not infrequently also to be found in severe cases of senile dementia, was missing here, although the plaques were of a size and frequency never seen before in the other cases. So, although one might be tempted to do so, one cannot relate plaques to fibrillary changes or vice versa" (in Möller and Graeber 39).

Tellingly, the second "case," that of Johann F., did not evidence the neurofibrillary tangles (NFTS) upon autopsy, and these were Alzheimer's main contribution in the description of the condition that Kraepelin named after him and are still regarded today as its hallmark (Whitehouse et al.). From the start, then, the cases that were used to establish the physical characteristics of the disease introduced contradictions. Moreover, they indicated that multiple and potentially mixed, rather than singular, histological changes were responsible for the clinical presentations of dementia. Researchers attest that Auguste D.'s brain also showed signs of mixed dementia. After the autopsy it was reported that the "larger cerebral vessels showed arteriosclerotic changes" (Maurer et al. 20). As these examples illustrate, mapping the brain has repeatedly proven limited and, at times, distorting. Here, too, the distinction between what we discover and what we construct remains unclear.

Alzheimer also explicitly raised the question of whether "the cases of disease which I considered peculiar" [those of Auguste D. and Johann F.] are sufficiently different clinically or histologically to be distinguished from senile dementia or whether they should be included under that rubric" (in Möller and Graeber 37). In stark contrast to Kraepelin, in the most extensive report on the illness that was named in his honour, Alois Alzheimer writes: "As similar cases of disease obviously occur in the late old age, it is therefore not exclusively a presenile disease, and there are cases of senile dementia which do not differ from these presenile cases with respect to the severity of disease process. There is, then, no tenable reason to consider these cases as caused by a specific disease process. They are senile psychoses, atypical forms of senile dementia" (41). I draw attention to Alzheimer's disagreement with Kraepelin's position to emphasize the basic controversy concerning Alzheimer's disease that continues to haunt the disease category.[20] This fundamental controversy stems from the fact that senile dementia was, and remains to this day, a puzzling problem closely aligned with normal aging. Indeed, as Kraepelin himself attests: "The imperceptible transition of the distinct forms of senile dementia to the common psychological alterations of old age makes any precise description of the limits of health impossible. To a certain degree therefore the identification of the illness is arbitrary here" (80). His comments suggest that our concept of "health," like the Lockean notion of identity as a remembered biography, is itself a fantasy or fiction. Kraepelin's acknowledgement of the arbitrary separation between senile dementia and old age also recalls Corey's warning cited in the introduction that "through an inappropriate pursuit of the good [or the fiction], we lash out at our doom and cause harm" (7).

Despite Kraepelin's intention to establish a new disease concept, both Alzheimer and Perusini were violently opposed to Kraepelin's plan. Even Kraepelin himself was uneasy about his most basic claims. In the conclusion to the now famous essay in which he introduces Alzheimer's disease, he makes the following confession: "The clinical interpretation of this Alzheimer's disease is still confused" (77). At bottom, Kraepelin was torn between the two basic approaches to categorizing phenomena – lumping and splitting. While it was tempting to lump the disorder Alzheimer identified in his patient Auguste D. under senile dementia, her age made him hesitate. "While the anatomical findings suggest that we are dealing with a particularly serious form of senile dementia," Kraepelin writes, "the fact that this disease sometimes starts already around the age of 40 does not allow this supposition" (77). To preserve his theory of involution – the view that old age itself was linked to dementia, particularly in women – Kraepelin was perhaps reluctant to align the appearance of dementia in middle-aged individuals with what was then termed "senile dementia." Yet, immediately after drawing the line between age and youth – senile dementia and Alzheimer's disease – Kraepelin recants his position and again blurs the line: "In such cases," he writes, "we should at least assume a 'senium praecox,' if not perhaps a more or less age-independent unique disease process" (77).[21] Kraepelin's use of the word "perhaps" followed by the phrase "more or less" underscores his prevarication. Taken as a whole, the sentence contradicts itself since the first part argues that scientists can identify senility upstream, in middle-aged individuals, whereas the second part reasserts the well-known, contemporary view that Alzheimer's is not akin to senility, but in fact constitutes a "unique" and "age-independent disease process" (77).

In addition to their inability to align the disease with either the "presenium" (age forty-five to sixty) or the senium, nineteenth-century clinicians and researchers wrestled with an even more basic and troubling inability to reconcile the appearance of disease processes – the characteristic plaques and tangles – in the bodies of demented individuals with the same symptoms in the brains of non-demented individuals and individuals suffering from other diseases. This finding remains a conundrum for Alzheimer's researchers.[22] In "Histology and Clinical Findings of Some Psychiatric Diseases of Older People," Perusini writes: "I call attention above all to the link of the fibril changes with plaque formation. However, with regard to the actual fibril condition, I have observed more often than in any other experimental material, single absolutely identical changes – even if in not so great an extent – in some old persons who were not reported to have been mentally ill. This circumstance must obviously be attributed a certain value in the interpretation of our cases" (117). In "The Nosographic Value of Some Characteristic Histopathological Findings in Senility," Perusini again emphasizes the ambiguous implications associated with the presence of "senile plaques" in normal and demented elderly individuals. As he explains, neurofibrillary alterations (tangles) were "described for the first time in Italy by Bonfiglio, and later, by many others" (132). Perusini points out, however, that Cerletti "was the first to observe them in normal elderly" (132). Their presence in cases of both healthy and demented people prompted Perusini to assert: "Therefore, even the presence of neurofibrillary alterations can be considered, for the time being, merely as one of the histopathological findings occurring in the involution of the brain during old age. The inherent character of the relations existing between these alterations of neurofibrils and senile plaques is not yet known" (132; emphasis removed). In his concluding summary, Perusini again insists:

1) The Redlich-Fischer plaques represent one of the findings related to the senile involution of the brain and only in this sense do they represent a characteristic finding in aging;

2) In some cases, both in the "normal" elderly and in the senile demented patients, as well as in the atypical forms of senile dementia characterized by Alzheimer, the particular alterations of neurofibrils described by this Author are found; this finding, too, is no more than one of those which accompany senile involution of the brain;

3) The study of the Redlich-Fischer plaques, of the particular neurofibrillary alterations described by Alzheimer and the

vascular alterations described by Cerletti, together with other and clinical data confirm that *no clear-cut distinction exists between senile dementia and normal aging as far as the clinical and anatomo-pathological elements are concerned.* (144–5; emphasis added)

In sum, early researchers were reluctant to view Alzheimer's as distinct from normal aging. Moreover, they were not even certain that the plaques and tangles were specific to illnesses associated with "involution," since these phenomena were not always discerned in tandem.

As Perusini observes, "in some cases of dementia cited by Alzheimer, although senile plaques were extremely abundant, the peculiar alterations of neurofibrils ... were completely missing" (142). He is referring, in this instance, to the case of Johann F. cited above. Plaques and tangles were also observed in patients with diseases other than dementia. Plaques, for example, had been described in 1882 by Blocq and Marinesco in the brain of an epileptic patient (Berrios, "Alzheimer's" 358). Redlich also described them in two elderly epileptics in 1889 and called them "miliary sclerosis" (in ibid.). The term "miliary" comes from the Latin word for the grain millet and was used to describe lesions or tubercles that had the size and shape of millet seeds. Perusini likewise recalls that "Dr Alzheimer found these plaques in a 31-year-old patient affected with dorsal tabes [syphilis], who appeared to be mentally intact" ("Histology" 123). To add to the confusion, some contemporary Alzheimer's researchers propose that plaques, far from constituting "the bad guy, actually play a protective role" (Ingram 164). Mark Smith argues, for example, that plaques are actually "generated by the brain to corral the real bad actors, the small precursor molecules, toxic versions that tend to aggregate into plaques" (ibid.). Taken together, the controversies associated with the nineteenth-century origins of the disease concept support my earlier insistence that from the start, Alzheimer's disease constituted an enigma and it continues to serve as the site for powerful personal, familial, and national projections.

In light of these controversies many scholars remain puzzled as to why Kraepelin – a senior and well-respected scientist and clinician – hastily baptized Alzheimer's disease, particularly in light of the fact that very few cases had been reported. When Kraepelin made the claim to having discovered Alzheimer's disease, "only five cases had been reported" (Berrios, "Alzheimer's" 360). Moreover, Perusini's first case – he reported four in his 1909 paper – was in fact the same as Alzheimer's first case, "in which some features have been changed"; most notably, the postmortem results "no longer showed arteriosclerotic changes" (360). Likewise, in the same paper, Perusini replicated of one of Bonfiglio's cases (1908) (ibid.). In view of these facts, Berrios draws the following conclusions:

1. Alzheimer was not particularly keen to see his "peculiar" form of dementia described as a new disease; he in fact believed that it was simply an atypical form of senile psychosis. Perusini (1911) also thought this was the case.
2. There were surprisingly few cases described after the original one and before Kraepelin decided to baptize it as a separate disease. All except one were reported by men working in Alzheimer's lab. Furthermore, there was some double-reporting which is surprising in view of the fact that these workers had in all probability large numbers of dementia cases at their disposal; in addition none of the cases was pure [i.e. the cases illustrated symptoms of other diseases such as arteriosclerosis] either clinically or pathologically.
3. There was little reason (on purely scientific grounds) to elevate this "peculiar" form of dementia into a disease, particularly since during this period clinical and histopathological variations upon current "diseases" were often reported. (ibid. 359)

In fact, Kraepelin's staff did not have "large numbers of dementia cases at their disposal" because at the new urban university clinics Kraepelin "sought to admit, diagnose, and discharge as many patients as possible in order to gather clinical data across the entire spectrum of psychopathology" (Engstrom 409). As Engstrom writes: "For him the university clinic was a diagnostic transit station that admitted large numbers of patients, diagnosed them, and then distributed them to an array of secondary institutions for specific care or treatment" (409). In essence, the clinics were focused on treating "acutely ill patients over chronic patients" – a practice in keeping with the clinic's mandate to train prospective physicians "to recognize early and acute symptoms, not chronic, assertedly incurable states" (407). Because of the slow progression of their illnesses, patients suffering from senile dementia "were simply shunted through academic clinics to second-tier custodial institutions. Consequently, when it came to clinical observation of cases of senile dementia, there loomed a gaping hole in the empirical evidence base" (410).

To date, scholars remain at a loss to explain Kraepelin's "hurried baptism" of the disease (Berrios, "Alzheimer's" 362). Several hypotheses have been put forward. The first is that he did so "for *scientific* reasons, that is, he genuinely believed that Alzheimer had discovered a new disease" (362). Another is that his department was involved in a rivalry with "Pick's in Prague (which included the great pathologist Fischer)" (362). Yet another speculation is that Kraepelin was keen to triumph over Freud by showing that there were mental disorders that were organically rather than psychologically based (362). As Ingram observes, "the problem was that Freud, using psychoanalysis, was actually having success, while Kraepelin and the twenty pathologists in his lab were not" (28). Kraepelin's battle with Freud recalls my earlier point that illusions of mastery, including our attempt to master Alzheimer's disease, often and perhaps inevitably entail repressing or "forgetting" the gaps in our knowledge. Freud was a threat to Kraepelin in this regard because he insisted on recognizing forgetting as intrinsic to human consciousness. According to Freud's theories, forgetting was a given and not simply a failure experienced by the cognitively challenged non-elect.[23]

Finally, some scholars suggest that Kraepelin coined the new disease in an attempt to justify "the creation of an expensive pathological laboratory in Munich" (Berrios, "Alzheimer's" 362). Yet most historians concur that Kraepelin was "too good a clinician to believe himself in arguments such as those which he had put forward in favour of the 'independent' view" (ibid. 362–3) – that Alzheimer's disease was distinct from senile dementia. The repeated and voluble shock and dissent from Alzheimer himself and from those who worked with him as well as the critical views expressed by other scientists certainly support the view "that he had little justification for creating a new disease" (ibid. 363).

Although Kraepelin's motivation remains a mystery, it is evident that he was dedicated to dividing and classifying mental diseases as part of an overarching desire to "classify the multitude of psychiatric clinical states in accordance with their origin, their clinical manifestation and their course in order to form groups of diseases and to introduce a clinically useful nosology" (Maurer and Maurer 113). During the annual meeting of the German Association for Psychiatry in Munich in 1906, Kraepelin's efforts at categorizing mental illness

– what was then termed "anatomical dogma" – were firmly rejected
by a group of psychiatrists led by Hoche and Bonhoeffer, the so-
called anti-Kraepelians, who argued that it "is impossible to explain
mental symptoms on the basis of anatomical findings" (in ibid. 114).
At one point, Kraepelin's opponent, Bonhoeffer, insisted that there
"can be no question of a nosological specificity" (133). Hoche was
even blunter: "The search for types of diseases is the futile chase after
an illusion" (133). In his defense, Kraepelin retorted, "what you are
referring to as an illusion, Mr. Hoche, is an ideal which, although we
may not reach it, we must nonetheless endeavor to achieve" (113).
Kraepelin's response can be considered as an important aspect of the
ironic stance – a recognition that crucial information may remain
hidden. In addition to its humility, Kraepelin's response acknowledges that some attempt at knowing (however flawed and partial)
remains indispensable if scientific enquiry is to proceed at all. Yet
as we have seen it was extremely difficult for these early researchers, including Kraepelin, to draw firm boundaries between normal
and pathological adulthood and old age, and between healthy and
pathological aging.

Taken together, the findings in this chapter demonstrate that
understandings of age-related dementia and of Alzheimer's disease,
in particular, cannot be prised apart from their historical context. In
the late nineteenth century, demented individuals did not merely lose
their intellects, but, more problematically, they also lost their proper
"place," and the ability to play appropriate social roles. Psychiatrists
responded with particular fascination and offered unique ovarian
forms of therapeutic treatment when their female patients seemingly
forgot their place and proper relations to their husbands, households,
and the social world at large. As we have seen, in the writings of
both Charcot and Kraepelin – the two leading neurologists in the
nineteenth century who helped to lay the foundations for geriatric medicine – "the pathology of bodily aging is repeatedly associated with the female body" (Katz, *Cultural* 46). Whether conceived
of as hysteria or as Alzheimer's disease, pathological memory loss
was most readily "seen" in the bodies of women. Moreover, as Katz
observes, in those cases when illness strikes an elderly man, "the old
man is, as it were, feminized, and old age for both men and women is
divorced from adulthood, thus implicitly infantilizing the older person" (46). Although Alzheimer participated in these associations in
his treatment of Auguste D., he also promoted Johann F.'s case as one

of his most significant cases, thus disrupting the association between dementia and women's involution. Despite Alzheimer's writings on Johann F., most early researchers share the long-standing gendered association between women's bodies and pathological memory loss. These views are reinforced by the way later accounts emphasize Auguste D.'s role and her more perfect representation of the conventional idea of Alzheimer's pathological plaques and tangles.

Having surveyed the complex origins of Alzheimer's disease in Germany, in the next chapter I turn to Upper Canada – what is now known as the province of Ontario – in the 1850s. As noted in the introduction, in the 1850s, Upper Canada was a crucial site for the creation of asylums. During this period in Canadian history, people with dementia became "patients" within the newly constructed asylums. Within the walls of these Canadian institutions, as in Germany, the biomedical model of dementia was simultaneously created and contested.

2

The Rise of the Asylum in Ontario and Its Impact on Canadian Families

As medical historians observe, despite Kraepelin's hasty baptism Alzheimer's disease did not gain widespread attention until the 1970s. In effect the disease "lost its way for four decades" (Lock 36). Disinterest in the new disease – a latency period of sorts – can be attributed to four factors. First, senile dementia continued to be viewed as part of the process of normal aging; "the matter of early age of onset alone did not prove to be sufficiently convincing evidence for pre-senile dementia to be accepted as a distinct disease" (ibid.). Second, as noted in the previous chapter, plaques and tangles had been found in the brains of individuals other than those with dementia, and at least one case of Alzheimer's did not show plaques and tangles (Johann F.'s), so the disease lacked adequate specificity (Katzman and Bick 9–10). Third, the outbreak of the First World War diverted resources from laboratory work to the war effort (Lock 36). Finally, leading physicians at the time argued convincingly that arteriosclerosis and cerebrovascular events – in essence, small strokes – were the leading cause of later-life dementia. Drug companies thus concentrated their efforts on combating arteriosclerosis, in the hopes that they would discover pharmacological agents to address this problem (ibid.).

Given the pervasiveness of our current Gothic fears, the lack of sustained interest in Alzheimer's disease on the part of physicians and the public before the 1970s is quite remarkable, and it raises a basic question that provides the focus for my study: how and why did the understanding of Alzheimer's disease transform from a rare medical condition – a subset of dementia that strikes relatively younger people, as outlined by Kraepelin in 1910 – to its current Gothic and apocalyptic status as a "dread disease" that supposedly stalks every elderly person?

Rather than focusing on the rise of Alzheimer's disease solely as a biomedical concept – the subject of several excellent scholarly works by Jesse Ballenger, Robert Katzman and Katherine Bick, and, more recently, by Canadian anthropologist Margaret Lock and by Canada's well-known science writer Jay Ingram – this chapter takes a broader, socio-historical and literary approach to trace the roots of our contemporary panic. In what follows, I analyze how, from the end of the nineteenth century to the early twentieth century, increasingly negative views of aging, old age, and dementia played a role in shaping Canadians' current Gothic fears. To explain this current dread associated with old age and dementia, it is necessary to explore the relationships amongst increases in longevity, the rise of the asylum, and early iterations of the myth of the "menace" of the aging population. As we will see, the dread has precedents; this is not the first time the aging population has been cast this way.

This chapter begins with an exploration of this persistent myth and the version disseminated at the fin de siècle in Ontario. I follow this section with a detailed examination of several fundamental and interrelated factors that contributed to the increasing medicalization of age-related dementia – essentially, the pathologizing of senility – in the late nineteenth and early twentieth centuries: (1) the gradual shift from acceptance of old age within the context of religious notions of transcendence to an increasingly scientific approach that distinguished between a healthy and a diseased old age; (2) the creation of purpose-built asylums to house individuals suffering from mental illnesses; and, finally, (3) the disputes among asylum superintendents, politicians, and concerned families about who should look after the elderly in their "dotage." Owing to the mounting costs accrued by the newly built asylums, debates raged as to whether people with dementia should be admitted or cared for at home by their families. My aims in this chapter are threefold: to trace the roots of the persistent myth of the "menace" of the aging population. I also want to help readers to develop a more nuanced understanding of the historical context and influence of this myth on elderly people and their families in Canada. Finally, I endeavour to analyze how this myth dovetailed with the waning reliance on more elegiac, religious forms of consolation, the increasingly Gothic medicalization of dementia, and the rise of the asylum in Ontario at the end of the nineteenth and the beginning of the twentieth century.

From our current vantage point, it may be difficult to conceive of a time when age-related dementia did not arouse Gothic terror – a difficulty that raises the following question: why should we explore socio-historical contexts prior to the late 1970s when Alzheimer's disease came to be understood as a menacing biological disorder? In this chapter, and throughout the book, I argue that a consideration of the historical periods prior to the crystallization of the current disease concept allows us to appreciate that dread and evil do not reside within the illness itself, but instead are largely shaped by how society constructs the meanings and experiences of mental deficiency and, more specifically, late-onset dementia. As we will see, the terror and dread now associated with the illness spring from the social transformations that made it possible to view dementia as an intractable medical problem (rather than a regrettable, albeit natural and expected, facet of the life course). These transformations entailed shifting the burden of caring for individuals suffering from dementia from the community to the family, and, as a result, exacerbated the shame and guilt associated with institutionalizing a loved one.

SECTION I: THE MYTHIC MENACE OF "THE AGING POPULATION"

An individual in Canada who reached the age of sixty-five in 1851 could expect to live to about seventy-six, whereas in 1981 she could look forward to living into her early eighties (Dillon, *Shady* 146). In the nineteenth century, childhood diseases claimed many lives. Those who made it to sixty-five had a good chance of living for another decade. In the twentieth century, diseases of older age including cancer and heart disease were being treated, leading to an even longer life. Statistics Canada, citing average longevity, offers the following figures concerning life expectancy in their study of seniors in Canada: "In 1901, a woman born in Canada could expect to live, on average, until the age of 50, and a man until the age of 47 (Martel and Belanger, 2000). In 2003, the life expectancy at birth for a Canadian was about 80 years. Progress in increasing life expectancy has not ended yet; in a period of only four years between 1997 and 2001, the life expectancy at birth increased by about one year" (Turcotte and

Schellenberg 44). Surprisingly, however, this achievement of longevity has not been greeted with delight.

As British historian Pat Thane observes: "The twentieth century has achieved what earlier centuries only dreamed of: in developed countries, and increasingly in many less developed ones, the great majority of people who are born live to old age. They mostly do so in reasonably good health, in conditions which bear no comparison with the miserable destitution of the aged poor in most past times and places. Yet, surprisingly, this change is greeted, not with relief and pleasure, but with apprehension, even panic" (1). Our panic springs from the belief that, due to the ravages of age-related illnesses – most notably Alzheimer's disease – elderly individuals will not live out their golden years enjoying health and happiness. Instead they will become a burden on a shrinking population of workers, "imposing upon younger generations new and intolerable costs of pensions, health care, and personal care" (1). Yet as historians demonstrate, our current dread is neither new nor entirely rational. More important, despite the myth, elderly individuals have never constituted and likely will never represent an undifferentiated, cognitively impaired mob – a grey tsunami – that, due to the inexorable effects of cognitive decline, will overwhelm the economic and social resources of the Canadian nation-state.

The term "apocalyptic demography" (sometimes also termed "alarmist demography"[1] or "voodoo demography") characterizes this pessimistic and irrational mode of thinking: "the over-simplified notion that a demographic trend – in our case population aging – has catastrophic consequences for a society" (Chappell et al. 24; see also Evans et al., and Gee and Gutman). As scholars observe, this model is highly prevalent in the mass media, which reduces the complexity of aging "to a one-sided negative view that our society cannot afford increasing numbers and percentages of older people" (Chappell et al. 24). As researchers from the University of British Columbia explain: "In these apocalyptic scenarios, continuing increases in life expectancy, combined with a low birth rate, lead to steady increases in the average age of a population and an increasing concentration in the older age groups. Per capita, then, health and functional capacity decline and care needs and costs increase. This places an ever-growing burden on the shrinking proportion of the population that is economically productive. Overall well-being declines as a larger and larger share of collective resources have to be devoted to supporting

an ever-older, ever-sicker population" (Evans et al. 161). Although
this apocalyptic scenario has "a powerful face validity – since older
people do retire, do have, on average, significantly higher health care
costs, and are more likely to be dependent" – detailed analysis of the
projections shows that these factors are "not sufficient in themselves
to sustain the scenarios of apocalyptic demography, which rest on
a more extensive set of implicit assumptions that are neither self-
evident *a priori*, nor consistent with existing research or emerging
evidence" (ibid. 162).

Apocalyptic demography typically consists of five interrelated
themes or constructs (Gee). First, aging is viewed as a social "problem." Second, the model reductively and inaccurately homogenizes
older people. The third entails age blaming: seniors are singled out
for overusing social programs and, consequently, for government
debt and deficits. The fourth theme concerns "intergenerational
injustice," conveyed by rhetoric suggesting that older people are getting more than their fair share of societal resources. The fifth theme
involves the intertwining of population aging and social policy, so
that social policy reform rests on the idea that deep cuts have to
be made to accommodate the increasing numbers of seniors in the
Canadian population. If the public accepts the view that seniors will
bankrupt society due to their demands on the health care and pen-
sion systems, then it is a simple step to move towards a dismantling
and privatizing of the old age welfare state – and the whole welfare
state, for that matter – to counteract the societal burden of an aging
population (Gee; see also Evans et al. 187, and Chappell et al. 24).
In other words, this rhetoric is employed particularly by those with a
conservative social agenda.

Rebuttals of apocalyptic demography use empirical evidence to
prove that it is totally unfounded and they insist that there is an
"extreme disconnect between evidence and rhetoric" (Evans et al.
166). For example, fixating solely on the age dependency ratio without looking at the total dependency ratio – which includes children
and older, non-working individuals – in a given society creates the
illusion of a problem that, in fact, does not exist. Currently, Canada's
overall dependency ratio is at an all time historical low (Chappell
et al. 26). Moreover, when Canada and other Western countries ran
into trouble with government debt/deficit – trouble that was widely
attributed to increased spending on social programs, particularly
those for seniors – a host of Canadian economists showed that the

debt/deficit was not due to over-spending on social programs, but instead could be traced to Canada's monetary policy, specifically the Bank of Canada's decision in the late 1980s to reduce inflation (ibid.). In fact, social scientists and economists agree that Canada "will be able to afford the aging population with little difficulty as long as we experience at least moderate levels of economic growth" (see ibid. 26–7; see also Beach). Researchers also concur that "population aging itself will account for only a small part of future health care costs and will require little, if any, increase in public expenditure for health care" (Chappell et al. 26–7; see also Evans et al. 166).

Apocalyptic demography is overly simplistic because health care costs are influenced not only by demographic trends by themselves but also by rates of hospital use, reliance on increasingly expensive technology, and the prescription rate and price of pharmaceuticals (Evans). With respect to the latter, there has been "a very large increase in de facto prices resulting from shifts in prescribing from less to more expensive agents without evidence of therapeutic benefit" (Evans et al. 181). Simply put, spending more "per person under treatment for particular illnesses, rather than treating more people for more illnesses is the main story behind increased drug expenditures for older persons" (ibid. 179). Viewed in light of the evidence, concerns that the aging of the baby boom generation will bankrupt the universal health care system "are simply unfounded" (Chappell et al. 428).[2] Turning the tables on the mass media's Gothic representation of elderly individuals as a monstrous unsustainable burden, Evans et al. suggest that the apocalyptic demography itself is the monster: "the claim that attempting to meet the health care needs of an aging population will bankrupt modern societies, or make universal health care systems unsustainable ... is a 'zombie,' an idea or allegation that is intellectually dead but can never permanently be put to rest" (186).

My research on media representations of senility, dementia, and Alzheimer's disease from the mid-nineteenth century to the present enabled me to see the dramatic ebb and flow of apocalyptic demography in Canadian magazines and newspapers. As I explain in greater detail in this chapter, fears of the menace of the aging population in Canada were disseminated primarily at the end of the nineteenth century. By and large, however, these fears were eclipsed by what society at the time perceived to be a far greater threat posed by the feeble-minded, a concern that occupied society from the end of the nineteenth century to the Second World War.[3] For roughly fifty years, from 1927 to 1979, the media calmly acknowledged that life expectancy was rising. Yet for the most part society remained optimistic about the future of the elderly.[4] By the end of the 1970s, however, this type of optimistic future-mindedness was abruptly extinguished and apocalyptic demography returned with a vengeance,[5] dominating the Canadian media for twenty-five years. In 1983, Alzheimer researcher and president of the Alzheimer Society of Canada Arthur Dalton prophesied that Alzheimer's would "soon be labelled the 'disease of the century'" (Hollobon, "Is" 5).[6] From 1990 to 2015, newspaper headlines repeatedly warned Canadians about the threat posed by Alzheimer's. In the 1990s, the media began referring to Alzheimer's as "epidemic" (Kaellis and Kaellis B3).[7]

As historian Edgar-André Montigny argues, the government's approach to the dependent elderly in nineteenth-century Ontario provides a generative foundation from which to interrogate North American society's most recent iteration of the so-called "crisis of the aging population" (*Foisted* 4). Contrary to the popular media's view that our current crisis is unprecedented, in keeping with other social historians, including Thane, Montigny convincingly demonstrates that there have, in fact, been several notable periods in history in which population aging has been cast as a "social problem" (ibid. 24; see also Thane 332–51). According to Montigny, a particularly notable "crisis" occurred at the turn of the century in Canada:

> During the depression in the 1890s, government officials decided that, instead of increasing the space available in institutions to keep up with the growth of the aged population and the increasing poverty and need of their families, access to institutional care would be restricted to those old people with no relatives to care for them or to those aged individuals who were actually dangerous. One result was that aged people who had families, or who were senile but supposedly "easy to care for at home," found it increasingly difficult to gain admission into an insane asylum or house of refuge. Another was that families found themselves shouldered with an increasing burden of care as people once considered legitimate subjects of public institutional care became the sole obligation of their relatives. (*Foisted* 144)[8]

Montigny argues further that in the 1890s *and* in our current era, "the growing size of the aged population would not have attracted much attention in the legislature had it not been for the fact that in these periods the government faced a fiscal crisis" (ibid.).[9]

In 2017, as I write this chapter, far more elderly individuals are living to a greater old age in Canada, yet as Thane rightly asks: "If so many features of the experience of older people are less novel than has been thought, do they by reason of their undoubtedly unprecedented numbers, and projections that these will rise higher still, constitute a wholly new and troubling burden?" (13). In considering answers to this question, the pronounced panic at the end of the nineteenth century and its illusory basis remain highly instructive. In the case of the latter "crisis," statistics demonstrate that "the majority of the population over sixty-five did not require government support" (Montigny, *Foisted* 146). Citing Montigny's findings, Canadian demographer Lisa Dillon concludes from her extensive analyses of nineteenth-century censuses that "the majority of elderly persons lived independently and were no more or less financially secure than younger persons" (*Shady* 10). Nevertheless, the negative stereotype prevailed that *all* aged people were "poor, ill, and dependent," and it helped to fuel "panic over population aging and the burden such trends represented to public resources" (Montigny, *Foisted* 146). In effect, by arguing that it was "impossible to provide care for every old person in the province," the government was able "to justify reducing or eliminating public support for the minority of the aged population that was truly dependent" (ibid.).

In his study of the Toronto Hospital for the Insane, Geoffrey Reaume likewise attests that in the late nineteenth century by far the largest number of patients – 25 per cent in Ontario and 55 per cent in 999 Queen Street West, the "Provincial Lunatic Asylum" as it was known – suffered from what was then termed "dementia praecox" (what is now termed schizophrenia);[10] approximately 15 per cent were diagnosed with "depression"; and 10 per cent each were committed due "to senility, involutional melancholia, general paresis (syphilis), and exhaustion"; and finally, 5 per cent each were institutionalized "for epilepsy, 'imbeciles,' alcoholism, and other drug and toxic problems" (17). Senile dementia was thus not a drain on the public purse.

In 1876, twenty-one years after the official opening of the Toronto Lunatic Asylum, it was "estimated that about 86 per cent of the asylum population were chronic" (long-term and often committed for life), and by the turn of the century, "81.5 per cent of all admissions to the asylum were in this category. By 1940, over 85 per cent of the inmates were not considered fit for discharge" (Reaume 7). In his study of mental health policy in Ontario from 1930–89, Harvey G. Simmons observes that, in 1940, there were "14,314 people listed on the books of all Ontario hospitals, including Orillia. Of this total, 364 patients were diagnosed under the heading 'senile psychoses,' and 337 under 'psychoses with cerebral arteriosclerosis'" (4). This translates as roughly 4.6 per cent of the elderly patient population exhibiting symptoms of dementia. Simmons argues further that it is "likely that if the province had provided suitable accommodation for the elderly, numbers in the latter categories would have been substantially reduced" (4).

The statistics cited above indicate the extent to which chronic care was the primary feature of the patient population of asylums in Ontario. In assessing the data concerning the late nineteenth and early twentieth century, it is also crucial to appreciate that "rather than representing the aged and demographically marginal, as has been found in case studies of Houses of Industry that were gradually being created in the province in the late Victorian period, the majority of admissions to both institutions [in Hamilton and Toronto from 1851–1891] were in their so-called prime of life – in their twenties, thirties and forties" (Wright et al. 113). These figures emphasize what a host of contemporary Canadian medical historians have repeatedly asserted, namely, that Victorian asylums were "hardly a refuge for the elderly or the senile" (Warsh in ibid. 115).

If elderly people suffering from dementia were not incarcerated in great numbers in insane asylums, then where were they living? Unfortunately, it is difficult to answer this question with precision since, as Susan Morton observes, "of all the groups in the community, the aged were the most invisible to the social historian" (in Snell 476). To make matters worse, in the nineteenth century "disability was the least thoroughly recorded category in the census," so "no firm conclusions can be drawn" (Montigny, "The Economic" 470). Thanks to the efforts of Carl Ballstadt, Elizabeth Hopkins, and Michael Peterman, the editors of *I Bless You in My Heart: Selected Correspondence of Catharine Parr Traill* (1996), we do have a singular, riveting account of Traill's sister Susanna Moodie's experience of dementia.[11]

In a series of letters (nos 79–80) written in March, April, and June of 1885, Catharine recounts that toward the end of Susanna's life, the latter was utterly transformed: she played with dolls,[12] suffered terrible delusions and hallucinations that she had been robbed and that her head had been cut off,[13] and she could not recognize her own daughter who, along with a patient nurse, cared for Susanna until she died in the spring of 1885 (Ballstadt et al. 284–8). Catharine insisted, however, that Susanna had "lost her own *identity*" and was thus "not responsible" for her strange and wilful behaviour because in dementia "the powers of the mind are shaken" (285). Catharine's frank account of her sister's illness is significant for several reasons: first, the letters offer a detailed account of the symptoms of age-related dementia. Second, they provide insight into Susanna's perspective and poignantly highlight the latter's fears that she has been robbed and murdered. Third, they convey her belief (and potentially, her wish) that her murderer was facing execution and would thus pay with his life for "cutting off" her head. Finally, the letters demonstrate that Catharine dealt with Susanna's illness and death by viewing it as a metamorphosis to "a higher state" – a return to "The Lord."[14] Although Catharine relied on faith for consolation, she turned to medical science to explain the nature of her sister's disease. In the final letter to her son William, dated 18 June 1855, Catharine relates that the disease that claimed Susanna's life "was softening of the brain ... *Senile decadence* of the *brain* – the Doctor said it was" (288; emphasis in the original). In light of the insight Traill provides into her sister's illness, it is unfortunate that it is the only published report my colleagues and I found of a family's experience with dementia in the late nineteenth century.

Despite the dearth of information concerning the nineteenth and early twentieth centuries, historians have nevertheless offered crucial insights into the living conditions and treatment of elderly people during this period. For instance in 1871 census records indicated that three quarters of Canadian individuals aged sixty-five or more lived with their children (Dillon, "Parent" 441). Statistics also demonstrate that "aged men, whether they were married or widowed, always lived with their children in larger numbers than their female counterparts" (442).

Generally speaking, nineteenth-century society dictated that elderly individuals suffering from dementia lived with their children, were inmates of the poorhouse, or were incarcerated in the asylum since private old age homes "did not exist in Canada at the turn of the century" (Snell 501–2).[15] In her study of elderly individuals[16] at

the Wellington Country House of Industry from 1877–1907, Stormie
Stewart reminds us that the fate of children was the primary concern
at the time; hence the poorhouse offered asylum to children, deserted
wives, and unwed mothers.[17] By the turn of the century, however,
"inmates under forty-five had all but disappeared" (421). These changes were not due to concern for the elderly; instead, they "resulted
from the passage of an amendment in 1895 to the 1893 Children's
Protection Act of Ontario which stated that children could not be
placed or allowed to remain under the same institutional roof as
dependent adults" (421). Poorhouses were transformed into old age
homes "largely as an unintended consequence of reformist zeal for
saving children from the stigma and 'contamination' of pauper institutions" (421). By 1900, the only acceptable inmates were "elderly,
infirm, or feeble-minded" (421).[18] For the purposes of my study, the
co-mingling of elderly and so-called "feeble-minded" individuals is
highly significant. As I explain in more detail in chapters eight and
nine, an important yet elided foundation for the present panic concerning the Gothic "tide" of demented elderly is late-nineteenth and
early twentieth centuries' obsession with the newly constructed category of "the feeble-minded."

    In addition to countering the Gothic myth that asylums were
flooded by waves of demented elderly individuals, it is important to
refute the equally erroneous belief that older women were disproportionately confined to Canadian asylums (Wright et al. 111–12) – a
belief which may have circulated because of the prevalence of women
in European asylums, most notably the Salpêtrière. In fact, women
in Ontario were more "commonly kept in the extended household,
especially if they could contribute to the household economies by
childminding" (Wright et al. 104). Although neither of these myths
was true and the "majority of nineteenth century aged population"
– of both sexes – "did not require government support," due to the
persuasive rhetoric of asylum superintendents and the government,
the myth of the "crisis" has repeatedly been cited as fact (Montigny,
Foisted 146). To date, the "menace" of the aging population remains
a highly persuasive rhetorical trope.

    In the service of debunking this persistent myth, it is helpful to
appreciate that in Britain, by the end of the twentieth century, although
people were living longer, they were not making greater demands on
medical care. In short, as Thane points out, "a longer life does not
mean a longer period of illness before death; rather, as people live

longer, the onset of serious ill-health occurs later in life, if at all, since most older people, including those who live to be very old, do not experience a period of protracted, serious ill-health before death" (15). Equally important, longevity is also not necessarily correlated to longer periods of non-productivity or retirement. Current predictions, for example, suggest that "fifty per cent of the children born since the year 2000 will live to one hundred years of age"; equally crucial, there is no reason to believe that this new cohort will depend completely on society for their existence (Ingram 82). Such fears are "misplaced" since "a sample of the (admittedly small) group of Americans over 100 years old revealed that 40 per cent were independent" (ibid.).

As researchers observe, retirement is evolving into a process without a clear beginning or end. In the US, for example, it is estimated that between 30–50 per cent of the population do not retire all at once and some do not retire at all. Instead, many people move into final retirement via partial retirement or use "bridge jobs" from their career into retirement. In Canada, in a recent study, 8 per cent of seniors polled stated that they had no intention of retiring (Chappell et al. 319). In addition, many people with low-paying or part-time jobs simply cannot afford to retire; hence, the image of a monolithic block of retired elderly individuals draining the public purse is largely a dystopian fiction.[19] Hard data confirms that longevity does not correlate to longer or more critical forms of illness or to a non-productive lifestyle. Equally important, as a host of scholars persuasively argue, "in periods of financial recession, the threatening image of the aged put forward by the state often has more to do with justifying policy decisions than with providing an accurate image of the true circumstances of the elderly" (Montigny 143; see also Thane 350; see also Chappell et al. 27–8).[20] As Thane argues:

The prevailing pessimism in public discourse about the ageing of society may appear to be an expression of wholly rational economic fear. At least as probably it may be less transparently rational, as societies at the end of the millennium perceive themselves as ageing and declining, failing to renew themselves, just as ageing bodies decline. Similar fears of "degeneration" gripped European societies at the end of the nineteenth century, as birth rates fell and high rates of "physical deterioration" were perceived especially in developed urban societies. The population panic of the 1930s resonated with fear of international conflict and loss of Empire. Such fundamental fears, as least as much as informed investigation and rational evaluation of the social and economic consequences of demographic change, have shaped the popular and the political discourses about population ageing throughout the century. (16)

In Britain from the 1920s to the 1950s, similarly alarmist views concerning the "menace of an aging population" were promoted by gloomy demographers. Insisting on the overwhelmingly negative effects of the declining birth rate and the aging of the population, Richard Titmuss, for example, prophesied in the 1940s what he termed "national suicide" (in Thane 338). In later life, Titmuss recanted his earlier pessimistic view, and came to believe "with good reason, that arguments about the financial burden of aging had become part of the growing armoury of weapons deployed in the 1950s by enemies of the welfare state against its supposedly excessive costs" (in ibid. 350). Recently, studies from Britain announced the analyses from three regions in England "showed 25 percent less dementia than had been expected" (Matthews et al.). Rather than celebrate the positive news, a proponent of the Gothic view of dementia, Dr Barry Greenberg – the US-born director of the newly established Toronto Dementia Research Alliance and the director of neuroscience drug discovery and development at the University Health Network in Toronto – wrote: "For some reason, reading this article triggered a vision of Neville Chamberlain reassuring Britain that Hitler represented no significant concern, just about one year before the Nazis drove their tanks into Poland" (in Sherman, "Dementia Researcher").[21]

In the conclusion of her account of the post-Second World War iteration of the myth of the "menace" of the aging population in Britain, Thane reminds readers that the future is neither predictable nor "inexorably and solely driven by demography" (13). As it turns out, at the end of the twentieth century in Britain, unemployment among younger people proved "a larger and more expensive source of welfare dependency than old age"; in addition, the falling birth rate had the unforeseen consequence of reducing "the very considerable public and private costs of childrearing, which are greater than the costs of supporting older people" (ibid. 13–14). In fact, the birth rate rose again while the panic was in progress, and from the 1950s onward "wholly unforeseen numbers of young migrants arrived from the Commonwealth" and "larger numbers of women were in paid work than had previously been known or predicted, further undermining prophecies of a perilous imbalance between workers and dependents in the economy" (13). In view of these ironic reversals, Thane concludes that "there are few direct lessons to be learned from history, but some have been forgotten from the last time politicians, economists, and demographers were panicked by the 'menace' of an ageing population, in the 1930s and 1940s" (13). Although the fears disappeared, so, too, did "the lessons of this episode, which had been wholly forgotten when the menace of the ageing re-emerged in public discourse in the 1980s" (13). Knowledge, and more precisely our construction of history as a narrative, is predicated on a process that includes forgetting, repeating, and remembering.

To summarize: despite claims to the contrary, in Ontario at the end of the nineteenth century hordes of elderly demented individuals were not flooding the newly built asylums. As I explain in the next section, the myth that they were was largely promoted due to the rise of Western biomedicine, which privileged *curing* individuals over *caring* for them. Equally important, at the end of the nineteenth century elegiac, religious attitudes toward aging, old age, and dementia – which viewed illness as part of life's mysteries to be endured with the aid of religious narratives of consolation – were increasingly challenged by empirical approaches that sought to explain these mysteries. The latter viewed aging and illness as biological problems – Gothic evils – to be resolved and, wherever possible, to be cured by medical practitioners.

SECTION II: CHANGING RELIGIOUS AND SCIENTIFIC APPROACHES TO AGING, OLD AGE, AND DEMENTIA

Approaches to later-life dementia reflect a culture's prevailing views of aging and old age; in the nineteenth century, religious narratives offered an important framework that imbued the life course with meaning. As Ingram observes, "for centuries religion had been the only significant thinking about the passage of life ... Religion provided motivation: for instance, to counter the view that aging simply draws one further and further from usefulness and closer and closer to death, the Puritans argued that old age actually had an important purpose. It brought one nearer to salvation, something that no forty-year-old could experience. Therefore, there was an incentive, and a powerful one, to live every last day of one's life in a moral way" (12–13). Yet religious attitudes toward the elderly changed in the nineteenth century. Tracing the shifts in the conceptualization of aging that occurred during the Victorian period is crucial because the fin de siècle laid the foundations for our current views of normal and pathological aging. According to Thomas Cole, "before 1800, when most people in Europe and North America lived in families and communities regulated by religious and social principles of hierarchy, dependency, and reciprocal obligation, acknowledgement of the intractable sorrow and infirmities of age remained culturally acceptable" (230). Increasingly after 1800, physical decline and age-related infirmity were no longer understood as part of God's design – punishment for original sin. According to this dwindling religious perspective, earthly punishment is more than compensated for by the pious individual's spiritual return to God and transcendence upon death. Believers implicitly upheld an approach to life imbued with dramatic irony – one in which God, the spectator, was alone privy to a broader perspective on human living and dying.

By the end of the century, due to the rapid "aging of urban immigrants, perceptions of an accumulating scrap heap of older industrial workers, the recognition of old age as a clinically distinct period of life, and the early stages of an epidemiologic transition from infectious to degenerative diseases," earlier religious views of aging, which acknowledged and reconciled deterioration within a spiritual narrative, had receded in the face of Victorian society's growing anxieties associated with aging (ibid. 163). Unlike their predecessors, middle-class Victorian Americans increasingly relied on "the psychologically primitive mechanics of splitting images of a 'good' old age of health, virtue, self-reliance and salvation from a 'bad' old age of sickness, sin, dependency, premature death and damnation" (ibid. 230). Within this emergent dualistic framework, born of the capitalist "drive for unlimited individual accumulation of health and wealth," the aged decaying body and demented mind "came to signify precisely what bourgeois culture hoped to avoid: dependence, disease, failure, and sin" (ibid.). In keeping with my earlier analysis of the elegy and the Gothic, aging, old age, and dementia were increasingly aligned with dread and evil. According to Cole, the "primary virtues of 'civilized' morality – independence, health, success – required constant control over one's body and physical energies. The declining body in old age served as a constant reminder of the limits of physical self-control.

It also triggered fears associated with loss of psychological and economic control and independence.

Cole's work, like that of most historians, has been focused on the US whereas my study focuses on both the narrative construction and the lived experience of age-related dementia in Canada. As noted, however, there is a paucity of nineteenth- and early twentieth-century historical accounts concerning the condition of the aged, in general, and the dependent aged, in particular, in Ontario and the rest of Canada. Due to the overwhelming focus on children and youth in the Victorian period (Dillon, *Shady* 59), in Ontario neither physicians, nor asylum superintendents, nor historians felt the need to document the experiences of elderly suffering from dementia or those of their families. This was not due to ageism but simply indifference. As a result, the lives of the frail and dependent elderly – those who fell under the category of the "chronic" or long-term cases in asylum records – have largely been forgotten; this is yet another instance of forgetting associated with our understanding of late-onset dementia.

The questions addressed in this chapter reflect my attempt to remedy this oversight: first, what factors determined whether elderly people suffering from dementia were cared for by their families or committed to the newly built asylums? Second, if and when individuals were committed, how were they treated in these institutions? More precisely, what was life like on the back wards and which therapies were directed to elderly people with dementia at the close of the nineteenth century? As noted earlier, my aim in analyzing this historical information lies in exploring the increasing medicalization of dementia and its ramifications for individuals with cognitive decline and their families in Canada. Debunking the myth factually is essential. Analyzing the experience of demented elderly individuals exposes the human cost of the myth, and demonstrates why tracking the prevailing paradigms associated with aging, old age, and dementia also remains a crucial political and ethical endeavour. Although mastering or narrating the absolute Truth about dementia remains an impossible goal, it is nevertheless crucial to gain insight into prior models that have been elided and people's experiences with these models. Ideally we can use this information to reflect on the benefits and limitations of whatever models we adopt.

As the previous chapter's analysis of the encounter in the Frankfurt asylum between Alzheimer and Auguste D. suggests, scholarly investigations of scientific approaches to dementia from the nineteenth century to the present must contend with the rise of the asylum in Europe and North America. In this section, I turn to the rise of the asylum in Ontario and, more specifically, to the treatment given to people with age-related dementia. Not surprisingly, many of the historical controversies that arose in the nineteenth century continue to haunt discussions of Alzheimer's disease to this day. Asylum superintendents and government officials debated what are now familiar questions: is age-related dementia a medical problem, or an inevitable facet of the aging process? Should people suffering from dementia be housed in mental institutions or should they be cared for at home by their families? What factors might necessitate institutionalization? Finally, and equally important, what treatments should be offered to people with dementia – and are they beneficial?

As demonstrated in the previous chapter's analysis of the ironic – albeit largely elided – elements of the story of Alzheimer's disease, it is necessary to consider the geographical and historical context when discussing any era's approach to age-related dementia. More specifically, a historical approach illustrates that the answers to these questions are never determined solely by empirical, medical knowledge; instead, they are inflected by broader socio-political and economic considerations.

SECTION III: THE ASYLUM IN ONTARIO

In this section, I analyze the rise of the asylum in Ontario – not because elderly demented individuals were disproportionately confined to asylums, but because unlike "the great majority of people who left no intentional traces or records" (Darroch and Ornstein in Dillon, *Shady* 21), these institutions kept detailed records of their therapeutic practices and of their patients. As we will see, an analysis of these records attests to the ambiguous status of age-related dementia at the end of the nineteenth century – an illness that hovered between the normal and the pathological. The historical records also offer insight into the various treatments directed toward elderly, demented individuals, and shed light on the repeated concern raised by superintendents that Canadian families were heartlessly shirking their responsibility to provide economic and emotional support to their senile relatives. Most of these chronic cases remained in the asylum until their death, and superintendents repeatedly complained that they lowered overall "cure rates," thereby tarnishing the reputation of the asylum.

Canadian medical historian Edward Shorter argues that the rise of the asylum in the late Victorian period is "the story of good intentions gone bad" (*History* 33). The "dreams of the early psychiatrists failed," according to Shorter, since by the First World War, "asylums had become vast warehouses for the chronically insane and demented" (33). As Shorter explains: "In 1800, only a handful of individuals were confined in asylums. Beds in even the most famous of historic asylums, such as Bedlam in London, Bicêtre in Paris, or the "fools" tower" (*Narrenturm*) in Vienna, numbered in the dozens or low hundreds. In the nineteenth century, these numbers exploded. By 1904, there were 150,000 patients in US mental hospitals corresponding to a rate of almost two for every thousand of the population" (*History* 34). In Canada, at the close of the First World War, mental hospitals were "in a deplorable condition" – all were "badly overcrowded and under-staffed; some held hundreds of soldiers suffering from psychiatric disorders associated with active service" (Tyhurst et al. 5).

Initially, facilities for the insane in late-nineteenth century Canada were constructed in the provinces of Newfoundland, New Brunswick, Ontario, and Quebec. My analysis, however, focuses on approaches to seniors with dementia in Upper Canada, which became the province of Ontario after 1867.[22] Generally speaking, historians – particularly those influenced by the work of Michel Foucault – agree that during the late-Victorian period, the state's exercise of power became "increasingly focused on organizing, controlling, and administering the human body," and, at this time, medicine supplied a scientific standard of optimal functioning and of deviance (Cole 196). As Dillon insists, our understanding of aging cannot be prised apart from nineteenth-century discourses that "lauded rationalization, classification, and counting" (*Shady* 15). When elderly, impoverished Parisians "came to live and die in gigantic hospitals like Salpêtrière and Bicêtre, their bodies and corpses supplied the research material for the first geriatric treatises" (Cole 196). As Stormie Stewart observes, this was true in Ontario as well.[23] In other words, at this time, earlier elegiac views of aging, old age, and dementia were becoming Gothicized as the medical paradigm gained legitimacy. In essence, this model identifies a disease process and "locates it physiologically within the body, assuming that there are specific causes for diseases that can be discovered through biomedical research and that discovering them will lead to a cure" (Chappell et al. 416). As Carroll Estes explains in *The Aging Enterprise* (1979), old age itself was viewed as a biomedical problem that could be treated by medical doctors. Also gaining traction was the modern assumption that promoted the view that the elderly should not be integrated into the main culture, but instead housed in distinct facilities such as old age homes and asylums. Citing Carol Haber's insights, Sharon Anne Cook writes: "No attempt is made to confer new power or prestige on those who have reached old age. Rather, our society seeks to ensure the "separation of the old from work, wealth and family." One way this is accomplished is to force the elderly to sever their ties with the rest of the community by establishing a separate residence for them out of town" (28). The legacy of these decisions is palpable in the stigma associated with the threat of institutionalization, which constitutes a central preoccupation in modern and contemporary literary works focusing on aging and dementia.

The rise of the asylum dovetailed with scientists' and clinicians' tendency to challenge the previous generation's acceptance of life's mysteries. In *Clinical Lectures on the Diseases of Old Age* (1881), Jean Charcot insisted that physiology "absolutely refuses to look upon life as a mysterious and supernatural influence which acts as its caprice dictates, freeing itself from all law" (13; in Cole 197). Rather than accept that God alone possesses the breadth of perspective necessary to fathom both life's mysteries and its dramatic ironies, Charcot was bent on replacing the consoling narratives of Religion with the forensic discourse of empirical Science. In adopting this perspective – essentially a refusal of life's central irony that we do not and cannot have all the answers – Charcot was representative of a paradigm shift and not just positing his own idiosyncratic view. The elevation of physicians' status was predicated on the objectification of human subjects, such as Auguste D., whose bodies served as raw data. In this case, refusing irony – the limits of knowing – entailed evacuating other human beings of their subjectivity to transform them into objects of knowledge. Equally significant, despite Charcot's confidence in his ability to resolve life's mysteries, clinicians such as Charcot and Kraepelin, who were instrumental in developing our current understandings of senescence and senile dementia, had a difficult time drawing the line between health and illness, and, ultimately, viewed aging itself as "a quasi-pathological process of cell and tissue degeneration" (Cole 196), as I noted in the previous chapter. Ironically, both men eventually conceded that "normal aging was not always distinguishable from disease" (ibid. 201).

As historians who have studied conceptions of aging and old age observe, disparate models have been used to conceptualize the life course and the complex relationship between aging and illness. During the fourteenth and fifteenth centuries, for example, few individuals knew exactly how old they were, but "measured life, if they did at all, in terms of ages or stages" (Ingram 10). Acceptance of the stages of life and of good and ill health, including age-related dementia, is evident, for example, in a German poem of 1578, which divides a woman's life into eight phases: "At age 10 she was a child, at 20 a maid, at 30 a wife, at 40 a matron, at 50 a grandmother, at 60 'age-worn,' at 70 'deformed,' at 80 'confused and grown cold'" (in Thane 47). Prior to the nineteenth century, attitudes toward mental decline were not necessarily or uniformly pessimistic (see Ballenger *Self*). In the mid-nineteenth century Florence Nightingale wrote to her father about her mother's mental decline; owing to the historical shift in attitudes toward dementia, Nightingale's optimistic approach to her mother's condition may strike contemporary readers as odd: "While my dear mother loses her memory (conscious, alas! To herself) she gains in everything else – in truth of view, in real memory of the phases of the past, in appreciation of her great blessings, in happiness, real content and cheerfulness – and in lovingness. I am quite sure that, during the nearly half-century in which I have known her, I have never seen her anything like so good, so happy, so wise or so really true as she is now" (in Thane 311).[24] Nightingale's account of her mother is significant because it counters the Gothic discourse. More precisely, it suggests that something may potentially be gained when the Lockean biography is lost: people may become strangers to themselves and others, but this is not necessarily a tragic or horrific transformation. Even if readers are skeptical of Nightingale's overwhelmingly cheerful account, it nevertheless demonstrates the existence of alternative, consolatory fictions.[25] Acceptance – and, in the case of Nightingale's letter cited above, outright optimism in the face of cognitive decline – was as Cole suggests grounded, for the most part, in religious faith. This faith, however, waned in the light of scientific pessimism stoked by the growing awareness of the irrevocable nature of brain damage and of the intractable nature of inherited defects. European and North American physicians alike rapidly assimilated Charcot's and Kraepelin's theories with the result that, "in England and America, the word *senile* itself was transformed in the nineteenth century from a general term signifying old age to a medical

term for the inevitably debilitated condition of the aged" (Cole 196).
Aging and old age were thereby discursively conflated with the dread
of cognitive decline. As Mark Jackson explains: "During the long
turn between the nineteenth and twentieth centuries, mild forms of
mental deficiency were reconceptualised as pathological and as more
dangerous than severe forms of deficiency" (3). As we will see, in
Canada, Victorian approaches to aging together with new forms of
institutionalized care had equally profound, and not entirely positive
implications for individuals suffering from dementia later in life and
for their families.

SECTION IV: THE RISE OF THE ASYLUM IN NINETEENTH-CENTURY ONTARIO

In late-nineteenth-century Ontario, mentally ill individuals were being
removed from the local, district jails and confined within newly constructed asylums. During this period, the mandate for a gentler, less
invasive, or "moral" treatment of insanity largely shaped the custodial,
non-interventionist approach that prevailed until the Second World
War. Provisions for the insane in early Ontario among European
populations prior to the construction of asylums followed the traditions of settler families and communities and included "boarding out, warning out, family care and management, and treatment
by local medical practitioners" (Wright et al. 106; see also Warsh
7). "Boarding out" entailed housing destitute lunatics in private
homes at parish expense (Warsh 7). "Warning out" referred to the
banishment of the unwanted outside municipal or county boundaries (Wright et al. 106 n28). At the time, authorities were concerned
primarily with "segregation of the insane and protection of society
and property" (Tyhurst et al. 2). The dependent elderly were viewed
as both a familial and community responsibility, and "public opinion and the courts upheld and accepted this situation" (Montigny,
Foisted 86). Since Upper Canada did not adopt the English poor-law
system – a form of poor relief practiced in England and Wales that
was based on late-medieval and Tudor-era laws, which were codified
in 1587–98 – there was neither organized outdoor relief nor workhouses for the maintenance of the poor insane" (Wright et al. 106).
This partly explains why, in 1810, legislation was passed making the
town of York's local jail a site of confinement – a practice that was

made explicit in an 1830 act supporting the maintenance of "insane destitute persons either in the jail or some other place" (ibid.). As a result, in addition to the evils associated with dementing illness, families had to cope with the additional burden and shame of incarcerating a loved one, as if he or she were a criminal.

Segregation was later transformed to more humane forms of custodial care largely because "reform-minded notables both inside and outside of Upper Canada" abhorred this situation and lobbied for "the establishment of a publically funded lunatic asylum that would approximate the emerging institutional ideal in other North American colonies, the Unites States, and Britain" (ibid. 107; see also Tyhurst et al. 2). In the United States in the 1840s, reformer and activist Dorothea Lynde Dix conducted a thorough investigation of the treatment of the poor suffering from mental illness in her home state of Massachusetts. Her efforts led to widespread changes: most notably, the bill to expand the state's mental hospital in Worcester. Dix continued her efforts across North America, eventually visiting Nova Scotia in 1853. Whereas Dix's efforts met with success, the Upper Canadian reformers' hopes were not realized until a permanent Toronto Provincial Asylum was established in 1850 (see Theodore M. Brown; Garraty and Carnes; David L. Goldman). Lunatic asylums were initially constructed in "the principal cities, in Toronto, Kingston, London, and then Hamilton" (Wright et al. 110). Such was the demand that the Toronto asylum found itself "overcrowded with patients soon after its doors were opened" (ibid. 108). Whereas historians typically cite these developments as evidence of progress, Montigny maintains that the opening of the Toronto House of Industry in 1837, followed by the Toronto Lunatic Asylum in 1838, marked "the first steps in a process that eventually eliminated what outdoor relief existed" (*Foisted* 89–90). Outdoor relief took the form of money, food, clothing, or goods given to alleviate poverty, but did not require that the recipient enter an institution.

Furthermore, these developments "emphasized the notion that the aged were properly a familial as opposed to a community responsibility, and forced the aged poor who could not be supported by kin to segregate themselves from their communities in order to receive public assistance" (ibid.). As I explain in chapter three, arguments in favour of allowing the community to support vulnerable individuals prevailed in the 1950s and played a role in the deinstitutionalization movement. The shift in responsibility from the community to the family, together with the waning of religious forms of consolation, altered both the meaning and the experience of caring for a person with dementia. Rather than remaining a facet of the life course, dementia was transformed into an intractable medical problem that was increasingly foisted solely on the individual's family.

Historians concur that during the nineteenth and early twentieth century, "looking after the mentally ill fell in the first instance to the family"; it was "the family that decided to keep an afflicted individual at home or to seek care" (Shorter, *History* 49). As long as the community provided support, families were able to care for vulnerable elderly individuals. Changes occurred, however, at the turn of the century, when community support was withdrawn and families started seeking alternative outside care (ibid. 51). At the time, government regulations stipulated that there were "two methods by which a family could have a difficult person admitted into an insane asylum: ordinary process and warrants" (Montigny, *Foisted* 120). Ordinary process dictated that three physicians had to certify that the person was insane, but even if the person were certified, he or she "would be eligible for admission into a hospital only after a bed became available" (ibid.). Yet, owing to "the crowded state of the provincial asylums during the nineteenth and early twentieth centuries, it was almost impossible for a person to gain admission to an asylum in this way" (ibid.). By far the more expedient method involved acquiring a warrant, which was obtained as follows:

> Public authorities such as justices of the peace, magistrates,
> and jail doctors could confine a person in a local jail and issue
> a warrant testifying that the person was a "dangerous lunatic,"
> meaning that he or she posed a threat to self or community.
> Asylums were forced to admit warrant patients regardless of
> the number of free beds ... "Many families were forced to have
> their kin imprisoned and declared insane and dangerous in order
> to secure them admission to an asylum under warrant." Under
> such a system it was almost impossible for a family to send
> a loved one to an asylum in a humane manner ... Thus, aside
> from the stigma attached to being treated for mental illness,
> the "indignity" of being committed to an asylum often included
> being confined in one of the province's "squalid and inhumane"
> district jails. (ibid.)[26]

For example, almost one third of the elderly people committed to the Rockwood asylum, established in Kingston, Ontario, in 1858, arrived "from a cell in a county jail after having been labeled 'dangerous lunatics' – many of them so designated merely because that was what was necessary to get them into the asylum" (ibid. 121). As the information above indicates, the reduction of care provided by the community coupled with the stigma of being treated for mental illness, which involved confinement in the district jail, negatively affected the meaning and experience of the illness, exacerbating its status as a dreaded evil.

SECTION V: LIFE IN THE ASYLUM

Although the myth promoted by asylum superintendents and the Canadian government that asylums were being flooded with elderly people in their dotage was false, as noted earlier it is still important to examine how people with dementia were treated in the asylum, in order to demonstrate the human costs associated with the biomedical model at that time. Thanks to the painstaking work of Canadian social historians, we now have intimate and detailed accounts of life at the Toronto Hospital for the Insane from 1870–1940 (see Reaume, and Montigny, *Foisted*) and Homewood, a private asylum in Guelph (see Warsh). The Toronto Hospital, for example, "had a total of 16 wards, eight each for men and women. Six wards were reserved for paying patients, who were charged from two to six dollars per week. The largest number of beds, however, was on the public wards" (Reaume 8). In practice, asylum superintendents tended to differentiate between acute and chronic cases of mental illness. For example Joseph Workman, the Superintendent of the Toronto Provincial Asylum and reputedly "the most powerful alienist in English-speaking Canada at the time, prioritized Toronto as a curative institution, and seems to have redirected or transferred several score of incurable patients to the Hamilton Asylum" (Wright et al. 124). Due to superintendents' increasing ambition to cure rather than care for people with mental illness, age-related dementia was increasingly perceived of as a shameful and costly inconvenience.

In keeping with my goal to examine the repercussions of biomedicine's tendency to disavow the subjectivity of individuals suffering from dementia, in what follows, I attempt to provide an answer to the question raised above: what was it like inside the wards of the hospital for the elderly? Geoffrey Reaume prefaces his explanation by noting that the "rise or decline in the quality of the living environment for patients depended on which ward an individual was on and how much was paid, or not paid, for room and board" (9). Even for well-to-do people, conditions "could be unpleasant, but accommodations for the poor were miserable, overcrowded, smelly, and dirty" (9). For decades, the asylum was infested with rats, and many patients legitimately feared falling asleep in their beds, anticipating that they would be bitten; in addition to the rodents, all manner of vermin plagued the inmates (9).

By the 1930s, however, asylums were "considerably cleaner than half a century previous" and, as Shorter states, discharge rates "for younger patients were actually quite high" (*History* 191; see also 278). Ironically, some of the changes associated with the Depression, including the fact that the asylums "were reasonably well staffed with physicians and nurses, were due more to the depressed state of the country than to the altruism of those concerned" (Rae-Grant, *Images* 14). Simply put, during the Depression more people were willing to work on staff at asylums for lower wages. Although Shorter repeatedly cites the high discharge rates for younger patients, virtually without exception, elderly patients with "senile dementia" were relegated to the back wards, where they languished until they died. According to the pathologist Bernard Tomlinson, as late as 1960, chronic geriatric patients were "the most ill-housed (not ill-treated). They were given the least attention … than any other group … They were literally imprisoned by their circumstances" (in Katzman and Bick 80–1). As my analysis suggests, however, such imprisonment was a byproduct of the prevailing attitudes associated with mental illness, specifically the waning faith in religious modes of consolation and the rise of biomedical discourses that viewed age-related dementia as an intractable medical conundrum. Indeed as researchers observe, "for reasons that were more political (regarding the mentally ill) and economic (for the impoverished elderly) than anything else, institutional care became the accepted form of treatment for both populations" (Chappell et al. 218).

Although the two groups were cared for in institutions, clinicians viewed them as incurable. As noted earlier, when the "scientific method" was introduced in the late nineteenth and early twentieth century, physicians and researchers increasingly "explain[ed] mental illness on the basis of disease, damage to the brain, and congenital and hereditary defects" (Tyhurst et al. 2). Since damaged brain tissue cannot be regenerated and since little can be done to correct inherited constitutional defects, the scientific approach led to an era of pessimism in treatment (ibid.). Ironically, then, in contrast to the earlier period of elegiac religious acceptance, the late-nineteenth-century Gothic pathologization of dementia may well have made life more difficult for elderly individuals coping with cognitive decline. This is one of the central ironies associated with the paradigm shift from a religious to a biomedical approach to dementia: Charcot's aim of revealing God's mysteries, gaining total knowledge, mastery, and control in an effort to cure the disease resulted in objectifying and expelling those whose experience rendered this goal impossible.

Not only could doctors not cure dementia, the care they offered their patients was also limited and, at times, harmful. In effect, the majority of patients, including elderly individuals suffering from dementia, did not receive anything beyond food and shelter. This attitude persisted until the 1970s as some physicians also withheld basic medications such as antibiotics from people suffering from "senile dementia" (see Katzman and Bick 187). With respect to the treatments offered in the late nineteenth century, it is important to recognize that dementia alone was not cause for active intervention. However, if the patient suffered from what were deemed disruptive behavioural symptoms – and, like Auguste D., many, in fact, became agitated, noisy, and violent toward themselves and others – they were subjected to a variety of treatments listed below.[27] While "moral treatment" entailed that active treatments and manual restraints were rarely used, asylum staff responded to noisy, agitated, and violent patients with therapies that ranged from hydrotherapy to sedation. The cost of drugs was always a consideration, and funds were rarely spent on chronic cases. Before the advent of the physical (drug-based) therapies in the 1930s, however, hydrotherapy, which was cost efficient, was one of the few means of calming agitated patients (Warsh 121). This method "generally adopted in North America was devised by Joel Shew, leading New York hydropath and editor of *The Water-Cure Journal*" (ibid. 48). Shew determined that water "functioned best when administered gradually through the skin," and he promoted the use of a wet sheet pack, in which the patient would be wrapped, then secured and topped by a feather bed; the patient "remained in his cocoon for twenty-five minutes to several hours, depending upon the seriousness of his condition" (in ibid.). As noted in chapter one, Auguste D. was given therapeutic baths, "sometimes with cold water, sometimes with hot, nearly every day" (Lage 18). Indeed, as we saw, water therapy was also Kraepelin's preferred method for treating dementia of the Alzheimer's type. As he explains in his chapter on dementia, when drugs failed, and patients would not stay in their beds, "water therapy, frequently also wet wrappings were well tolerated" (42).

In addition to immobilizing and calming patients using hydrotherapy – an aqueous straitjacket, if you will – asylum staff also relied on injectable sedatives (to calm patients) and hypnotics (to put them to sleep). From 1803 onward, chloral hydrate – or "knock-out drops," as they were known – was the drug of choice. After 1903, barbiturates, most notably phenobarb, became "a favourite in asylums well-off enough" to afford them (Warsh 122). As Cheryl Warsh attests, in Ontario "the most-favoured hypnotics of the nineteenth century were chloral hydrate and sulphonal"; these drugs were used in asylums for "the purposes of restraint and control" (123). In practice, then, for people suffering from dementia who were deemed disruptive or dangerous, "moral treatment" entailed that chemical restraint replaced mechanical restraint (ibid.). In 1878, a patient at York "charged that chloral was being used to 'quench the poor sufferers into quietness'" (ibid.). In 1899, the alienist Dr Hitchcock similarly decried the pervasive use of these sedatives in a report to the British Medico-Psychological Association: "At almost every asylum with which I was connected ... I have seen two 16 oz bottles [of sedatives] made up for the males and females, given night after night to be used at discretion for patients who were noisy. I have seen this most detrimental treatment pushed until many patients have been at death's door" (in ibid.).

In addition to being noisy, restless, and violent, elderly patients suffering from dementia were also prone to depression and psychosis. Upon exhibiting these symptoms, patients were treated with various "shock" therapies, which were popular from the late-nineteenth century until the 1950s – when the new anti-psychotic drugs such as chlorpromazine came on the market (Shorter, *History* 48–55). Electroconvulsive therapy (ECT), in particular, was "aimed at lessening the confusion of patients with dementia and restoring their ability to function socially, [and] was said to produce the most favorable results'" (Ballenger, *Self* 50). The popularity of ECT waned, however, after the introduction of anti-psychotic drugs. When Heinz Lehmann, at the Verdun Hospital in Montreal, first administered chlorpromazine (also known as Thorazine) to his patients in 1953, he assumed it was merely another sedative. To his surprise and delight, however, "it acted like a chemical lobotomy" (in Shorter *History*, 252).[28]

Given the paucity of therapeutic treatments available for mental illness in general, and for people with dementia in particular, contemporary readers may conclude that asylums were inhospitable places for elderly individuals with dementia to spend their final years. Indeed, as historian R.A. Houston observes, contemporary observers are quick to condemn "late-nineteenth- and twentieth-century institutions as dumping grounds for society's victims: 'warehouses of the unwanted'" (27). Yet as Houston also points out, during this period "a range of attitudes toward care co-existed," and the decision to send a person to an asylum "was not taken lightly" (27). Moreover, in contrast to the claims made by asylum superintendents, "those who took this course cannot simply be written off as uncaring or failing" (27). Ultimately, "in the absence of proof that one regime or location of care was superior to another," Houston cautions that it is "better to try to understand the reasons why an option was chosen rather than to judge" (27). As I explain in the next section, despite the claims on the part of superintendents that a host of families were heartlessly shirking their responsibilities, a small number of families were driven to incarcerate their loved ones due to the financial, physical, and emotional burdens associated with caring for an elderly person suffering from dementia – burdens that were once shared with the community as a whole. The fact that a few families were forced to put their loved ones in an asylum does not substantiate the myth of the geriatric as a social burden.

SECTION VI: NINETEENTH-CENTURY DEBATES CONCERNING THE APPROPRIATE LOCUS OF CARE FOR THE DEPENDENT ELDERLY

Frustrated by their inability to cure dementia – a goal motivated by the emergent biomedical paradigm championed by Charcot – asylum superintendents sought to rid their institutions of the burden of elderly demented individuals. As medical historians observe, although asylums "have been seen, quite rightly, as midwives to the psychiatric profession," the latter has "not always been unanimous in its attitude to the proper locus of care" for elderly people suffering from cognitive decline (Bartlett and Wright 15). From the start, there were heated debates "within the ranks of medical superintendents of

asylums over which groups should be confined, and battles between
alienists and other medical professionals over clientele" (ibid.). In
their official reports, for a host of reasons, which included a desire
to enhance their cure rates, asylum administrators forcibly and regularly conveyed the view that asylums were not suitable places for
people suffering from senile dementia, and they chastised families for
abandoning their aged in asylums. In 1899, Daniel Clark, Medical
Superintendent of the Toronto Hospital for the Insane, lamented one
family's treatment of their mother, Gloria D., "a 69-year-old widow
with two children" (Reaume 47). Gloria D. suffered from delusions
and believed herself to be "very wealthy, talked to people who were
not present, charged others with trying to swindle her, and threatened
her daughter-in-law" (47). Her son initiated the admission process.
As Clark wrote in his report to the Inspector of Asylums:

> The statement of Dr Machell's is not that she is excited and
> unmanageable but that she is quiet and harmless and has been
> left alone for days and days. This is another illustration of the
> attempt to make this a place for incurables to save the friends
> the trouble of looking after them ... It always seems to me a
> great pity that an elderly person should be sent to the asylum
> for the insane to die, especially when such are quiet and manage-
> able as this woman seems to be. This woman ... never attempted
> to injure herself nor others ... The only delusion she has is that
> she has an immense amount of money at her disposal. Even if
> we had room for a patient of this kind I would resist the admis-
> sion of a person who seems to be only in the dotage of old age.
> (in Reaume 47)

Despite Clarke's opposition in his report, Gloria D. was admitted to
the asylum in 1899 and remained there until her death in 1907, a
year after Auguste D. died in Frankfurt am Main.

Clark's comments concerning Gloria D. are significant for two reasons: first, he articulates the overarching desire to ensure that the asylum not be conceived of as a "place for incurables." Second, in a bid
perhaps to ensure that elderly people were cared for at home, Clark
drew on the waning historical attitude that "dotage" or "senility" in
"old age" was "normal." One is led to assume, however, that Gloria
D.'s family felt otherwise. Put somewhat differently, the definition of
"insanity" – which rests on the diagnosis of a pathological condition – was challenged, if not entirely undermined by the enduring,

elegiac notion of "senility"; this was true for both Alois Alzheimer and Daniel Clarke. Simply put the term "insane" was reserved for individuals suffering from a pathological condition or disease. The term "senile," however, was applied to people who were negotiating an unavoidable facet of the life course.

Clarke's assertions also illustrate asylum superintendents' repeated yet unsubstantiated claims that their institutions were being inundated by elderly incurables. As Montigny explains,

> These documents [the reports of asylum superintendents] are replete with examples of "helpless old dements," who could be "easily cared for at home," if only their families were not so willing to heartlessly shirk their responsibilities and send their aged relatives to an insane asylum. In the view of most administrators few of the old people sent to asylums were insane; most were merely suffering from the ravages of senility. As the inspector of the Hamilton Asylum reported in 1899, "many (patients) are old people suffering from mental senility; the family may be unable to provide the means of caring for them. They are sent to the asylum simply for safe keeping and to ease the burden upon the friends." (Montigny "Foisted" n.p.)

As Montigny asserts, however, asylum officials would frequently "argue that the patient was 'quiet and harmless' and did not need asylum care"; this practice was especially common in England where asylum officials "tried to release quieter patients to workhouses or to the care of their families" (ibid.). But many of these patients "'lost their tranquility' and had to be returned to the asylum" (ibid.). Moreover, the fact that aged people were merely "in their dotage" did not actually mean that they could be "easily cared for at home"; quite the contrary, many families "had great difficulty then and now copying with symptoms of paranoia, especially delusions of persecution and unrealistic jealousies, which caused a person to become unpredictable, violent, abusive and frequently dangerous" (ibid.).[29] In his research on the Kingston Asylum, Montigny also notes that nineteenth-century asylum superintendents actually exaggerated the numbers of aged in their institutions as a means of exculpating themselves for low cure rates (ibid.).

Thus at the end of the nineteenth century, to enhance the reputation of the asylum and to cut costs in a period of financial recession, asylum superintendents (as well as governments in Europe and the North America) decried the practice of "granny dumping" and put the onus entirely on families to care for their loved ones. In contrast to this myth, medical historians who study asylum records are repeatedly "struck by the distance families went to try and accommodate insane family members within the community, before turning to the asylum as a measure of last resort" (Wright et al. 105).[30] Far from being uncaring, families only reluctantly committed a family member to an asylum when his or her behaviour "became intolerably disruptive to the family, or dangerous to the community, or where there was a lack of resources, both human and financial, to care for the individual in the home" (Warsh 10).

Rather than attempting to offer a definitive diagnosis as to whether or not these patients were indeed "insane" or merely "senile," my aim here, and in the study as a whole, is to explore the divergent stories concerning late-onset dementia and Alzheimer's disease, and to analyze the basis for the tensions among them. Due to the gradual shift away from a more accepting, faith-based attitude toward the increasing medicalization of dementia in Ontario, as in Germany at the turn of the century, "senility" was paradoxically viewed as both "natural" and "pathological." In Ontario, however, this ambiguity was exacerbated by the fact that the goals of scientific classification were frequently at cross-purposes with asylum superintendents' desires to enhance cure rates and thereby secure their asylum's reputation and its revenues. Both asylum superintendents' and the Canadian government's desire to cut costs underlay the prevalent use of Gothic images of asylums as warehouses for hordes of senile, dependent elderly individuals. This rhetoric, which ignored the efforts of well-meaning families to care for relatives with dementia, was strategically deployed, as it is again today, to persuade the public of the wisdom of reducing support services for the dependent elderly. But to appreciate the broader, complex responses to dementia in Canada, it is necessary to look beyond the biomedical framework and the history of asylums to popular and literary accounts. Maintaining the temporal and geographic parameters of my study, the next chapter turns to media reports and fictional works to trace the fascinating shift in Canada from elegiac to Gothic approaches to dementia and Alzheimer's disease.

Popular Perceptions of Aging and Dementia in Canada: The Theory of Waste and Repair from the 1860s to the 1960s

To complement the previous chapter's analysis of the biomedical views of aging and the controversies associated with the rise of the asylum at the end of the nineteenth century, this chapter investigates the media[1] and literary treatments of dementia during that time. Whereas in the previous chapters, discussions of research and asylum culture were foregrounded, in this chapter medical theories of the day serve primarily as contextual, background material. Although media accounts of dementia for this early period in Canadian history were plentiful, the same could not be said for fictional portrayals.

To help me in my search for literary accounts of dementia in the late nineteenth and early twentieth centuries, I enlisted the aid of a dozen scholars in early Canadian literature. To everyone's surprise, the group could only come up with two examples:[2] Susie Francis Harrison's short story "The Story of Delle Josephine Boulanger" (1886) – a Gothic tale featuring a psychotic and traumatized elderly woman from Quebec, who is, as it turns out, not cognitively impaired – and Catherine Parr Traill's brief, non-fictional account of her sister Susanna Moodie's dementing illness (see the discussion of Susanna's illness in chapter two). Rather than feel discouraged, the group suggested that the dearth of fictional materials highlights several issues relevant to my research. First, healthy older characters were required by the plots in the fiction of this period; second, English-Canadian writers tended to represent Francophone people from Quebec as insane or, more accurately, tinged with a Gothic eccentricity; finally, they speculated that alternative discursive and knowledge frameworks were available during this period that allowed society to interpret dementia or "senility," as it was known at the time, very differently.[3] Ultimately, our futile search confirmed what my prior research had already suggested: the biomedical diagnosis of dementia as we now understand it (as applicable to elderly individuals and, by and large, irreversible) was constructed in the late 1970s. As noted in the introduction, in Canada the word "Alzheimer's" was first cited in 1977, in a death notice that invited people to donate to the Alzheimer's Disease Study.[4] References to both dementia and Alzheimer's surfaced again, far more forcibly, in both media and literary accounts in the 1980s and 1990s, when scientists joined forces with the Alzheimer's Association and pharmaceutical companies to promote the need for research funds. At the end of the twentieth century, the baby boomer generation also began caring for their aging parents and contemplating their own impending status as elderly Canadian citizens, which increased interest in the topic of dementia and Alzheimer's, in particular. As table 1 indicates, there were no references to Alzheimer's disease in the fifteen-year period from 1960 to 1975. In the next ten years, there were fewer than eighty references. The number of references increased dramatically in the five-year period beginning in 1985. From 1985 to 1990, the number grew to more than 2000. In the next ten-year period, this number more than tripled. During the next five-year period from 2000–05, the number close to tripled again, approaching more than 19,000 references. In the next five-period the figure increased more moderately to 20,000. From 2010–15, references began to taper off by roughly 5,000.[5]

I begin with a detailed account of my futile search for early Canadian literary accounts and of the paucity of media references to Alzheimer's prior to 1977 to explain why this chapter juxtaposes the media accounts from the 1860s to the 1960s, in section one, with the fictional narratives written in the 1960s that reflect on this earlier period, in section two. Owing to the temporal diversity of the texts under consideration, there are obvious challenges associated with relying on them to elucidate the lived experience of dementia at the end of the nineteenth to the mid-twentieth centuries. My goal in comparing media and fictional accounts, however, is not so much to elucidate the Truth about the experience over a century as it is to trace the workings of two competing and enduring theories concerning dementia, which relied on the opposing concepts of "waste" and

Table 1 Media references to "Alzheimer's" in *The Globe and Mail*

1960–70	0
1970–75	0
1975–80	3 (two death notices – 1977 and 1978 – inviting people to contribute to Alzheimer's studies)
1980–85	75
1985–90	2,156 with 372 in the title
1990–95	3,822 with 662 in the title
1995–2000	7,885 with 1,142 in the title
2000–05	19,184 with 2,570 in the title
2005–10	20,054 with 2,218 in the title
2010–15	15,720 with 1,837 in the title

"repair." Before turning to the texts under consideration in what follows, I offer a brief overview of this Victorian theory.

The nineteenth-century view of waste as a physiological principle derived from the discovery in the 1860s of the second law of thermodynamics, which understood "unusable energy" – waste – as an inevitable, dissipative force; in other words, it revealed the process of entropy (see Charise 158–234). Whereas the majority of accounts of dementia – particularly those conveyed by the media in the late nineteenth century – adopted the view that aging and old age represented unmitigated decline or "waste," the literary accounts from the 1960s offer a fascinating, albeit belated application of the lesser-known Victorian theory of "waste" *and* "repair."

In *Physiology of Common Life*, published between 1859 and 1860, George Henry Lewes challenges the prevailing theory of entropy and "waste" in a lengthy discussion of age and aging, in which he envisions life not solely as an entropic movement toward death, but instead as an oscillation between two contrasting and dynamic forces, waste and repair (see Charise 165). In volume two of his study, Lewes refers to waste and repair as the two reciprocal nodes underlying the fate of the living "fabric of the body" (Lewes in ibid. 169). More precisely, Lewes proposes that old age occurs when "the balance [of waste and repair] begins to lean; the movement of Assimilation slackens, and Death slowly advances" (ibid. 174). In essence, waste begins to overtake repair. Rather than view this shift in the balance between waste and repair as inevitable or pre-determined, however, Lewes insists that "the limits of this epoch are the most variable of all" (ibid.). In saying this, Lewes emphasizes that this state of transition or "epoch" of flux is not predetermined by biology, but, instead, is based on a host of extrinsic factors, including the quality of care. Lewes's insistence on variability "complicates longstanding striations of childhood, youth, manhood, and old age" (Charise 174). Equally important, in contrast to traditional models of bodily temporality like the "ages" or "stages" of life, as Charise observes, for Lewes it is the shifting preponderance of waste and repair, and not the passage of chronological time as such, that really determines bodily age and the time of one's death (174).

What is most striking about the Canadian media and literary accounts analyzed in this chapter, and what links them thematically, is their mutual reliance on the concept of waste in their discussions of aging and illness as well as their references to the historical period of modernity. Among other changes, the industrial revolution, which spanned the period between the 1840s and the 1930s in Canada, "caused a momentous transformation" from a "rural agrarian society to an urban, industrialized society" (Chappell et al. 311). Simply put, modernity was seen as a negative entropic force that accelerated aging and dementia. In addition to highlighting the longstanding relationship between narratives of aging and dementia and Victorian theories of waste and repair, the comparative analysis of media and literary discourses offered in this chapter reveals a variety of contrasting views of aging, old age, and dementia that persisted until Alzheimer's was reinterpreted as a single disease in the late 1970s. A study of these contrasting views also underscores the difference between our current Gothic view of dementia and the range of religious and scientific beliefs that prevailed in earlier periods of Canadian history. For the purposes of my book, the comparison is extremely useful because it illustrates the existence of multiple approaches to dementia, many of which have been forgotten.

As I argue in section one, during the late nineteenth century the Canadian media promoted both idealized and stigmatized views of elderly individuals, particularly as it suited the newspaper editors' religious and/or political agendas. Although literary works maintain a negative view of aging and dementia, with a few exceptions, they explore the more personal experience of illness. Equally critical, the literary texts highlight the potential, albeit often unrealized, for repair. Their approach recalls Cole's view cited in my introduction that "growing up and old is not only a *process* ... it is also an *experience*, an incalculable series of events, moments and acts lived by an individual person" (xxxii). Fictional treatments of dementia repeatedly emphasize the physical and emotional challenges associated with caring for a loved one suffering from cognitive impairment – challenges that are exacerbated due to the stigma associated with mental illness and that also reflect growing anxieties about the negative impact of modernity and urbanization.

In the literary works considered in this chapter by Stephen Leacock, Mordecai Richler, Alice Munro, and Margaret Laurence, waste and repair are tied to the experience of age-related dementia in the context of modern, industrialized society. More precisely, their texts interrogate "the modern assumption" that the elderly "should not be integrated into the main culture" but instead should be encouraged or forced, if necessary, "to sever their ties with the rest of the community by establishing a separate residence for them out of town" (S.A. Cook 28). As we will see, the fictions of Leacock, Richler, Munro, and Laurence rely on images of old age and dementia to decry this view and, at times, to ponder the wastefulness of modern lives dedicated to the selfish pursuit of material gain – a wastefulness that is symbolized both by dementing illness and also, in some cases, by the unethical treatment of people coping with dementia, who are viewed as "waste." Although they adopt a fatalistic and pessimistic view of aging and dementia, the fictions under consideration emphasize that suffering and loss are exacerbated by modernization, which has physically separated and estranged individuals from their loved ones and made caregiving, which was once the responsibility of the entire community, a crushing burden that falls on individuals – primarily women. In this sense, Canadian fiction reflecting on this period diagnosed not merely the individual, but also the impact of modernization on the meaning of aging.[6] The connections drawn by Canadian writers between the illness and the changes brought about by the industrial era vividly demonstrate that the "meaning" of senile dementia is inflected by specific locations and historical moments.

In addition to reflecting on the theory of waste and repair, in their accounts of dementia that recollect the interwar years, Leacock, Munro, Richler, and Laurence repeatedly underscore how the disease of forgetting exposes prior and more foundational, repressed instances of forgetting – the inherent inconsistencies and gaps in our self-knowledge and our knowledge of others. Both forms of memory loss thwart our attempts to construct a coherent sense of self. Literary narratives also often express profound anxiety and doubt concerning the meaning of and appropriate ethical responses to dementia. Due to their acknowledgment of doubt and their portrayals of divergent views of and responses to dementia, the texts under consideration undermine the Lockean fantasy of identity as a seamless, coherent narrative predicated on total recall. Equally critical, rather than represent dementia solely as a Gothic horror, literature exposes what the Gothic represses, namely that our attempts at winning the "war" against dementia – by uncovering its secrets and thereby finding someone or something to blame – is futile, particularly in the case of an illness whose origins are multiple, mysterious, and seemingly linked to normal aging, and whose cure remains equally elusive.

SECTION I: DEMENTIA IN THE MEDIA – THE INEXORABLE LAW OF DECLINE AND WASTE

Although for the most part the media accepted the view that the waste associated with aging was unavoidable, in the late nineteenth century some Ontario newspapers confidently promoted religious, elegiac modes of consolation in the face of mortality and age-related dementia. Articles in the *Christian Guardian*, for instance, maintained an overtly religious and elegiac acceptance of aging and death. This approach is perhaps best expressed by theologian and preacher Nathanael Emmons who, as Ingram explains, "offered sermons in New England for more than sixty years, dying in 1840 at the impressive age of ninety-five. According to his theology, people could influence to some degree whether or not they might ascend to heaven, but above all, they were dependent on God and God had absolute authority over who died and when. In the timing of death, human behaviour would not influence Him" (15). Not surprisingly the *Christian Guardian* upheld equally firm and explicitly religious views of dementia, as evidenced by the obituary for the minister William Mitford, who suffered from "a softening of the brain" before he passed away (12). In the lengthy obituary, the author, J.D., explains that Mitford's condition induced "a decay of memory, and a want of power to keep up an intelligent recognition of men and things" (12). Nevertheless, he insists that Mitford's faith never wavered and that, miraculously, his memory of his religious teachings remained untouched by disease:

> There were frequent seasons of clearness of mind, when he would speak of the things of God, and hold short religious conversations with his family. A kind minister, who made frequent visits during his affliction, says, – "His responses in prayer were very appropriate, and even to the last, if any portion of a favourite hymn had been quoted in his hearing, he would have continued the quotation for a few lines, or verses, repeating them in their order."
>
> He spoke but little at times, but what he did speak was to the praise of God, and an evidence of the happy state of his mind ... His friends were often surprised at the fulness [sic] and correctness with which he repeated several of our excellent hymns. He always delighted in singing the praises of God; and while confined to his room on his last Sabbath on earth, he joined with much feeling and interest while the family sung around his bed. On the Tuesday following, the day of his death, he appeared some better, and his medical attendant expressed an opinion of a favourable turn of his disease. In the morning he appeared unusually happy, and sung the doxology ... But in the evening when his mind appeared unusually clear ... suddenly he ceased to breathe. (12)

In portraying Mitford's final days, the author illustrates that in the face of degeneration and death, Mitford and, by extension, readers are consoled by the enduring presence of religious faith. Although faith could not alter the degenerative teleology of the life course or wholly dispel the view of decline and waste, the repeated references to Mitford's "happy state of mind" afford the possibility of complicating the theory of bodily waste by affirming the potential for psychological modes of repair.[7]

Despite its own generally positive approach toward mortality, on occasion the *Christian Guardian* conveyed its readers' negative view of aging – as, for example, when addressing public concern about the minister William Ryerson's decision to enter into politics at the ripe old age of sixty-four. The paper's stance on this issue was not unusual since newspapers at the time uniformly relied implicitly and explicitly on the theory of waste when they insisted that many politicians were too old to govern.[8] On the whole, the Methodist paper was supportive of Ryerson and defended his decision to become involved in politics and insisted that it was not wrong for a minister to engage in worldly matters. In fact, the paper castigated other religious groups, specifically the Baptists, for thinking that they were *not* involved in politics. A letter published in the paper on 31 July 1861 took issue with a matter that the paper published about Ryerson. The writer, J. Spencer, mentions the latter's profession as a minister, but also cites Ryerson's advanced age as an equally important factor mitigating against his fitness for political office.[9] A similar cautionary note concerning the drawbacks associated with age was sounded by the *Toronto Telegram* in its coverage of the heated mayoral race in December 1885 between the sixty-six-year-old incumbent Alexander Henderson Manning (b. 1819) and the forty-one-year old challenger William Holmes Howland (b. 1844).

Although Manning previously served two terms as mayor, the *Toronto Telegram* maintained that Holmes, the younger man, was far and away the "fittest man for mayor" (26 Dec. 1885, 3). Editor J. Ross Robertson repeatedly cited the benefits of "energy" over "experience." In an article published on 31 December 1885, he asserts that the "electors have a better guarantee for the advancement of the reforms outlined in [Howland's] 'inexperienced' energy than in the decaying vital forces of his opponent" (2). In his reference to "the decaying vital forces" Ross echoes the prevailing theory of entropy and its emphasis on waste. In a subsequent article, Robertson argued that it "is no fault of Mayor Manning that he has outlived his usefulness as a public man, but the fact itself is patent to all, and the comment is universal that while he was competent enough as mayor ten or fifteen years ago, he is totally unsuited to the altered condition of things that now obtains" (2 Jan. 1886, 4). Manning did, however, find a defender among readers of the *Daily Mail*. The ex-mayor of Toronto, who served from 1883–85, Arthur Boswell, quipped in the latter paper that Mr Howland "did not know any more than a baby" (31 Dec. 1885, 8). The *Christian Guardian*'s, the *Toronto Telegram*'s, and the *Daily Mail*'s comments were tepid, however, in comparison to the vitriol unleashed at aging politicians in the *Globe*.

The *Globe*, which later joined with the *Mail* to become Canada's national newspaper in the late twentieth century, was far more aggressive in aligning dementia with the process of aging and the theory of waste. The *Globe* also blamed aging and dementia for feminizing and infantilizing the country's once powerful and rational statesmen. The paper's investment in using accusations of "dotage" to tarnish the reputations of politicians is perhaps most evident in its attempt to prevent William Ryerson from entering politics. A letter to the editor dated 29 June 1861 entitled "Ministers of God on the Field of Politics" objects to Ryerson's decision to run for a seat at the age of sixty-four and oust the incumbent, Mr Biggar. The writer opens by stating that Ryerson is "in his dotage" and concludes by warning readers that he "can at best be among us only a few years more" (C.M.D., *Globe* 2). Dismissing his detractors, Ryerson, who was "always interested in politics" ran as an independent candidate for the West Riding of Brant and won, "defeating Herbert Biggar, despite the vigorous opposition of George Brown and the *Globe*" (Symons). As late as 1869, *The Globe* was still on the attack. In "Dr Ryerson's Last Pamphlet," editor George Brown responds to Ryerson's insistence that he was not in his dotage for the past ten years: "We have examined our fyle [sic] for 1859 and cannot find any reference to the dotage of which the Dr speaks; though, no doubt, a good many of his sayings and doings at that time intimated 'dotage' more than anything else" (2).

An article entitled "A Sad Ruin," dated 5 May 1886 likewise relies on accusations of "senility" to decry the poor performance of then Finance Minister Mr McLelan, blaming his supposed shortcomings on his age and the decline of his mental faculties:

We will not attempt to define accurately the degree in which Mr McLelan is a failure. To do so would be very painful to us, for who can wish to expose the sad incapacity of a man whose weakness is made almost venerable by senility! White hairs entitle the merest mumbler to a certain reverence, but public duty is paramount, and we must call on the government to relieve Mr McLelan of tasks in the attempted discharge of which he is compelled to expose himself most piteously. To his credit it must be said that he tries to do his work, and that he does it as well as he knows how. Not feebleness of intention but a pathetic decadence of the mental faculties renders his parliamentary performances so remarkable ... It is very improper to keep an Ancient One, who might well be enjoying the evening of life in prattling with grand-children, in the forefront of political battles ... Let him depart, let him be provided for if necessary,

no provision on his behalf can be so costly and so dangerous
to the country as that now made for him. When gone, we may
charitably say of him in the paraphrase of Heinn, "Take him
for all in all, he was an old woman – we shall not look upon
his like again." (4)

McLelan was sixty-two years old when the article was written and
although there were older statesmen who played a significant role
in public affairs, the media attack was highly successful; Archibald
Woodbury McLelan ended his tenure as minister of Finance in
January 1887. This defamatory passage recalls the observation cited
in the previous chapter that in the late nineteenth century, the pathology of bodily aging was "repeatedly associated with the female body"
(Katz, *Cultural* 46). In addition, by suggesting that children are the
best company for the elderly and by parodying Hamlet's description of his father – "Take him for all in all. He was a man" – the
article also supports the related insight that in those cases when illness strikes an elderly man, "the old man is, as it were, feminized, and
old age for both men and women is divorced from adulthood, thus
implicitly infantilizing the older person" (ibid.).

Similar attacks linking aging to dementia and the theory of waste
were launched in the *Globe* at Canada's first prime minister, Sir John
A. Macdonald. His detractors cited his waning powers as a threat
to good governance and called his status as a rational, adult male
into question. On 3 September 1886, an article entitled "He Has No
Policy" warned, "The country is in a dangerous situation and needs
a serious, painstaking Man at the head of affairs, instead of an old
garrulous Boy who chatters about himself with senile frivolity" (4).
Later that same year, Macdonald likened himself to a comet, and his
opponents made great sport of the analogy. As one writer quipped,
"his hearers doubtless reflected that a comet is a useless old thing
with a diminishing head, moving in an eccentric orbit, and followed
by a gaseous and most inconsequential tail" ("Comet or Nurse" 4).
At the time, Macdonald was seventy-one years old. His response to
these attacks was documented in the *Daily Mail*.

The attacks were launched when Sir John A. was embarked on a
tour of the province. When he stopped in Orillia on 1 December 1886,
the *Daily Mail* printed his response to the "systematic attacks made
on his public and private character by the Toronto *Globe*" ("The
Premier" 8). In his reply, Macdonald dismissed the references to his

supposed senility on the grounds that that the paper was merely the tool of the Liberal government:

> The *Globe* is the paid servant of the Liberal party. It is in the hands of Mr Edgar, the Henchman, the Whipper-in, the Lieutenant of Mr Blake. Every word appearing in that paper emanates from the Opposition. They are responsible for every attack on myself or on my colleagues, and if the language is base, if the insinuations are cowardly, and the conduct is ungentlemanly, upon the leader of the Opposition, and upon the miserable tools who print and publish it, must the stigma rest." It was said the camomile [sic] flourished more the oftener it was tradden [sic] on; so he had gone on increasing in strength and power the more he was attacked. (in "The Premier" 8)

When a few days later, on Friday, 3 December, Sir John A. was indisposed and had to rest because of his health, he was quoted in the *Daily Mail* as saying that his illness was "owning to an indisposition which had overtaken him that afternoon. He said that it was one of the penalties for being an old man, but he generally got over these attacks and was able to resume his labours once more" ("Sir John" 8). In light of this chapter's focus on waste and repair, it is worth noting that on the one hand Macdonald acknowledges his bodily weakness, essentially the operations of entropy and waste – what he terms "the penalties for being an old man." Yet on the other hand, he also implicitly argues that he possesses the capacity for repair. The battle between the opposing and oscillating forces of waste and repair are likewise evident in letters published in the *Daily Mail* from the Prime Minister's supporters such as "the Liberal Conservative students of Victoria University" who wrote as follows: "It is with the deepest indignation that we read the calumnious, malignant and unprincipled attacks of your opponents, but our indignation is turned to contempt when we look upon your venerable and distinguished presence, and recognize the master intellect that flashes from an eye bright with the light of a thousand victories" (8). Unlike McLelan, Macdonald refused to be bullied into resigning; he died in office five years later.[10]

As the quotations cited above suggest, during the late nineteenth century the media registered the shift from religious to increasingly secular and scientific views of aging, old age, and dementia – the latter views stressed waste over repair. Whereas the *Christian Guardian* upheld a religious view of dementia that posited God's absolute power over the life course, scientific views of the life course were gaining traction, as evidenced by the *Toronto Telegram*'s use of the phrase "the fittest man for mayor." As the vociferous attacks on Sir John A. Macdonald attest, the emerging modern, Darwinian, scientific model portrayed aging as a monolithic narrative of degeneration and decline.

During the late nineteenth and early twentieth century, media, biomedical, and literary discussions increasingly adopted the scientific theory of waste and viewed the body in these modern, secular, and scientific terms. In contrast to our historical moment, however, they typically cited vascular changes as one of the causes of dementia – a view that was in no way distinctively North American (Shorter, *History* 15). In his vast psychiatry textbook, published in 1812, Philadelphia physician Benjamin Rush – officially acknowledged by the American Psychiatric Association in 1965 as the "father of American psychiatry" ("Dr Benjamin") – stated that the "cause of madness is seated primarily in the blood-vessels of the brain, and it depends upon the same kind of morbid and irregular actions that continues other arterial diseases" (in ibid.).

An article in the *Globe* dated Saturday 13 October 1888, echoes Rush's theory, and states that the hardening of the arteries encouraged "the formation of clots, which, sooner or later, shut off all blood supply in the region to which the vessel is distributed" ("The Advance" 7). The article asserts further that "the effect of depriving a part of the brain of its supply of blood is to cause its destruction by softening. Most cases of softening of the brain occur in old age" (7).[11] In 1946, Walter Alvarez, gastroenterologist and a pioneer geriatrician who headed the gastrointestinal division at the Mayo Clinic for twenty-five years (1926–50), similarly echoed Rush's views in his paper entitled "Cerebral Arteriosclerosis with Small Common Unrecognized Apoplexies." "One of the commonest diseases of man," Alvarez wrote, "is a slow petering out toward the end of life, and one of the commonest ways of petering out is that in which the brain is slowly destroyed by the repeated thrombosis of small sclerotic blood vessels" (in Katzman and Bick 6–7). Alvarez's influence on American physicians was profound; "for the next three decades his explanation was readily accepted by practicing physicians who would attribute progressive dementia in the elderly to 'stiff pipes' and small strokes" (Katzman and Bick 7).[12] For example in 1940, in his regular column

"The Doctor Talks," Dr Herman N. Bundesen likewise emphasizes the links between the hardening of the arteries, the wasting of the body, and memory loss: "Old age is called senescence which does not indicate disease but merely indicates the changes which occur in the body with increasing age. Among these changes is the wasting of various parts of the body. The metabolic rate, that is, the rate with which the chemical activity in the body goes on, is lowered. There is a tendency to poor appetite, poor nutrition and loss of weight. The walls of the arteries become hardened, the heart muscle is weakened and the amount of water in the body is decreased. Elderly persons are less emotional and less imaginative than younger ones, and frequently there is some disturbance of memory" ("Simple Living" 11). As Bundesen's statements suggest, this theory persisted into the mid-twentieth century.

In addition to promoting the popular "sclerotic" theory of "hardening" arteries and "softening" brains (Ballenger, *Self* 18), physicians in early twentieth-century North America also held the theory that dementia was the result of "shattered nerves." This approach represented a move away from the purely biological and toward the psychosocial. After the First World War dramatically exposed physicians to the reality of shellshock (see Tyhurst et al. 2), the diagnosis of shattered nerves – a variant of hysteria – was distributed frequently to men as well as women. The theory of shattered nerves was especially popularized by the writings of the influential New York neurologist George Miller Beard, although he termed it neurasthenia. According to Ballenger, the theory of shattered nerves was "emblematic of late-nineteenth-century American anxiety about the pace of modern industrial society" (*Self* 20). In perhaps his most famous work, *American Nervousness* (1881), Beard offers his theory concerning the supposedly inexorable impact of age on the mental faculties – what he termed "the law of the relation of age to work" (a direct reference to the second law of thermodynamics) – and insists that aging brings about "a catastrophic decline in productivity" (ibid.). In keeping with the increasing pathologizing of the aging process in the nineteenth century, Beard did not believe in natural death from old age; for him "death in old age was not a gentle cessation of unimpaired function, but a ten- to fifteen-year period of decline beginning with cerebral disease" (Cole 166). Rather than promote a purely somatic view of decline, however, Beard argued that the pressured work environment contributed to age-related dementia, and that modernity was partly responsible for our ills. His views concerning the toll exacted by modernity are, as we will see, taken up by writers such as Munro, Richler, and Laurence, who more forcibly adopt a bio-psychosocial approach to challenge the view that modernization is synonymous with progress, and to interrogate the social ramifications of shifting the burden of caring for people with dementia from the community to the family.

In 1907, the same year that Alzheimer gave his brief yet infamous report on Auguste D., the *Globe* cited an article on insanity in Britain that warned readers that senile dementia accounted "for over 38% of last year's fresh lunacy cases," and insisted that "we live too long for the kind of work most of us do" ("Senile" 5). Although lengthy, I cite this article in full because it highlights several key factors associated with modern views of dementia, namely, the concern that health technology was prolonging "useless" lives, the theory of neurasthenia, increasingly associated with urban life in North America, and, finally, the mythic image of senile demented individuals crowding the local asylums: "'The advanced medical knowledge of today,' said the authority referred to, 'keeps a multitude of persons alive whose minds are practically worn out. The present age demands more brain work and nerve strains from everyone than was demanded only a few years ago. There is less and less demand for people who can only use their hands. The physical wear and tear has decreased while the brain work and the strain on the nervous system have increased. The result is that the mind dies first and the body is kept alive by medical science, which thus adds to the growing list of senile dementia cases in our asylums'" ("Senile" 5). The persistence of this view, with its Gothic rhetoric, is evidenced by former American Psychiatric Association president Abraham Myerson's suggestion more than three decades later, in 1944, that "progress in longevity brought with it the distressing fact that more people ... outlive their brains" (in Ballenger, *Self* 40). Thus from at least the mid-nineteenth century until the 1950s, a popular image of old age portrayed the period as "a dreary waste, unproductive and cheerless, characterized chiefly by rheumatism, imbecility, and decay" (Wentworth in Cole 143).[13] In a letter to the editor entitled "The Man of Fifty," a writer commented in the *Globe* on his odd predicament:

But is it not strange that the man of fifty, who is active, and has a maturity of experience far beyond that of the average young man, should be set aside while a school kid takes a place of responsibility which he is not capable of filling, because he can be secured for a somewhat smaller salary?

That as it may, the man of fifty is apparently considered a dud, not fit for the work of life, a worn-out vessel, to be set upon the shelf as a has-been. Still is it not significant that the only places where these duds, these fossils, who have reached the dotage period, are in demand and can command the highest salaries, should be upon the Judge's seat of our judicial courts or within the exalted precincts of the Senate Chamber? – A Curious Fossil. (4)

The growing abhorrence of old age at the turn of the century in North America, in part the product of the theory of waste, is equally apparent in the American physician Ignatz Leo Nascher's 1914 textbook *Geriatrics*. The Viennese-born Nascher, who grew up in America and obtained his medical degree in 1855 from New York University, coined the term geriatrics and is widely regarded today as the founder of the field. Recalling the German poem from 1578 cited in the previous chapter, and its acceptance of dementia as one of life's inevitable eight stages, Nascher conceived of four ages of life: childhood, maturity, old age, and senility, and he argued that the transition "from old age to senile generally took place in the individual's late 70s or early 80s, a critical period known as the 'senile climacteric'" (Cole 202). Previously physicians such as Kraepelin and Alzheimer had relied on the distinction between "senile," after 65, and "presenium," spanning the ages of 45 to 60, "although some later writers upped the age to 65" (Katzman and Bick 1). In keeping with an earlier Victorian moralistic dualism, however, in 1914 Nascher described old age as wholly repugnant, and he went so far as to proclaim that the "appearance of the senile individual is repellent both to the esthetic sense and to the sense of independence, that sense or mental attitude that the human race holds toward the self-reliant and self-dependent" (v–vi). The force of Nascher's repulsion recalls Kristeva's discussion of society's dread of the "abject" – a dread that was increasingly expressed in the early twentieth century.[14] The general view of entropy is perhaps best expressed by the Canadian physician Herman N. Bundesen, cited earlier, in his article entitled "Memory Loss and Fatigue Hit Old Folk":

Mental changes often take place as a person becomes aged. Loss of memory is a common example of this condition. These

mental changes may occur along with the general aging of all
body tissues. It is called senility and comes on at about 75 years
or older. Also mental changes may come as a result of hardening
of the arteries.

   The earliest symptom, in most cases of senility, is easy tiring.
Then develops failure to concentrate. A variety of other symptoms may occur. The patient may become set in his ways, and
may avoid any new methods or ideas. Irritability, anger, depression and suspicion occur in many of the persons. At one time
the patient may be relatively clear and coherent. Then, in a few
hours, he may not be able to recognize his best friend or speak
in a coherent manner. Disturbance of the memory is typical of
the mental disturbance of elderly people. (11)

Of note is Bundesen's repeated insistence that memory loss is a common problem among elderly individuals, that the symptoms of senility include both somatic and psychological changes, and that typical
symptoms range from "tiredness" to the inability to recognize one's
"best friend or speak in a coherent manner."
   To a limited extent, the media occasionally challenged the dominant view that old age was a period governed by waste by sporadically
publishing articles that suggested it might be possible to forestall the
indignities associated with old age and senility. One headline proclaims that "Improvement in Diet Will Delay Senility" (*Globe and
Mail*, 28 July 1927). Another claims "Simple Living Habits Best
Old Age Treatment" to prevent memory loss and "the neutritis of
old age" (Bundesen, *Globe and Mail*, 25 Nov. 1940, 11). In addition to promoting vitamins and minerals, physicians recommended
sleep as a strategy for repairing the effects of aging. "Are you growing senile prematurely?" one article enquires; if the answer is yes,
"try Professor Braines' elixir – sleep" ("Growing" 15). In his article
on "Memory Loss and Fatigue," Bundesen likewise observes: "The
tiredness and fatigue and lack of concentration which develop early
in these mental disturbances [affecting elderly people] may often
respond quickly to such simple treatment as more rest in bed, a vaca-
tion, regulation of the bowel habits and improvement in the general
nutrition" (11). Positive thinking is also evident in Sally Townsend's
article "How Never to Grow Old," which cites Dr Martin Gumpert,
author of the recently published book *You Are Younger Than You
Think* (1944). According to Gumpert: "There is not truth either to

the formula that we must die at 70, or to the belief that we must necessarily be tortured in old age by the humiliation of senility" (Townsend 8). Buoyed by Gumpert's optimism, Townsend concludes on an upbeat, prophetic note. "The time seems to be close at hand," she asserts, "when we all can say happily with [Robert] Browning: 'Grow old along with me! The best is yet to be, the last of life, for which the first was made" (8). In 1960 the *Globe and Mail* published another article promoting the potential for healthy aging, which featured the advice of Dr Wilder Penfield, "world-renowned brain surgeon and physician" ("Penfield Says" 17). In contrast to the previous doctors who advocated rest and sleep as conducive to "repair," Penfield emphatically states that rest "is not what the brain needs. Rest destroys the brain. Retirement is the proper time to change the harness, reduce the physical load and increase the mental challenge" (ibid.).[15] Despite the occasional optimistic article, the theory of waste continued to dominate in the Canadian media.

Thus far I have explored the diverse approaches to aging, old age, and dementia conveyed by four Canadian newspapers in the late nineteenth and early to mid-twentieth century. I have also analyzed their relation to the medical theories of the day concerning the supposed inevitability of dementia due to the natural effects of dotage, which were exacerbated in many cases by small strokes and shattered nerves. The next sections turn to fictional portrayals of the latter stage of the life course and the dementing illnesses associated with them to determine how Canadian writers responded to, and in some cases revised, the theory of waste and repair. Since, as we have seen, Alzheimer's disease was not viewed as the primary cause of dementia until the early 1980s, section two includes detailed analyses of texts that portray age-related dementia as instigated by a variety of causes ranging from strokes to shattered nerves to problems associated with very old age. Section two also includes Alice Munro's portrayal of Parkinson's disease, a terminal dementing illness that, like Alzheimer's, instigates cognitive impairment; whose symptoms can be similar; and which may coexist with Alzheimer's disease (see the Alz.org website). Individuals with Parkinson's, their caregivers, and the researchers and clinicians who study the disease know that one of its later primary symptoms is dementia. For this reason, "Parkinson's disease dementia" is described at length on the Alzheimer's Association website. In drawing connections among conditions that are strongly correlated with dementia, my goal lies in deconstructing the monolithic, Gothic notion that dementia is the result of a singular, monstrous entity: Alzheimer's disease.[16]

An analysis of early media and fictive accounts of various forms of dementia in relation to the theory of the dynamic relationship between waste and repair is instructive because first, it reminds us that historically, in addition to accepting dotage in old age, other illnesses were understood to play a role in causing late-onset dementia. Second, both the media and, to a greater extent, literary depictions adopt a broader bio-psychosocial approach to suggest that dementia is exacerbated by factors associated with modernization and, at times, becomes a repository for our fears concerning modern life – urbanization, increasing industrialization, and capitalism – that result in "shattered nerves." Equally important, fictional representations of dementia emphasize that the difficulty associated with coping with the illness and enhancing the body's potential for repair springs largely from the stigma associated with mental illness and the lack of support offered to caregivers looking after a relative suffering from a dementing illness. On the whole, fictional portrayals adopt an elegiac approach that turns readers' attention to the human losses associated with the illness – losses that, as depicted in literature, affect the individual and her family, and which call for rituals of consolation.

SECTION II: DEMENTIA IN CANADIAN LITERATURE: THE SATIRE OF STEPHEN LEACOCK

In keeping with the diversity found in the media's treatment of dementia, fictional accounts ranged from satirical to elegiac portrayals of dementing illness. On the whole, fictional accounts also tended to adopt a bio-psychosocial rather than a purely biological explanation, repeatedly linking dementia to both somatic origins and to broader political, economic, and socio-cultural factors. Interestingly, Canadian writers frequently suggested that the accelerated mental decline, exhaustion, and waste associated with modern life played a role in aggravating both the condition and care of dementing illness. As I argued in section one, in the late nineteenth century the media expressed responses ranging from religious/elegiac to more pessimistic biomedical/Gothic views of cognitive decline. Yet Leacock's and, more overtly, Munro's, Richler's, and Laurence's more unequivocally elegiac texts, which reflect on the later interwar period, poignantly consider how society's treatment of the dependent elderly registers a loss of humanity. Their works also question whether there is any way to avoid or, at the very least, repair what the forces of modernity have destroyed.

Trends associated with modernization in Canada[17] led to the chafing against traditional familial and communal structures – which, as noted in the previous chapter, were "regulated by religious and social principles of hierarchy, dependency, and reciprocal obligation" (Cole 230). These trends are perhaps best expressed by Canada's beloved comedic writer Stephen Leacock in his satirical short story cycle *Sunshine Sketches of a Little Town* (1912). Leacock's narrator characterizes Dean Drone, the elderly reverend of the town of Mariposa, as a useless failure of a man, stricken with both shattered nerves and vascular dementia. As the narrator, a local Mariposan, explains, Drone suffers a stroke after realizing that his hair-brained scheme – "the Whirlwind campaign" (Leacock 89) to raise money to build a new church – proved an abysmal failure. Tongue planted firmly in cheek, Leacock's narrator insists, however, that Drone remains utterly unaffected by his recent stroke:

Dean Drone? Did he get well again? Why, what makes you ask that? You mean, was his head at all affected after the stroke? No, it was not. Absolutely not. It was not affected in the least, though how anybody who knows him now in Mariposa could have the faintest idea that his mind was in any way impaired by the stroke is more than I can tell. The engaging of Mr Uttermost, the curate, whom perhaps you have heard preach in the new church, had nothing whatever to do with Dean Drone's head. It was merely a case of the pressure of overwork. It was felt very generally by the wardens that, in these days of specialization, the rector was covering too wide a field, and that if he should abandon some of the lesser duties of his office, he might devote his energies more intently to the Infant Class. That was all. You may hear him there any afternoon, talking to them … so you will understand that the Dean's mind is, if anything, even keener, and his head even clearer than before. (ibid. 107–8)

The narrator slyly insists that Dean Drone's head is so clear – read "empty" – that, to the reverend's delight, he finds he can read works in the Greek that "seemed difficult before. Because his head is so clear now" (108). Viewed in terms of the theory of waste and repair,

Leacock pokes fun at those naive enough to believe that the force of
entropy can be opposed by the force of repair.

Although Leacock's narrator repeatedly and overtly mocks the
aged, demented Reverend, using familiar nineteenth-century rhetoric
that infantilizes the elderly man, the collection's final section betrays
a far more ambivalent and complex response to aging and decline
– one that resonates with a newfound, elegiac sense of the decline
and waste increasingly associated with capitalism, urbanization,
and modernity. In the final section, entitled "L'Envoi," the narrator
directly addresses a nameless Mariposan who left town as a young
man to seek his fortune in the city. Now an older man, the prodigal
returns home by train at night. Addressing him in the second person, the narrator chastises him for abandoning his antiquated, rural
town, its inhabitants and, in the process, his own youthful innocence:
"What? It feels nervous and strange to be coming here again after all
these years? It must indeed. No, don't bother to look at the reflection of your face in the window-pane shadowed by the night outside. Nobody could tell you now after all these years. Your face has
changed in these long years of money-getting in the city. Perhaps if
you had come back now and again, just at odd times, it wouldn't have
been so" (186). In addition to stressing the degenerative influence of
"these long years" – which alters the prodigal's reflection and recalls
Oscar Wilde's uncanny, Gothic portrait of Dorian Gray – this passage
implicitly insists that maintaining one's identity, figured in Leacock's
fiction partially in economic terms, is implicitly tied to aging in the
small, pastoral town of Mariposa. Succumbing to the lure of urban
life, and abandoning one's rural home and its elderly inhabitants,
ultimately entails rejecting a crucial facet of oneself. For Leacock this
disruption of the Lockean identity had a profound moral valence.
Put somewhat differently, as a result of rushing to the city for the
purposes of "money-getting" – by participating in crude, immoral
urban businesses where money changes hands – the prodigal himself
is changed. While not demented, his physical health (figured as and
aligned with other forms of "capital" in Leacock's work) is squan-
dered, and he returns to his abandoned home, an unrecognizable,
wasted figure. As one of the many former Mariposans who haunt
the Mausoleum Club in the city, he mirrors his demented double:
the equally spent figure of Dean Drone, whose vitality was lost in a
similarly greed-driven enterprise, the Whirlwind campaign.

To a great extent Leacock's pessimistic and moralistic view of aging echoes the sermons of ministers in the late Victorian period, who similarly insisted that "sin was neither innate nor entirely voluntary but developed inevitably from the world's corrupting influence" (Cole 129). In keeping with Canadian literature's distinctly conservative approach to modernity and to literary modernism, Leacock's fiction adopts and adapts elements of the conservative, moral imperatives of earlier religious discourse. In this sense Leacock's work is foundational to my argument that Canadian literature's inherently elegiac approach to dementia is the inheritor of prior elegiac, religious discourses.

Leacock valued "community over the individual, organic growth over radical change, the middle way over extreme deviation. Such values form the basis of Leacock's satiric norm, the authorial position from which he attacked rampant individualism, materialism, and worship of technology" (Lynch n.p.). I argue further that Leacock's attack against modernization and his tendency to blame it for accelerating the wasting process laid the foundation for subsequent conservative literary portrayals by Laurence, Munro, and Richler, which likewise incorporated religious views and resulted in a distinctly moralistic approach to the avariciousness of the modern era and its treatment of the frail elderly.

In a sermon to young men at the Brooklyn YMCA published in 1870, the preacher Henry Ward Beecher explicitly warned his audience that migration from the country involved the "greatest loss that the young can sustain ... the loss of home ... God's natural training ground" (in Cole 132–3). Ministers such as Beecher believed that in the city "the struggle for advancement discouraged fidelity, honesty and thoroughness"; worse, in the absence of these virtues, "alcohol, tobacco and sexual indulgence abounded" (ibid.). "And this is a course," Beecher prophesied, "that grows worse with the years, and must in the end of life leave a man hopeless in old age" (ibid.). Leacock's narrator's pronouncements can also be usefully read in light of the more pervasive nineteenth-century sentimentalism that "was part of the self-evasion of a culture at once committed to and disturbed by capitalist values of efficiency and productivity" (Cole 136). As Leacock's fiction intimates, modernity's promise of efficiency and productivity was shadowed by the Gothic threat of "spiritual corruption and mental disintegration," evidenced by cognitive decline (Botting 2). For the writers under consideration, dementia alone did

not constitute a dreaded evil; instead, capitalist values – which sanctioned the mockery of a community's vulnerable elders and dismissed
them as shameful, wasted failures – represented a far graver moral
threat. In contrast to the biomedical model, Canadian literature
resisted the increasing valorization of and emphasis on the individual, the unequivocal embrace of progress, and the rejection of seemingly outdated spiritual views and traditions along with the elderly
individuals who embodied these seemingly outmoded belief systems.

Such resistance is evident in Alice Munro's "The Peace of Utrecht,"
a semi-autobiographical story about her mother's struggle with
Parkinson's disease. In keeping with Leacock's *Sunshine Sketches of a
Little Town*, "The Peace of Utrecht" poignantly conveys the concerns
in the Depression years about aging, mental illness, and the fracturing
of generational bonds exacerbated by modernization. Rather than
focus on the mother's perspective, Munro's story, like Leacock's, directly addresses the experience of the younger generation. "The Peace
of Utrecht" deftly portrays the intimate and conflicting emotional
responses of two daughters, Helen and Maddy, to their mother's
neurodegenerative illness. Their responses, in turn, are juxtaposed
to those of their elderly aunts, Annie and Lou. Whereas Helen, the
narrator, leaves home to study at college, and eventually marries and
has two children, her sister Maddy remains in the small Ontario
town of Jubilee. Never marrying, Maddy dedicates herself to caring for their mother for ten years until she dies.

The story unfolds during Helen's brief visit to the family home.
Helen recalls the shame she and Maddy felt as teenagers when forced
to witness their mother's decline:

> We tried both crudely and artfully, to keep her at home ... not
> for her sake, but for ours, who suffered such unnecessary humili-
> ation at the sight of her eyes rolling back in her head in a tempo-
> rary paralysis of the eye muscles, at the sound of her thickened
> voice, whose embarrassing pronouncements it was our job to
> interpret to outsiders. So bizarre was the disease she had in its
> effects that it made us feel like crying out in apology (though we
> stayed stiff and white) as if we were accompanying a particularly
> tasteless sideshow. All wasted, our pride; our purging its rage in
> wild caricatures we did for each other (no, not caricatures, for
> she was one herself; imitations). We should have let the town
> have her; it would have treated her better. (195)

This passage recalls the shift between the loci of care noted earlier, which saw the transfer from quasi-communal to solely familial responsibility for looking after individuals suffering from mental illness. As Munro's story suggests, during the Depression, it was no longer appropriate for the mentally ill to wander "freely about their communities" (Chappell et al. 220). As the story painfully illustrates, at this time, the family was expected to bear the entire burden of caring for their loved ones, to the detriment of all concerned. Unlike a social science essay or a medical case study, which abstractly outlines the facts, Munro's fiction immerses readers in the lived experience of a dementing illness. Her narrative unfolds over time and describes characters with whom the reader can identify. As a result, her fiction conveys the emotional weight of the situation, and invites readers to ponder the characters' moral dilemmas – dilemmas that spring from a socio-political situation from which neither caregivers nor their loved ones emerge unscathed.

Unlike Leacock's chatty, intrusive narrator, who acts as the reader's tour guide and satirizes the town's inhabitants, Munro's narrator remains uninvolved and refrains from judging the various characters' responses to dementia. In opting for a detached narrative perspective that simply dramatizes the influence of dementia on a family, "The Peace of Utrecht" reinstalls what other media and biomedical discussions of dementia defend against, and, in the process, implicates readers in the experience of abjection and loss instigated by the illness. In Munro's fiction, helplessness and failure attend any attempt to rely on simplistic narratives that feature a clear villain or a cure. Kinship roles and identities are likewise fraught and in flux as mothers become both childlike and monstrous, and children are unwillingly thrust into the adult role of caregivers, who are understandably ashamed of and, at times, horrified by their monstrous charges. Compared to the chaos instigated by dementia in Munro's fiction, Leacock's satirical portrait of the demented Dean Drone seems like a quaint Victorian artifact. In "The Peace of Utrecht," characters and readers alike are forced to grapple with the uncertainty of meaning and identity, the limitations of narrative, and the necessity of holding seemingly incommensurable points of view without pronouncing judgment.

In Munro's narrative, the girls' shame also attests to the endurance of the values that dominated the Victorian period, which stressed the necessity of adhering to one's gender role and to playing one's proper part. As Munro explained in a recent interview: "I was brought up to believe that the worst thing you could do was 'call attention to yourself' or 'think you were smart.' My mother was an exception to this rule and was punished by the early onset of Parkinson's disease. (The rule was for country people, like us, not so much for towners)" (in Sterling and Brumfield). In keeping with the prevailing ideology, which Munro treats sardonically, her mother's illness could be interpreted as a punishment for leading a life considered morally unacceptable for a woman.[18] There is in fact a great deal of irony in this statement, given that Munro herself was recently awarded the Nobel Prize (10 November 2013) but was unable to receive the award in person, due to her own ill health; her daughter went on her behalf.

Owing to the prevailing views that the dependent elderly constituted a "useless burden" and that "the worst thing you could do was 'call attention to yourself,'" the voices of individuals suffering from dementia were rarely recorded. However, in Munro's fiction, the mother's experience and her voice resonate powerfully. In keeping with feminist elegies, Munro's stories frequently convey the voice of the dead mother using the rhetorical trope of *prosopopoeia* (a figure of speech in which an absent or imaginary person is represented as speaking). For example, Helen hauntingly recalls her mother's repeated plaints: "'Everything has been taken away from me,' she would say. To strangers, to friends of ours whom we tried always unsuccessfully to keep separate from her, to old friends of hers who came guiltily infrequently to see her, she would speak like this, in the very slow mournful voice that was not intelligible or quite human" (199).[19] Whereas the Gothic perpetuates fear in the face of a virtually unrepresentable evil, Munro's narrative restores the mother's "mournful voice." By engaging in acts of narrative remembrance, which bring the dead back to life, Munro's fiction insists on the difficult, yet necessary task of reconciling individuals to loss and death.

SECTION III: "THE PEACE OF UTRECHT" – AN ILLUSTRATION OF THE THEORY OF WASTE AND REPAIR

Toward the conclusion of Munro's short story, Helen visits the home of Aunt Annie and Aunt Lou. These elderly sisters serve as foils for Helen and Maddy and they underscore the story's governing metaphors of waste *and* repair. As Helen explains, she visited her aunt three times during her brief stay, and "each time they have been spending the afternoon making rugs out of dyed rags" (202–3). On Helen's third and final visit Aunt Annie takes her up to the attic and presents her with her dead mother's wardrobe, which Annie and Lou have lovingly and patiently repaired. As Helen explains, Aunt Annie "showed me where things had been expertly darned and mended and where the elastic had been renewed" (205). Aunt Annie offers Helen her mother's belongings as a gift, and castigates her niece for contemplating buying anything "when there are things here as good as new" (206). When Helen forcibly declines her aunts' gift, she realizes that she has run up against her aunts' most basic philosophy, "the rock of their lives," their hard-headed "materialism" that informed them that "things must be used; everything must be used up, saved and mended and made into something else and used again" (206).

Reading Munro's story in light of Lewes's theory enables readers to appreciate the existence of alternatives to the tragic view of the supposedly inevitable, corrosive forces of modernity and urbanization. More precisely, Lewes's approach helps to contextualize Aunt Annie's view that the mother's death was not inevitable, but instead was due to a failure of care. In "The Peace of Utrecht," the elderly aunts underscore that suffering from a dementing illness need not necessitate condemning a person to a meaningless, "useless" life or a lonely death.[20] In the confrontation between Helen and Aunt Annie, two diametrically opposing views of aging and illness – as an inevitable decline or an agonistic struggle between waste and repair mediated by the individual and her caregivers – come to the fore. After offering Helen her mother's newly mended clothes, Aunt Annie reveals a secret concerning Maddy's supposedly immoral treatment of their mother prior to her death. The references to textiles in the story echo Lewes's view of the forces of waste and repair as determining the fate of the living "fabric of the body" (Lewes in Charise 169). Even before Aunt Annie's revelation, Helen intuits the connection between the repair of her mother's clothes and the latter's death. As she says, "I wondered if the clothes had been the main thing after all; perhaps they were only to serve as the introduction to a conversation about my mother's death" (206). Aunt Annie then reveals that Helen and Maddy's mother suffered grievously and needlessly. Worse, she insists that she died prematurely because, rather than continuing to care for her at home, Maddy lied to their mother, lured her to the hospital, and then abandoned her there. Put somewhat differently

Maddy treated her mother, who suffered from a wasting disease, as "waste" and cast her aside. Weeping openly, Aunt Annie tells Helen that Maddy told their mother it was nothing but a check-up: "Your mother went in there and she thought she was coming out in three weeks ... Do you think she wanted to stay in there where nobody could make out what she was saying and they wouldn't let her out of her bed? She wanted to come home!" (207). Aunt Annie's condemnation of Maddy's behaviour conveys the former's implicit belief that ongoing care at home – in essence, the opportunity for regeneration and repair within a humane domestic sphere – could have forestalled their mother's rapid decline and death.

Helen, who defensively clings to the view of aging as inexorable decline, dismisses Aunt Annie's interpretation of events, insisting that "it was just time" (207). Their difference of opinion highlights the fact that the narratives mobilized or relied on by caregivers (as in the account of Gloria D. in the previous chapter) often reflect subjective motivations. Indeed, the evocative phrase "it was just time" invites us to consider *who* decides when and why the time is up, implicating us in a decision that can have no objective answer. Undaunted, Aunt Annie maintains her view that it was only after Maddy left their mother at the hospital that the latter "felt she would die" (207). "Don't you ever think," Aunt Annie insists, uncharacteristically angry, "that a person wants to die, just because it seems to everybody else they have got no reason to go on living" (207). In this scene, Aunt Annie comes closest to challenging the notion that disease alone reduced Helen and Maddy's mother's life to a mere "waste." Simply put, Aunt Annie angrily refutes the belief that Maddy and Helen's mother should acquiesce to death simply because she was suffering from the physical and mental ravages of a dementing illness – a belief that implicitly underlies Helen's comment that "it was time."

Aunt Annie goes on to emphasize that Helen's mother begged Maddy to take her home, saying she would die otherwise, but Maddy refused. Again Helen attempts to discredit her aunt's comments, this time by insisting that her mother did not always tell the truth. Ignoring Helen, Aunt Annie relates what proves to be the most emotionally devastating information, namely that Helen's mother was so desperate to escape the hospital that she fled at night in the middle of January, wearing only her slippers and a dressing gown. This information hits Helen hardest because Aunt Annie's Gothic account transforms the girls' mother from a demented Gothic monster into a helpless, innocent heroine desperate to escape incarceration and death. Indeed Aunt Annie's tale implies that anyone searching for the real monster must look elsewhere.

As noted in the introduction, one of the primary functions of the Gothic is to take the anger and fear experienced in the face of illness and death – two notable examples of the various evils we experience – and assign the blame for our misfortune to something or someone. In the Gothic, there is seemingly no escape from symbolizing a monster or from confronting the horror of the situation. Relating the conclusion of the mother's futile attempt to flee the hospital, Aunt Annie tells Helen that "they nailed a board across her bed. I saw it. You can't blame the nurses. They can't watch everybody. They haven't the time" (208). Ultimately, Aunt Annie pronounces judgment on Maddy: "we thought it was hard. Lou and I thought it was hard" (209). Although it might be tempting to side with the aunts and cast Maddy as the true monster, Munro's sensitive treatment of both the mother's and the girls' plights makes it impossible to irrevocably cast Maddy into that Gothic role. Instead, "The Peace of Utrecht" invites both its characters and its readers to see how the Gothic model of dementia – a model that views the illness as a crime to be solved – can impede the recognition of people's limitations and humanity and, as a result, obstruct the difficult work of reconciling ourselves to loss and death.[21]

In "The Peace of Utrecht," after returning from her visit with her aunts, Helen finds Maddy preparing supper in the kitchen. Although she admits to having visited Aunt Lou and Aunt Annie, rather than revealing what she has been told, Helen murmurs softly, "Don't be guilty, Maddy" (209). Seemingly aware of what Helen has learned, Maddy cries: "I couldn't go on … I wanted my life" (210). In the midst of her cryptic confession – with Helen's own children "running in and out and shrieking at each other" between Helen's and Maddy's legs – Maddy drops a pink, cut-glass bowl.[22] The shattered bowl represents the loss of physical as well as moral integrity; whereas the former loss may be inevitable, Munro's symbolism suggests that the latter is not. Simply put, socio-political forces put the family in a double bind that pitted the generations against each other – and neither emerged victorious.

In her perceptive study of the locations associated with old age in Munro's fiction, which range from home care to residential care facilities, Sara Jamieson clarifies that Munro's own family's experience looking after a mother with Parkinson's disease made Munro aware of the personal sacrifices associated caregiving (14). As Munro explained in an interview, as the eldest daughter it was her "job to stay home and look after [her mother] ... until [she] died" (in Ross 39). Jamieson observes that rather than stay home, Munro "accepted a scholarship to university." Citing Munro's biographer Robert Thacker, Jamieson explains that after "she got married in her second year and moved even further away, her mother's care became the responsibility of Munro's younger sister, and, finally, her father who was left to deal with his wife's worsening condition by himself, 'along with such assistance as his elderly mother and aunt ... and friends could provide'" (14)

Rather than resolve the competing claims of the older and younger generations, the story's conclusion maps this agonistic struggle, which is only worsened by being cast in the Gothic mode. Indeed, Munro's story raises the question as to why, in a civilized society, family members should be placed in this double bind. Instead of reductively locating a Gothic monster, "The Peace of Utrecht" suggests that changing demographic patterns, compounded by the lack of available resources to protect the frail elderly, resulted in the excessive suffering of both individuals coping with dementing illnesses and their families, and precluded any possibility of repair. To illustrate the symmetry and fundamental connection between individual and familial suffering, the story's conclusion juxtaposes the symptoms of the mother's paralyzing and dementing illness to her daughters' uncannily similar expressions of these symptoms: Maddy's existential paralysis and Helen's disorientation in her childhood home. After dropping the bowl, Maddy, who is barefoot, is rendered immobile. Although she tells Helen to get a broom and clean up the glass, Helen merely wanders helplessly around the kitchen. As Helen explains, "I seemed to have forgotten where it was kept" (210). Meanwhile, sorrowful and puzzled by her own existential paralysis, Maddy responds obliquely to Helen's suggestion that she leave, asking, "But why can't I, Helen? *Why can't I?*" (210).[23]

Like Leacock's *Sunshine Sketches*, Munro's "The Peace of Utrecht" illustrates the costs of weighing the claims of the frail elderly against those of the younger generation. Whereas Leacock's "L'Envoi" portrays the inevitability of aging and decline instigated by modernization, "The Peace of Utrecht" offers a more nuanced critique. More precisely, by questioning the legitimacy of the belief in the supposedly inextricable relationship between old age, decline, and death entrenched in the late Victorian period and by foregrounding the shared experiences of disorientation, cognitive impairment, and paralysis – experiences common to mother and daughters alike – "The Peace of Utrecht" effectively challenges the individualistic and dualistic view of good and bad aging. In the process, the story undermines the supposedly hard and fast boundaries between age and youth, normal and diseased.

Munro's story also suggests that moral transgressions occur when an individual's limited resources are utterly tapped and no broader communal or cultural supports are available. Without this social safety net, caregivers risk losing sight of the humanity of people suffering from dementia, and when this type of recognition is lost, a once-beloved family member can become objectified and viewed as waste. In Canada, demographic changes during the nineteenth century, particularly the steady decline in fertility throughout the century, led to smaller families (Dillon, *Shady* 281). Moreover, in keeping with Leacock's repeated references to trains, ships, and urban life, individuals also experienced greater geographic mobility due to the tendency to leave the countryside for work in urban centres. Such changes meant that there were "fewer people at home to care for sick or aged relatives" (Montigney, "Foisted" 826). Moreover as social historians remind us, "where caring is required, the responsibility is likely to fall disproportionately upon women, as it has always done" (Thane 12). Rather than simply casting blame on the younger generation, Munro's story highlights these changes and, in the process, underscores that coping with a dementing illness in the 1930s was "hard" for everyone.[24]

SECTION IV: BALANCING WASTE AND REPAIR: MORDECAI RICHLER'S "THE SUMMER MY GRANDMOTHER WAS SUPPOSED TO DIE"

The burden on female family members and the related difficulty associated with facilitating repair are forcibly conveyed by Mordecai Richler's short story "The Summer My Grandmother Was Supposed to Die," which was based on Richler's firsthand experience of his maternal grandmother's stroke-related dementia in the 1930s. His grandmother Sarah died in 1942, and Richler wrote the story in 1960 (Kramer 22–6). The narrative is told from the perspective of a young boy who watches his mother care for his demented grandmother

over a period of seven years. As the narrator explains, as his grandmother's illness "dragged on and on she became a condition in the
house, something beyond hope or reproach, like the leaky ice-box"
(330). As noted earlier, Canadian fiction about dementia is notable
precisely because of its uneasy mingling of the Gothic with the elegiac mode. In the case of Richler's fiction, the boy's father remains
skeptical of his wife's efforts to keep her mother alive, saying: "Some
life for a person ... She can't speak – she doesn't recognize anybody
– what is there for her?" (331). Whereas the father and the family
physician, Dr Katzman, discuss philosophy, the hard work of caring
for an elderly person with dementia relentlessly falls to the narrator's mother, who cares for her mother day and night, even "getting
up to rock her mother in her arms for hours" (331). In the fourth
year of the grandmother's illness, however, "the strain began to tell"
(331). The narrator's mother "took to falling asleep in her chair. One
minute she would be sewing a patch on my breeches ... and the next
she would be snoring" (331). Inevitably, we are told, there came the
morning "the mother just couldn't get out of bed" (331). At this point,
the family decides to put the grandmother in an old age home. For
two solid weeks, the narrator's mother rests in bed until "her cheeks
regained their normal pinkish hue" (332). After a month passes,
however, she visits the home and returns with her mother. Despite
her husband's protests that they are "recognized experts there. They
know how to take care of her better than you do," his wife dismisses
his views. "Experts?" she retorts. "Expert murderers you mean. She's
got bedsores ... they don't change her linen often enough, they hate
her. She must have lost twenty pounds in there" (332). Her criticism,
although embedded in a fictional story, recalls Auguste D.'s death,
which was instigated by an infection stemming from bedsores. In
Richler's fiction, the mother's dilemma mirrors the double bind outlined in Munro's "The Peace of Utrecht," in which Maddy has to
weigh the value of "taking her life" and gaining a measure of respite
and freedom against taking the life of her mother.

Richler's story, like Munro's, explores the largely unmapped
terrain of emotional impoverishment and bodily, rather than economic, exhaustion. Over the next two years, the narrator's mother
responds to this obligation and seemingly tips the balance in favour
of repair, but at the cost of her own ability to engage in acts of self-
care. As the narrator explains, "there was no significant change in

my grandmother's condition, though fatigue, ill-temper, and even morbidity enveloped my mother again" (333). One evening, turning to her young son, the mother asks, "Would you send me to the Old People's Home?" Despite the fact that he tells her he would not, she remains distrustful and mutters: "I hope that never in my life do I have to count on my children for anything" (333). Her doubt may spring from the fact that she is talking to her son rather than her daughter. Yet, as the story suggests, times are changing. Few male children in her son's generation would sacrifice their lives for their parents. As the father's behaviour in Richler's story suggests, adult males in the previous generation would not make this sacrifice, either. The mother's experience and despair refute the asylum superintendents' repeated and overly optimistic claims that "helpless old dements," benign elderly people "in their dotage," can be "easily cared for at home."

After seven years, the grandmother finally dies; the narrator returns to his house and finds his mother wearing "a black shawl" (333). Years of hard work caring for the grandmother are conveyed by a single image of the narrator's mother clenching "a knot of handkerchief ... in a fist that had been cracked by washing soda" (333). When the mother begins to weep, Dr Katzman quickly sedates her, plunging "a needle into her arm" (335), and the men return to their philosophical deliberations on the meaning of life. Their platitudes are interrupted, however, by the father, who urgently summons the doctor again, saying, "Dr Katzman, please. It's my wife. Maybe the injection wasn't strong enough. She just doesn't stop crying. It's like a tap" (336). As Richler's biographer asserts, in this instance the author sympathizes with his mother's views and as a result harshly satirizes the rest of the family and the moral bankruptcy of the community (Kramer 22). In the modern world depicted in Richler's fiction, the humanity of an elderly woman suffering from dementia goes unrecognized, to the extent that she is objectified and likened to a "leaky ice-box," and her sole humane caregiver, the narrator's mother, weeping in the face of her loss, is likened to "a tap." Taken together, the fictions explored in the preceding sections register concerns with the changes associated with modern society. Margaret Laurence expresses similar concerns in *The Stone Angel* (1964) but, as I argue in the next section, her novel promotes a return to elegiac consolation to mitigate the negative influence of modernity.

SECTION V: *THE STONE ANGEL*:
FROM GOTHIC RAGE TO ELEGIAC ACCEPTANCE

Laurence's novel *The Stone Angel*, related from the point of view of
the novel's ninety-two-year-old protagonist and "holy terror" (304)
Hagar Shipley, is perhaps Canada's most well-known portrayal of
age-related dementia.[25] Laurence's novel stands out for its unflinch-
ing account of the perils of aging and mental decline in a society
that views both as shameful instances of failure. The novel opens
with an epigraph from Dylan Thomas's famous elegy to his dying
father: "Do not go gentle into that good night. / Rage, rage against
the dying of the light." Although readers may be tempted to take
these words at face value and assume that, in keeping with Hagar's
stubborn nature, the novel counsels battling to the end against sickness and death – the abject waste that attends aging and old age – I
argue virtually the opposite. The epigraph represents Hagar's point
of departure, the first step on a long and complex existential journey
that begins with her terrified and enraged struggle against human
frailty, femininity, and mortality and ends with her elegiac acceptance of loss and death and, equally important, an understanding of
the rituals that assist in the process of mourning. Viewed in terms of
the theory of waste and repair, *The Stone Angel* extends and complicates Lewes's initial conception of the two opposing forces. On
the one hand, Hagar's body succumbs to the force of waste. On the
other hand, her mind is healed by the reparative forces of storytelling,
imagination, and fantasy,

The novel spans several weeks, during which Hagar, who is ter-
minally ill, runs away from her son Marvin and daughter-in-law
Doris. Marvin and Doris, who are in their sixties, are overburdened
and mentally and physically exhausted from caring for Hagar, who
is frail, ungrateful, and defiant. The novel oscillates between past and
present because Hagar's physical quest to find a space of safety and
autonomy is mirrored by a psychic quest, in which she reviews memories. The reader learns of her childhood, marked by the death of her
mother and the pride of her father, a self-made man who identifies
with the Currie clan; her marriage against her father's will to the
lower-class Bram Shipley; and the birth of her two sons, Marvin and
her favourite, John. Crucial memories are awakened when Hagar
runs away. While sifting through her memories, Hagar ultimately recognizes how her pride and defiance instigated many of the profound

losses she experienced in her life – the end of her marriage to Bram and, later, the death of her younger son, John. In keeping with her biblical namesake[26] Hagar flees into the wilderness, but the flight is brief. She is quickly discovered by Marvin and taken to hospital. The novel ends with Hagar's death in the institution.

As a devout Christian who lost her own mother when she was four years old and her father five years later, Laurence offers her heroine Hagar the chance, late in life, to experience a moment of communion and epiphanic insight that releases her from a protracted war against loss and death. Hagar's epiphany takes place toward the novel's conclusion. Fleeing the nursing home, Hagar has a chance encounter with a stranger, Murray F. Lees. After drinking to excess, both Hagar and Murray lose their inhibitions; for the first time Hagar admits her guilt and grief concerning the loss of her son John. Commiserating with Lees about the tragic deaths of their sons affords Hagar an opportunity to commune with a fellow human being on the basis of their mutual vulnerability and loss, rather than on the basis of an illusion of invulnerability and strength. By staging a secular version of communion and by relying on other biblical and elegiac intertexts, Laurence's novel reinscribes traces of religious discourses that, as noted earlier, were integral to an elegiac approach to death that was increasingly being abandoned in the modern era. Thanks to this moment of insight, Hagar is able to distance herself somewhat from her culture's relentless pathologization of the female body and its misogynist conflation of femininity with mental and physical weakness, ranging from hysterical displays of emotion to bodily illness and mental degeneration.[27]

In keeping with the anxieties about the spiritually destructive facets of modernity noted in the previous stories, *The Stone Angel* contrasts the empty accumulation of material capital with the unproductive yet healing elegiac ritual of recollecting and narrating stories about the dead for the consolation of the living. Hagar's father, Jason Currie, epitomizes the former, buying the most expensive marble funeral monument for his wife, building and furnishing the new church with pews that bear his name, and boasting that as a self-made man, he was a more successful businessman than his own father (15). By the end of the novel, however, Hagar finally manages to distance herself from her father's proud, solitary, and taciturn ways.

Like Munro's quasi-biographical story "The Peace of Utrecht," *The Stone Angel* traces the various tactics people use to defend against loss. Indeed as Christian Riegel observes, all five texts in Laurence's Manawaka cycle underscore "the pain of loss and the struggle to come to grips with it"; they also function "as a significant commentary on the relation of the individual in the western world to the discourses of death and mourning in the mid- to late twentieth century" (6). As noted above, Leacock's narrator mocked aged and demented characters such as Dean Drone. He also blamed modernity for fracturing and corrupting identity, and urged a return to more traditional, pastoral, and religious values – a return predicated on *remembering* one's humble roots. Although Laurence's narrative supports a similar religious vision that entails a doubling back to prior religious and elegiac narrative forms, in *The Stone Angel* consolation and redress – reparative forces – are not solely predicated on the process of remembering one's roots. They are equally dependent on forms of fabrication and imaginative play, ranging from role-playing to fiction-making.

From the start, Hagar, whose traumatic birth comes at the cost of her mother's life, learns to define herself against her greatest fear of feminine frailty and mortality.[28] Echoing her father's longing for immortality, Hagar experiences terror in the face of the glaring evidence of human mortality. Her terror is forcibly conveyed when, as a young girl, her brother Dan lies dying of pneumonia. In his delirium, Dan calls out for their dead mother. Desperate to console his sibling, Hagar's brother Matt begs her to impersonate their mother by putting on the latter's "old plaid shawl" and holding Dan in her arms (25).[29] Despite her desire to do what Matt asks, Hagar's fear of identifying with frailty and death, which she associates with femininity, makes her balk and leaves her petrified. As she explains, "all I could think of was that meek woman I'd never seen, the woman Dan was said to resemble so much and from whom he'd inherited a frailty I could not help but detest, however much a part of me wanted to sympathize" (25). Due to the longstanding associations among femininity, frailty, and death, supported by religious as well as biomedical discourses, Hagar finds herself unable to "play at being her mother" (25). "Crying, shaken by torments he [Matt] never even suspected," Hagar is emotionally petrified ("petra" meaning "rock" or "stone" in Latin). Although Hagar proclaims that on the night her son John died she was "transformed to stone and never wept at all" (243), readers thus recognize that she mirrored the stone angel at a much earlier age.[30] Although Hagar's Gothic view of death is instigated by her personal trauma, it is entirely in keeping with the more pervasive fear of old age and mortality propagated at the dawn of the twentieth century by individuals such as Leo Nascher. For Hagar, as for Nascher, death remains an obscene, evil facet of life.

The dreadful aspect of death is reinforced in *The Stone Angel* when Hagar recalls how, as children, she and her friend Lottie explored the town dump. On one of their expeditions, they stumbled across a scene whose grotesque conflation of birth and death recalls Hagar's own traumatic beginnings: "Then we saw a huge and staggering heap of eggs, jarred and broken by some wagoner and cast here, unsaleable ... We saw, with a kind of horror that could not be avoided ... that some of the eggs ... had hatched in the sun. The chicks, feeble, foodless, bloodied and mutilated, prisoned by the weight of the broken shells all round them, were trying to crawl like little worms, their half-mouths opened uselessly among the garbage. I could only gawk and retch" (27) Although Hagar remains characteristically paralyzed at the dump, her friend, Lottie – who, as a "bastard" child, throughout her life has been aligned with the abject – offers the chicks a merciful death. As Hagar recollects, at the time "it stung me worse, I think, that I could not bring myself to kill those creatures than that I could not bring myself to comfort Dan" (28). Due to her feelings of disgust when faced with frailty and death, Hagar believes that Lottie killed the chicks not solely out of pity, but also because they "were an affront to the eyes" (28). At this point in her life Hagar has yet to learn that death is neither solely a traumatic event nor a punishment for the wicked, but instead can constitute a merciful part of the life course – rather than a Gothic reversal of the birth process.[31]

Throughout the novel, Hagar experiences a series of mounting losses that include the deaths of her husband, Bram, and that of her cherished son, John. Clinging to her rage, she never once allows herself to grieve or mourn. In her last years, however, Hagar suffers from dementia, and thoughts of the dead return unbidden. Initially, Hagar represses her grief, which she finds shameful.[32] She maintains her stubborn dissociation from her own body, her emotions, and her inevitable physical and mental decline, until she encounters Murray F. Lees at Shadow Point. The reference to shadows links Hagar's journey to both the biblical story and to Walt Whitman's elegist, who likewise "fled forth to the hiding receiving night that talks not / Down to the shores of the water, the path by the swamp in the dimness / To the solemn shadowy cedars and ghostly pines so still" (ll. 123–5). Hagar describes her refuge in similar terms: "I'm standing among trees that extend all the way down the steep slopes to the sea. How quiet the forest is, only its own voices, no human noises at all" (150). In light of the explicit critiques of institutionalized care for the dependent aged mobilized by disparate individuals ranging from asylum superintendents to writers such as Munro and Richler, it is also significant that Hagar's flight is instigated by the threat of being incarcerated in a nursing home. Recalling Leacock's reference to the "Mausoleum Club," Hagar also likens the home, Silverthreads, to a "mausoleum" in which she will be "embalmed alive" (96). During the tour, Hagar pretends that she is deaf and blind, but nevertheless, in "this pyramid," she spies "several small, ancient women, white-topped and frail as dandelions gone to seed" (97). Desperate to avoid being uprooted and deprived of her home, like her biblical namesake, Hagar escapes the nursing home where her son Marvin and his wife, Doris, have taken her for a tour before committing her. Slowly and painfully, Hagar makes her way to an abandoned cannery by the sea where she encounters Lees, an alcoholic drifter who catalyzes her understanding of elegy and its power to console individuals in the face of loss and death.

Hagar and Lees's meeting is replete with Christian symbolism, including references to fish (an allusion to Christ) and the consumption of bread and wine (the elements of the Christian communion), and it is also studded with quotations from the Bible. In keeping with the scene's allusions to Christianity, readers also learn that Lees's grandfather was a Redeemer's Advocate, a circuit rider who travelled from town to town "preaching the Word." As Lees tells Hagar, when he grew up he too joined the Advocates, and met his wife at a Bible Camp, although he has since abandoned his faith and become a secular "life assurance" man (225–7). Taken together, the religious symbolism and biblical language set the stage for Hagar's first experience of spiritual consolation, and underscore the novel's movement away from a Gothic refusal of death and a return to prior, elegiac forms of communion and consolation. Significantly, this experience is predicated on Hagar first listening to Lees tell her a story about the tragic death of his infant son. Hearing Lees's story prompts Hagar to tell him of her own misfortune, suggesting that elegiac consolation is dependent on the hearing and telling of stories.[33]

Murray explains that while he and his wife attended a sermon about the coming of the world's end, their two-year-old son Donnie was left unattended and perished in a house fire.[34] After hearing about the tragedy, she confesses, "I can think of only one thing to say with any meaning. 'I had a son,' I say, 'and lost him'" (234). Although it is extremely curt, her acknowledgement of loss paves the way for her communion with Lees, and the release of her pent up rage and grief. "'Well,' he says, 'then you know'" (234). Before he hears Hagar's confession, however, Lees vents his need to allocate blame. As he tells Hagar, "I can't figure out whose fault it could have been" (234). After Lees lists all of the possible suspects, Hagar, in her characteristically impatient and blunt fashion, informs him that "no one's to blame" (234). In saying this, she affirms what, as noted earlier, becomes apparent at the end of Munro's "The Peace of Utrecht," namely that seeking the agent of evil is often a futile endeavour in the face of irrevocable loss. Whereas Munro's fiction leaves readers at an impasse, in *The Stone Angel* this recognition marks a crucial step in Hagar's shift from Gothic rage to elegiac and religious acceptance. In this way, Laurence's novel suggests that although the Gothic may be the appropriate genre when there is, indeed, a crime and someone is clearly to blame (in the case of abuse, neglect, or misdiagnosis), in cases when human agency is absent and individuals are helpless, then the elegy may be the more appropriate and, equally important, consoling and reparative genre.

At bottom, the cannery scene offers a restaging of Hagar's earlier, missed opportunity to play a supportive role for her brother Dan and for her husband, Bram. As an older woman suffering from dementia, Hagar now occupies the position of her dying brother Dan and her dying husband. She is now the one who is delirious and in need of someone to play the role of her lost beloved.[35] Hiding at the abandoned cannery with Lees, Hagar is shocked to discover that she has spoken her troubles aloud and she finds herself crying. She is equally startled when a voice speaks beside her: "Gee, that's too bad." As Hagar says, "I can't think who it is, and then I recall – a man was here, and we talked, and I drank his wine. But I didn't mean to tell him this" (245). For the first time, Hagar discovers that she is neither ashamed for speaking aloud nor for crying, which strikes her (and readers) as "remarkable" (245). Despite having uttered her confession, Hagar, like Lees, remains enraged. As she tells him, "It angers me, and will until I die. Not at anyone, just that it happened that way" (245). Yet rather than leaving Hagar in a state of helpless rage, *The Stone Angel* emphasizes the imagination's capacity to mitigate the pain instigated by the way things happen. The subsequent conversation between Hagar and Lees, which enables Hagar to release her

rage, suggests that elegiac play and role-playing are integral to healing and consolation. Although limited and overtly fictive, elegy may
be more effective in promoting healing than Gothic objectification
and dissociation.

In her delirium, Hagar confuses Lees with her deceased son John.
Initially, Lees is unnerved at being uncannily misidentified in this
way. "Heavenly days," he exclaims, Who do you think – ?" (247).
Despite his trepidation, he does not prevent Hagar from seizing the
opportunity to change the past, if only in fantasy. In her colloquy
with John/Lees, Hagar utters the words that she wishes she had
spoken. Her words express her love and desire to accommodate both
John and Arlene. Spoken in the context of her fantasy, they cancel
the harsh lecture that she did in fact utter, and which irrevocably
alienated her from John. To Hagar's relief, when her "son" speaks (in
the end, Lees gracefully acquiesces to play John's part and acts as a
surrogate son), "his voice is not angry at all" (247). In taking the part
of Hagar's dead son, Lees does what the younger Hagar could never
do; he identifies with the abject/other to offer consolation to the
living. "'It's ok,' he [John/Lees] says. 'I knew all the time you never
meant it. Everything is all right. You try to sleep. Every thing's quite
okay'" (248). Taken together, the early scene depicting Dan's death,
which foregrounds Hagar's inability to play the part of her mother,
and the later scene at the cannery, where Hagar finds herself in Dan's
situation, highlight the power of elegy and elegiac consolation and,
equally important, elegy's reliance on play and performance to console the living.

In *The Stone Angel* elegy is unequivocally, and some might argue
ruthlessly, oriented toward the living; John's experience and the real-
ities of his death are eclipsed by Hagar's need for imaginative consolation. In keeping with Zeiger's reservations concerning masculine elegy
outlined in the introductory chapter, Hagar's elegy rests on a dubious
and protracted process of substitution: John is, in fact, replaced twice
because in the scene noted above, John is replaced by Lees, but is also
ultimately replaced by his older brother, Marvin. On her deathbed,
Hagar consciously lies to her firstborn, telling him that he was "a better son than John" (304).

Unlike poets such as Matthew Arnold and Thomas Hardy, whose
works register a far more skeptical attitude toward the consolatory
powers of elegy, Laurence does not challenge the compensatory nature
of the traditional elegy, "aligning herself instead with the Miltonic

tradition of the genre" (Riegel 145). Viewed in the light of the tension between the Gothic and the elegy, Laurence's novel offers a model for a secular elegy that remains independent of biomedicine's promise of defying death. Laurence's model of secular elegy provides fictions that enable individuals in need of consolation to move beyond rage and futile attempts at allocating blame. Equally important, *The Stone Angel* suggests that individuals who have experienced the aesthetic rituals associated with elegy can offer consolation to others.

Having experienced role-playing with Murray Lees, Hagar finds herself able to similarly construct a consoling fiction for her son Marvin. Despite the latter's tireless efforts to care for Hagar, in his mother's eyes Marvin has always paled in comparison to his idealized dead brother John. When Hagar lies dying in her hospital bed, Marvin desperately seizes her hand, and Hagar realizes that Marvin, like the biblical Jacob, is wrestling with an angel and that she can only "release herself by releasing him" (304). Rather than remain a petrified, unreachable ideal, as she did earlier in life, Hagar acquiesces to playing, and she fabricates a consoling fiction. Although she tells Marvin a falsehood, she admits to herself that "it doesn't occur to him that a person in my place would ever lie" (304). Rather than cling to an impossible ideal of perfection – a reified stone angel that renders all human beings imperfect and abject – Hagar consoles her earthly son Marvin (and, in the process, herself) with the knowledge that he was good or, at the very least, good enough. Some readers may understandably be uneasy with the novel's traditional elegiac resolution – in essence, a retreat into fantasy and untruth – deeming it an unsatisfactory solution to the problem posed by the Gothic and, more precisely, by biomedicine's denial of death and assertions of omnipotence. Yet for Laurence, who returned to the subject of death and loss in all five of her Manawaka fictions,[36] a retreat into the imagination may have been a powerful form of consolation and redress.

To summarize, the literary works I have considered in this chapter underscore the legacy of the Victorian theory of waste and repair. In keeping with Lewes's initial, bodily formulation of the theory, Munro's and Richler's fiction emphasize the relationship between caregiving and physical health. In keeping with the description in *The Christian Guardian* of the minister William Mitford's happy death cited in the opening of section one, Laurence's portrayal of Hagar likewise holds out the possibility of prising apart the effects of repair on the body and the mind. Equally critical, the fictions under consideration emphasize the importance of moving beyond the Gothic paradigm, with its emphasis on blame and abjection. In Laurence's novel it is elegy, rather than the Gothic, that has the power to transform loss into something bearable for the survivors. In some texts, the carers for dementia patients are portrayed as survivors, while in Laurence's text it is the protagonist whose perception of survivorship changes due to her own experience of dementia. Hagar is transformed from a rigid, prideful survivor of trauma into a woman capable of engaging in creative and performative rituals of consolation.

Whereas at the end of the nineteenth century biomedicine increasingly consolidated a pessimistic view that linked aging, old age, and disease, the media at that time offered more diverse views of dementia that ranged from positive to deeply negative and satirical portrayals of old age. Of the four newspapers I surveyed, the *Globe* most emphatically and regularly embraced the negative, entropic view of aging. In keeping with the latter view, authors such as Stephen Leacock likewise saw fit to ridicule elderly individuals and to align aging with dementia. By mid-century, however, Canadian writers such as Richler, Munro, and Laurence portrayed the plight of individuals and families dealing with dementia in more compassionate and elegiac terms. Equally important, works by Munro, Richler, and Laurence demonstrate that the difficulties associated with coping with dementia and the tendency for the force of waste to overtake that of repair are not solely due to the ravages of the dementing illnesses themselves. Instead, an additional and perhaps even heavier burden springs from the prevailing shame and stigma – the legacy of earlier Victorian attitudes toward aging, class, and mental illness – combined with the lack of support provided by the government to caregivers, often middle-aged children, expected to cope on their own with the arduous task of caring for an elderly parent suffering from dementia.

In keeping with my book's oscillation between biomedical and imaginative models of dementia in Canadian culture, in the next chapter I explore how from the 1930s to the 1950s researchers and clinicians increasingly adopted the view that stress was the primary instigator of age-related dementia. During this period, largely thanks to the writings of Hungarian-born endocrinologist Hans Selye at the University of Montreal, stress-related theories of illness and disease profoundly altered medical views concerning the etiology and treatment of age-related dementia and Alzheimer's disease.

4

From Psychological and Stress-Based Theories of Dementia to the Triumph of the Biomedical Paradigm

As we saw in the previous chapters, in contrast to religious and bio-medical models that accepted "dotage" as part of God's plan and normal aging, a subset of biomedical approaches to dementia increasingly began to view the body as subject to the force of entropy and as responsible for instigating illness and suffering, owing to hardening arteries and softening brains. During this period, some scientists also promoted psychosocial explanations for dementia, tracing its etiology to "shattered nerves." Whereas the media articulated the range of theories circulating at the time, literary representations tended to emphasize the broader sociological and historical context, highlighting the corrosive influence of modernity, which put a particularly heavy burden on female caregivers. These nineteenth- and early twentieth-century views, which associated dementia with a wide range of causes, dramatically contrast with our current Gothic view of dementia, and Alzheimer's disease in particular, as the predominant "brain killer" (Khatchaturian 20).

At the first G8 Dementia Summit, at Lancaster House in central London, 11 December 2013, cognitive decline was portrayed in unequivocally catastrophic terms: "The world needs to fight the spread of dementia in the same way it mobilized against AIDS, a British government minister told a special summit on the disease on Wednesday, saying failure to tackle it would wreck state health budgets. Global cases of dementia are expected to triple by 2050, yet scientists are still struggling to understand the basic biology of the memory-robbing brain condition, and the medicine cupboard is bare" ("G8 Leaders").

At the summit, David Cameron, prime minister of the UK, made the following call to arms: "In generations past, the world came together to take on the great killers. We stood against malaria, cancer, HIV and AIDS and we are just as resolute today" (Hughes). Journalists covering the G8 Summit also observed that despite repeated failures to produce a pharmaceutical cure, drug companies are "still trying to crack the problem, since the potential prize would be sales running into many billions of dollars a year" (Hughes).

In this chapter, in an effort to understand how the Gothic model has come to dominate discussions of dementia, I explore how the tensions between biological and psychological approaches manifested themselves in geriatric psychiatry and shaped attitudes toward late-onset dementia in Canada from the 1930s to the 1960s. Whereas the previous chapter focused on the legacy of the Victorian theory of waste, this chapter pays particular attention to theories that link cognitive impairment to stress. In the late 1930s a highly influential model of stress was disseminated by the Hungarian-born Canadian physician and scientist Hans Selye (1907–1982), who became known as the "Father" of the field of stress research.[1] In essence, this chapter poses three basic questions: what led scientists and researchers from the 1930s to the 1950s to embrace and subsequently abandon the view that senile dementia was an illness with psychosocial origins? Second, why, beginning in the late 1950s, did scientists revise Kraepelin's view of Alzheimer's disease – a rare form of dementia that strikes relatively younger people – and construct the current model, which views presenile and late-onset dementia as one and the same disease? Finally, how did the increasing popularity of the biological approach to mental illness, in conjunction with the deinstitutionalization movement in the 1960s, affect people suffering from dementia and their caregivers?

Section one briefly explores the early nineteenth-century foundations for the debates between the biological and psychological approaches. Section two turns to the views of age-related dementia that prevailed from the 1930s to the 1950s. During this period, the psychological approach – influenced by the prevailing research on stress – profoundly influenced clinicians and researchers studying aging and old age. The "sociopsychiatric" approach, as it was termed, found one of its greatest champions in David Rothschild, a Canadian-American researcher, trained in pathology and psychoanalysis in Germany. Section three examines two British studies conducted in the 1950s – by neuropathologist J.A.N. Corsellis and psychiatrist Martin Roth, respectively – that profoundly re-oriented medical research on Alzheimer's toward our contemporary somatic approach. Section four focuses on the increasing popularity of the biological approach to geriatric psychiatry in Canada in the 1950s, which tempered Rothschild's emphasis on psychological factors and ultimately led to the collapse of Kraepelin's initial distinction between Alzheimer's and senile dementia. This approach traces its roots to the pioneering research of Dr Vojtech Adalbert Kral in Montreal in the post-Second World War era.[2]

In view of my overarching focus on the relationship between late-onset dementia and literary modes – specifically the elegy and the Gothic – as a response to loss, it is significant that both Rothschild and Kral concur that the origins of dementia can be traced directly to how an individual copes with loss and the suffering that attends it. Not surprisingly, both insist that what might best be described as a masculine elegiac acceptance of death is associated with cognitive health. By contrast, they maintain that individuals who lack the ability to respond to stress and suffering with detachment – people who, they argue, are emotionally labile, dependent, and melancholic – succumb to dementia in greater numbers.[3] In her book on AIDS, Sontag comments on this type of perspective on disease, what she terms a "characterological predisposition" (12) to illness. As she explains, "cancer is regarded as a disease to which the psychically defeated, the inexpressive, the repressed – especially those who have repressed anger or sexual feelings – are particularly prone" (12). She traces the emphasis on character in medical diagnoses such as tuberculosis and cancer (and I would add, late-onset dementia and Alzheimer's) to the shift from prior beliefs about an "exterior, contaminated environment to interior psychological contaminated ambiance that produced a disposition to mental illness" (43).

In promoting their characterological view of dementia, Rothschild and Kral reveal a debt to the nineteenth-century pathologizing of women's minds and bodies, as well as the hysteria diagnosis. In keeping with my emphasis on exploring and, where appropriate, calling into question the Gothic process of substituting the artifact for the individual, section five turns from Rothschild's and Kral's theories to actual accounts of clinical experience in Canadian mental asylums, which shed light on the day-to-day life of individuals with dementia in the 1950s. This section also outlines the results of the Canadian government's policies concerning mental illness, which laid the foundation for the deinstitutionalization movement.

SECTION I: THE EARLY DEBATES BETWEEN
SOMATIKERS AND *PSYCHIKERS*

In exploring the tensions between biological, psychological, and imaginative approaches to narrating aging, old age, and dementia in mid-twentieth-century Canadian society, it is helpful to appreciate that from Hippocratic times to the present, the pattern of thinking in Western medicine has been predominantly somatic or biological-reductionist. According to the biological narrative, illness and disease – or bodily suffering – are rooted in our material essence; in the case of late-onset dementia, the problem lies in our brains. When confronting bodily and mental illnesses, "physicians have regularly appealed to materialist and reductionist explanations in accounting for the clinical observations" (Brown 438). As we saw in the previous chapter, however, the materialist approach has always been shadowed by and, at times, intertwined with an alternative view that also runs through the history of Western medical thought. The latter traces the origins of illness not solely to somatic but also to "mental, non-material, psychological and socio-environmental factors" (ibid.). The latter factors are forcibly emphasized in much Canadian fiction, which draws attention to both the repercussion of words and ideas and the corrosive facets of modernization.

As I explained in chapter one, during the nineteenth and early twentieth centuries the predominantly psychological approach to treatment known as "moral therapy" held sway in Upper Canadian asylums. For the first time, Pinel directed attention "to the patient's 'story,' hoping to derive from it clues to precipitating emotional circumstances as well as ideas for possible behavioural interventions" (ibid. 442). Laying the foundation for Freud's "talking cure," Pinel rejected the somatic approach to mental illness because, as he explained, there was no solid empirical correlation between brain lesions and mental illness. "It is a general and very natural opinion," Pinel wrote in his *Treatise on Insanity* (1802), "that the derangement of the function of the understanding consists in a change or lesion of some part of the head ... But numerous results of dissection ... have shewn no organic lesion of the head" (in ibid.). Variations on Pinel's objections were repeated by psychologically oriented psychiatrists throughout the late nineteenth and early twentieth centuries. In essence, Pinel and his followers refused to substitute the artifact – or brain – for the person. In its current form, somatic or biological psychiatry "stresses the neurosciences, with their interest in brain chemistry, brain anatomy, and medication, seeing the origin of psychic distress in the biology of the cerebral cortex" (Shorter, *History* 26). By contrast, psychodynamic psychiatry "stresses the psychosocial side of patients' lives, attributing their symptoms to social problems or past personal stresses to which people may adjust imperfectly" (ibid.; see also Vidal 16).

Before turning to the debates concerning dementia in North America in the mid-twentieth century, it is helpful to briefly elucidate how the tensions between the biological and psychological approaches to mental illness were expressed in Europe in the previous century. In the early nineteenth century in Germany, for example, members of the mentalist or psychological school influenced by Pinel were labelled Psychikers and their opponents went by the name of Somatikers (Brown 443). In the 1820s and 1830s, Somatikers temporarily dominated the Psychikers. The line between the two camps was starkly drawn by one of the leaders of the Somatikers, Maximilian Jacobi (1775–1858), who insisted in 1830 that "there is no disease of the mind existing as such, but ... insanity exists solely as the consequence of disease ... in some part of the bodily system" (in ibid.). The struggle between the Somatikers and Psychikers persisted, and although attempts were made in the mid-century to reconcile the two sides, by the late nineteenth century the Somatikers had won the field. Organic neuropsychiatry, hereditarian theory, and the "brain pathology" of Theodor Meynert (1833–1892) represented the primary forms of "the new somaticism" (Brown 444).[4] By the turn of the twentieth century, thanks to the efforts of more psychologically inclined clinicians such as Richard Krafft-Ebing, Emil Kraepelin, and Adolf Meyer, the tide was again turning away from rigid forms of "brain mythology" (see ibid. 445). Although never entirely rejecting the somatic approach, these clinicians tempered the over-emphasis on brain pathology with attention to the bedside and to "the natural histories or life-courses of mental disorders" (ibid.).

By far the most successful attack on the "brain mythology" was launched by Freud who, like Pinel, focused on the patient's story. In the early decades of the twentieth century, psychiatrists in Europe and America readily adopted Freudian notions of repression, ambivalence, and unconscious wishes. Freud's psychoanalytic approach was introduced in Canada as early as 1908 by Freud's trusted friend and disciple, Ernest Jones. Before leaving Toronto in 1912, Jones served as an associate professor at the University of Toronto and was given responsibility for the neurology ward at Toronto General Hospital (Maddox 95–6). In the decade before the First World War, the new doctrines of psychoanalysis and psychotherapy spread rapidly among internists and family physicians in North America. In 1913, Charles Dana, professor of neurology at Cornell, wrote that "neurology has passed from the microscope and the autopsy suite to the study of psychoneuroses" (in Shorter, *History* 144). A neurologist now had to contend with "subjective states and the importance to all neuroses of environment, education, the character, temperament and social conditions of his patients" (144). Due to the reality of shell shock and the evidence of psychic trauma occasioned by two world wars, between 1930 and 1950 American psychiatrists increasingly embraced psychoanalytic theory.

SECTION II: DAVID ROTHSCHILD – A TWENTIETH-CENTURY, NORTH AMERICAN PSYCHIKER

In Canada, as we have seen, in the late nineteenth and early twentieth centuries the biological approach blamed the problem of later-life dementia on primarily somatic factors such as "hardening arteries" and "softening brains." However, proponents of this approach also recognized the psychological factor of "shattered nerves." With respect to the latter, as noted earlier, during the Great War, when "thousands of WWI shell shock casualties demonstrated dramatically that everyone is vulnerable to psychological, social, and physical stress," doctors also recognized the value and effectiveness of the psychological approach to mental illness (Tyhurst et al. 2). The psychological view was forcibly promoted during the 1930s and 1940s by psychiatrist David Rothschild, who investigated the relationship between Alzheimer's disease and senile dementia. Rothschild followed in Pinel's footsteps by rejecting purely somatic origins for what he termed the "psychoses customarily associated with aging – the involutional psychoses,[5] psychoses with cerebral arteriosclerosis, and the senile psychoses" (Rothschild and Sands 233). "Too exclusive a preoccupation with cerebral pathology," Rothschild argued, "led to a tendency to forget that the changes are occurring in living, mentally functioning persons who may react to a given situation, including an organic one, in various ways" (ibid. 49).

In support of his mentalist position, Rothschild, like Pinel, cited the contradictory findings shown repeatedly since Alzheimer's time – namely, the fact "that the presence and degree of dementia in a living patient often shows discrepancies with the presence and degree of pathological structures at autopsy" (Lock 60). In an attempt to account for the evidence of plaques and tangles in the brains of some cognitively normal elderly, Rothschild ultimately ascribed "part of the development of dementia in the elderly to psychological causes" (Katzman and Bick 6). Rothschild published nearly thirty papers on the psychiatric problems of aging, and championed a psychological approach to age-related dementia, first as research director of the Foxborough Hospital from 1927 to 1941 and then as clinical director at the Worcester Hospital from 1946 to 1956 (see Ballenger, *Self* 48). In addition to rejecting the somatic approach, Rothschild upheld Kraepelin's view that Alzheimer's disease was restricted to a rare, presenile form of dementia.[6]

At bottom, Rothschild's key contribution to debates about senile dementia lay in his emphasis on the debilitating influence of "stress," which highlights the role played by Hans Selye's theories.[7] "An individual's ability to withstand organic damage," Rothschild argued, "was decreased both by personality defects and by stress and life crises" (Rothschild and Sharp 53). His 1952 study, "Sociopsychiatric Foundations for a Theory of the Reactions to Aging," for instance, probes the origins of what he and his co-author Dr Sidney Sands term the "psychoses customarily associated with aging" (233). According to Rothschild and Sands, involutional psychoses typically occur between fifty to sixty years of age; psychoses with cerebral arteriosclerosis, between sixty to seventy; and senile psychoses, between seventy to eighty-nine (235).

In the introduction to their study, Rothschild and Sands posit that old age brings with it a fundamental set of stressors, which include the inevitable anxiety associated with the realization that the proverbial sands of time are running out. "Even those who successfully avoid speculation about the 'future beyond,'" they insist, "must contend with changes in themselves and in their roles" (234). As they explain, elderly individuals "suffer personal losses through the death of relatives and friends, there is a decrease in occupational activity and skill, their recreational pursuits are less lusty and far-ranging, their sexual powers and desires decline, and there is an increasing isolation from the main currents of life" (234). When these stresses are compounded by "organic damage to the central nervous system," they warn, "the organism suffers severe handicaps" (234).

Although their language, particularly terms such as "organism," gestures to biology, Rothschild and Sands ultimately located the etiology of age-related "psychoses" in psychology and, more precisely, in the individual's personality, which shapes his or her ability to cope with a variety of losses. After comparing the three groups with the control group of non-psychotic individuals comprised of fifteen men ranging in age from seventy-five to eighty at the Worcester State Hospital, the authors concluded that each group had a distinct psychological profile, which, they suggested, was causally related to their dementing illness. They divided their research subjects as follows: "the involutional psychoses" (group I), "psychoses with cerebral arteriosclerosis" (group II), "the senile psychoses" (group III), and the set of "nonpsychotic old men" – the control – (group IV).

With respect to group I, "the involutional psychoses" group, Rothschild and Sands explained that they were "almost uniformly vulnerable to evidence of personal decline in ability and status or to loss of outside support upon which they were dependent" (236). They argued further that members of group I showed "life-long evidence of egocentric object relationships and a rigid clinging to established habits of adjustment" (236). In keeping with Freud's emphasis on the sexual etiology of mental illness, Rothschild and Sands likewise asserted that "the involutional psychosis group" also "made a poor sexual and marital adjustment" (236). In comparison to group I, the personality profile of patients suffering from psychoses with cerebral arteriosclerosis – group II – was "not so clear-cut" (236). Despite group II's diversity, however, the authors found "a rather high incidence of lability in the emotional sphere and in the cardiovascular system" (236). According to Rothschild and Sands: "These people seem to have been more reactive to stress situations and not infrequently we found that the central psychologic [sic] problem appeared to be the attempt to deal with negative emotions, specifically, anger and hostility. They were much more prone to 'acting out' than our involutional group" (236–7). Nowadays, group II would be categorized as multi-infarct or stroke-induced dementia; yet Sands and Rothschild maintained that this group's illness was linked to their reactivity to stress and their tendency to manifest, rather than sublimate, negative emotions. Of all the groups, the "senile psychoses" (group III), proved to be the most diverse. Although in several cases "there was no evidence of any personality tendencies to distinguish them from their normal contemporaries," the authors nevertheless contended that they were "quite surprised to find that the premorbid personalities in this group were very similar to those of the involutional group" (237).

In other words, according to Rothschild an inability to adapt to stress due to character defects predisposes individuals to dementing illnesses in later life. As Sontag's comments cited earlier suggest, this approach is wrong since Alzheimer's is potentially exacerbated but not entirely caused by social factors. Worse, characterological approaches take on a troubling "blame the victim" approach that are repugnant. As noted above, Rothschilds and Sands suggest that senile psychoses can be traced to "the central psychologic [sic] problem – "the attempt to deal with negative emotions, specifically, anger and hostility." Their comments anticipate the erroneous notion that plagued Sontag while she struggled with cancer, specifically the view that breast cancer was due to repressed anger.

Viewed in this light, the doctors' findings concerning the non-psychotic control group are extremely revealing. As they explain, in addition to being less sensitive to disease and having escaped certain diseases that contribute to the morbidity and mortality rates of the general population, the control group was surprisingly even-tempered:

> Our subjects appear to have been much less dependent in their interpersonal relationships than even the so-called average. They had friends, held jobs, married, and raised children, but never seemed to become too deeply involved in these matters. They appear to have been more detached in facing emergencies and losses. With advancing years they look back on the past with good-humored indulgence and are able to accept their new limitations and dependence as a matter of course. It may well be that the possession of these special characteristics, rather than average characteristics, are what have permitted these men to reach advanced age with equanimity and relative freedom from disturbing symptoms related to deteriorative changes in the central nervous system. (235)

Ultimately, Rothschild and Sand's findings uphold their age's ideal of masculine independence and emotional detachment. They also invoke the flipside of the idealization of masculinity by implicitly locating the etiology of pathological memory loss in what society viewed as a more feminine tendency toward emotional volatility and dependence.[8]

From the 1930s to the 1950s, attitudes toward the aged and the frail elderly remained pessimistic and tinged with moral disapprobation. Whereas from the late nineteenth century on, "the dullness found in the senile, their isolation and withdrawal, their clinging to the past and lack of interest in worldly affairs were characteristically represented as the symptoms of senility – the social stigmata of the inevitable deterioration of the brain" – following the Second World War, gerontological discourse found a new target to blame, and "represented these as the *causes* of senility" (Ballenger, *Self* 58). As Ballenger explains: "The locus of senile mental deterioration was no longer the aging brain but a society that, through mandatory retirement, social isolation, and the disintegration of traditional family ties, stripped the elderly of the roles that had sustained meaning in their lives. When elderly people were deprived of these meaningful social roles, when they became increasingly isolated and were cut off from the interests and activities that had earlier occupied them, not surprisingly their mental functioning deteriorated. The elderly did not so much lose their minds as lose their place" (58). His comments recall Auguste D.'s repeated assertion, cited in chapter one, "I have lost myself." In the mid-twentieth century, clinicians were debating the reasons for this experience. In contrast to the purely biological, Gothic model, which focuses on the diseased brain, researchers cited prejudiced social attitudes and psychosocial factors as the primary instigator of dementia.

Media accounts published in Canada in the 1940s repeatedly suggest that senility, as it was known, can be avoided if people are given meaningful work and made to feel useful.[9] In an article entitled "The Question of Old Age," L.G. Stoner maintains that "the danger is of becoming static" (7 July 1944, 9) and he offers an anecdote to illustrate that people's failure to adapt rather than their chronological age contributes to cognitive decline:

One day to the writer's home came an intelligent gentleman soliciting subscriptions for a magazine. In the course of an interesting conversation he said he was 92 years of age – still useful while a woman contacted some years ago was worn and old mentally (not physically) at 42 years. Wherein was the difference, for both possessed intelligence? One was progressive the other out of touch with life and its possibilities. One danger lies in regarding the past and former conditions as desirable even for the present generation – which is unreasonable, for living facilities have changed through science, and life today cannot be carried on the same as of old. Let us aged people remember this and try to adapt ourselves to the changes effected. (9)

Variations of this anecdote are repeated in media accounts concerning aging and senility from the 1940s to the 1960s.[10] In an article published in 1962, for example, David Spurgeon cites Dr C. Keith Stuart, senior medical specialist of Ontario's Public Welfare Department, who argues that people's psychological and physical processes may well "shut down as a direct result of repeated rejection and thus end up in that state which is commonly known as senility" (17).[11]

As I argued in the previous chapters, and as evidenced by the media and by the fictive sketches of Stephen Leacock, at the turn of the nineteenth century, the senile man represented "the epitome of failure"; his decaying brain could not keep up with the demands or the pace of urban capitalism and "failed to produce anything of worth in a modern industrial society" (Ballenger, *Self* 58). By the mid-twentieth century the senile man was still considered a failure, yet it was no longer his aging brain that was the problem but rather his failure "to adjust to a consumer-oriented leisure society" (58).

In the 1950s a group of diverse academic, medical, social service, and business professionals – those who were of what Ballenger terms "the gerontological persuasion" (ibid. 56) – responded to what later came to be known as "ageism": "prejudice or discrimination on the grounds of a person's age; age discrimination, esp. against the elderly" (*OED*). They sought to improve the material circumstances attending old age through increasing public and private pensions, abolishing mandatory retirement, establishing a network of social and recreational services, and, perhaps most important, replacing the negative image of senility with positive images of successful aging (Ballenger, *Self* 59).[12] Although this shift from inevitable decline to "positive" aging might appear to be a beneficial development, it often came with its own implicit moral judgment – the legacy of Victorian moral dualism – that blamed senility on the elderly. As geriatrician Martin Gumpert, a champion of positive aging, wrote: "Old age and senility, nowadays almost identical, are no more necessarily related than infancy and rickets. With our aggregate of medical knowledge no child need suffer from rickets, and no elderly person need suffer from senility" (in Townsend, *Globe and Mail*, 23 Dec. 1944, 8). In Gumpert's writing, senility is aligned with disease; equally important, in his texts, the view that sickness in old age constitutes the result of individual neglect "rises at times to the level of a moral condemnation" (Ballenger, *Self* 68). At one point, Gumpert righteously insists: "People who suffer have to free themselves by their own power or they will never be free. Old people are neither morons nor infants ... Only the old man who grows to like being old, who knows no regret, who declines to make himself the object of endless self-pity, will succeed in being a 'modern' old man" (in ibid.).

Despite attempts to challenge ageism, the stigma associated with old age and, to an even greater extent, with senile dementia persisted. At the same time, however, research trends shifted dramatically. By the late 1960s both Rothschild's arguments concerning personality defects and Gumpert's individualistic, bootstrap philosophy seemed "archaic, at best, a throwback to the psychoanalytic hegemony that was fast receding" (Ballenger, *Self* 81). From the late 1950s onward, psychological explanations of dementia were increasingly countered by material evidence based on new technologies – most notably the electron microscope – by novel techniques developed in the neurosciences to analyze the brain, and by the belated recognition of the significance of earlier discoveries made in the 1920s. Important discoveries included the identification of senile plaque as composed of amyloid protein, the observation of plaques in the brains of young patients with Down syndrome who were dying, and, finally, the analysis of familial clusterings of Alzheimer's disease (ibid. 46). These findings, particularly the observation of the characteristic markers of Alzheimer's disease in young adults with Down syndrome, played a role both in the consolidation of the biological approach to dementia in 1950s and in the founding of the Alzheimer Society of Canada in 1978.

SECTION III: THE RISE OF THE SOMATIKERS IN THE 1950S – THE INFLUENCE OF CORSELLIS'S AND ROTH'S EMPIRICAL STUDIES ON ALZHEIMER'S DISEASE

The current Gothic narrative of dementia propagated by the media uses fearful, apocalyptic, and martial rhetoric and is grounded in developments in biomedicine that have made it increasingly possible to ignore the mind in favour of the brain – or, put somewhat differently, to substitute the artifact for the individual. As researcher and neuroscientist Michael Kidd recalls, in the late 1950s and even into the 1960s the sense of evil, dread, and helplessness associated with dementia was so prevalent that "if you raised the subject of senile dementia with doctors, not laymen, but doctors, they didn't want to know about it, they were so frightened of it, they would look the other way. They'd say, 'I don't want to discuss it. Look, we all grow old, we can't help it, it's a sheer, total, waste of time working on it'" (in Katzman and Bick 39). For the emerging group of biological psychiatrists in the 1950s whose goal lay in conquering this fear, the body constituted the battlefield: "brain pathology became the essential feature of senile dementia, the symbol of its grave reality and the object of cutting-edge biomedical research" (Ballenger, *Self* 81). Just as the development of silver-staining techniques, new dyes, and more precise microscope lenses enabled Alzheimer and his colleagues to view senile plaques and neurofibrillary tangles, the invention of the electron microscope by the Germans in the 1930s enabled bench scientists to view these same structures with even greater precision. Robert Terry, one of the first researchers to use automated counting methods to determine the degree of nerve cell loss in patients suffering from dementia of the Alzheimer's type, recalls his first experience working with the new electron microscope in the 1950s. "I had managed to get a Siemens electron microscope," Terry explains, "which was a great choice. It was a marvelous machine ... Everything worked. The pictures were good, and everything we saw had never been seen before. It was marvelous fun" (in Katman and Bick 23). For the first time, the cell's "ultrastructure" – the fine details within the cell, which can only be seen with the high magnification obtainable with an electron microscope – was revealed. "We had recognized the whole plaque," Terry explains, "all of the constituents that have subsequently come under extensive discussion ... And we reported all of these finding in our 1964 article" (ibid. 25–6). In Britain, the somatically oriented psychiatrists used the electron microscope to address what had consistently proven to be the Achilles heel of their argument that age-related dementia was a disease and not simply a facet of normal aging.

Two distinct research programs profoundly shifted the balance in favour of the disease model. The first study, undertaken by J.A.N. Corsellis – a neuropathologist at Runwell Hospital in Essex – and published in 1962, involved analyzing the clinical and pathological findings of 300 consecutive elderly patients who came to autopsy. Corsellis divided the population of his patients into two groups – those who suffered from organic mental disorders, characterized by the presence of physiological or anatomical changes to the nervous system, and those who suffered from functional disorders, characterized by the absence of any identifiable brain pathology. His study demonstrated that in the "overwhelming majority of cases, dementia was associated with pathological changes in the brain." Equally important, Corsellis's results demonstrated that although there was a clear tendency for cerebral degeneration of these various types to increase with age to an approximately equal degree in both categories, "the organic group showed a significantly higher degree – up to 80 percent – of all types of cerebral degeneration at every age" (see Weiner and Lipton 7). For Corsellis, the data offered evidence of a "well-ordered and demonstrable pattern for the common forms of cerebral degeneration"; in his view, the evidence effectively "demolished the psychodynamic model and restored pathology to its rightful place" (Ballenger, *Self* 85). This was a decisive moment in the consolidation of the prevailing Gothic model of dementia.

Like Corsellis, the authors of the second major study – led by British psychiatrist Martin Roth in the 1960s – viewed the psychological approach to age-related dementia with great skepticism and concern. In an interview Roth explained that the harmful influence of psychoanalysis "lay in its speculations and its emphasis upon the privacy of the analytic interview, which completely precluded any independent observation of what went on and the sacredness of the transference relationship, which destroyed any possible objectivity" (in Katzman and Bick 56). Like Emil Kraepelin who opposed Freud's views early on, Roth was deeply skeptical of the non-objective nature of psychoanalysis. Yet as I argued in chapter one, objectivity is an ideal that proves elusive even among well-intentioned scientists. More precisely, the fate of Auguste D. highlights the fact that supposedly objective methods contaminated the evidence. In confining and isolating Auguste D. in the asylum, Alzheimer and his colleagues unwittingly exacerbated Auguste's depression and anxiety. The structure of the "experiment" and its deleterious influence on her emotional and cognitive responses thus precluded any "objective" or purely scientific analysis of her organic brain disease.

To counter the claims of the Psychikers, Roth's group at Newcastle – which included the pathologist Bernard Tomlison and the psychiatrist Gary Blessed – had to overcome the research of influential pathologists who, in the past, had found what he termed "Alzheimer changes" in a "very high proportion of patients with perfectly normal personalities and intact minds" (ibid. 55). These findings, as Roth observed, "tended to wipe out interest in the Alzheimer lesions … they were unimportant, they were found in normals and Alzheimer's and in all sorts of states" (ibid.). In addition to lacking a unique and identifiable biomarker, Roth also had to counter the prevailing outlook that dementia was an inevitable part of the life course. As Roth lamented, at that time, people assumed "that everything in old age ultimately led to dementia" (ibid. 57).

Roth's Newcastle study proved to be "even more persuasive than that of Corsellis's because Roth's group followed patients in life and leading up to autopsy "rather than beginning with autopsy and retrospectively studying their clinical histories" (Ballenger, *Self* 84). In addition, Roth's Newcastle study used control patients "who were assessed as normal with psychological exams specifically designed to reveal dementia" (ibid.). Finally, and most important, the Newcastle researchers developed procedures for quantifying both their clinical and pathological descriptions: Blessed used standard psychological tests and a dementia scale he developed, and Tomlinson devised a standard method for counting plaques that could be verified objectively by others (ibid. 85). Although every pathological feature of the patients with dementia was found to a lesser degree in the patients without dementia, the study found a statistical difference between the two groups. In a series of influential articles appearing from 1966 to 1970, they argued that statistics proved that the amount of damage caused by the plaques in the brain corresponded to the severity of the behavioural changes – the clinical evidence of dementia – in their research subjects.

Although historians frequently cite the Newcastle study as the watershed moment for the Somatikers, at least one member of the Newcastle team cast doubt on their triumph. As David Kay explained in an interview, their approach to the problem largely determined their findings: "All of our efforts were put in to try to separate those [dementing] conditions from each other and from normal aging, whatever that is exactly. So, that was the whole thrust … rather than trying to show similarities between aging and various stages of dementia, we tried to demonstrate and concentrate on the differences between them. That was our philosophy, really" (in Katzman and Bick 248). Kay argues further that while dementia is clearly not inevitable, the question the Newcastle group attempted to determine, "whether it was clearly pathologically separate from old age," is "still unresolved" (ibid.). Simply put, researchers are still unsure whether Alzheimer's is a specific, discrete, *qualitative* disorder or a *quantitative* disorder, in which "an exaggeration and acceleration of the normal aging processes occur and dementia appears when neural reserves are exhausted and compensatory mechanisms fail" (Khatchaturian in Lock 54).

SECTION IV: BIOLOGICAL APPROACHES TO AGE-RELATED DEMENTIA IN CANADA — V.A. KRAL

Whereas the Newcastle group focused their efforts on demonstrating a statistically relevant correlation between brain pathology and clinical symptoms, in Canada, V.A. Kral's research addressed the related yet distinct problem of distinguishing between normal and pathological memory loss in the elderly. Kral trained in psychiatry and neurology in Europe. He and his wife, an ophthalmologist, were both concentration camp survivors. After the war, they worked briefly in Prague before immigrating to Canada in 1947. Initially Kral accepted a position at the Verdun Protestant Hospital in Montreal. Five years later he left, after receiving an invitation to work at the Allen Memorial Institute as director of their Gerontology Unit. During that period, he also served as a lecturer, then associate professor, at McGill University. Kral's contribution to geriatrics was formidable; he is credited with single-handedly founding psychogeriatrics in Canada (Merskey xv).

In the introduction to his 1959 paper, "Senescent Memory Decline and Senile Amnesic Syndrome," Kral poses three basic questions that clarify the fundamental and genuinely pressing problem that served as the focus of his research, and continues to haunt research on dementia and aging: "Does every aging individual suffer a memory deficit? Does it progress continuously and evenly as the years pass on? Is the memory loss quantitatively uniform in all aging individuals so affected or are there different types of memory dysfunction in senescence?" (32). Although Kral is lauded for initiating the renaissance of the biological approach in Canada, in fact his articles clearly reflect debts to both Roth, the Somatiker, and Rothschild, the Psychiker.

In his research on different types of memory disorders among aged individuals, Kral approvingly cites Roth's division of clinical subjects into five distinct groups according to their clinical symptomology, course, and outcome (34). Kral likewise divided his subjects into five groups: Group I, the control, was characterized by a "well preserved personality, appropriate emotional reactions, preserved judgment, preserved memory, no history or signs of functional psychosis"; Group II exhibited the same features but suffered from "mild" memory impairment, which showed itself in not "recalling, at times, names and data of the past which were available at other times" (34). Group II's memory loss, however, did not affect "remote" or "personal" memory and "confabulation" was entirely absent from their reminiscences (34). Group III had no memory defect, but suffered from "a definite history and/or signs of functional psychoses of either the affective or paraphrenic type" (34). Group IV showed "typical amnestic syndrome, namely: impairment of recent memory and immediate recall, disorientation, particularly in time, and loss of remote memory. Lastly, Group V was likewise characterized by an amnestic syndrome, but also showed additional psychotic signs, namely paranoid delusions, hallucinations, or depressive or manic mood swings" (34). In a series of papers that analyzed the findings drawn from these groups, Kral differentiates between "benign senescent forgetfulness" – as evidenced by Group II – and "malignant" forms of memory loss – as evidenced by groups IV and V. Whereas "mild" or "benign" dementia remains constant in character and is associated with the recall of non-personal data, the "malignant" type is progressive, affects both recent events and those of a personal quality, and, finally, is associated with a higher rate of mortality (48).

Strikingly, in later elaborations of his thesis, Kral explicitly drew on psychodynamic theories to argue that stress plays a key role in "disposing individuals to acute or chronic organic brain disease in old age" (79). Echoing the Psychiker Rothschild's description of stressors, Kral lists the following psychological catalysts:

The most important factors involved are the loss of prestige among family and friends, the loss of a life-long occupation, be it a job or housekeeping, decreased earning capacity and frequently a drastic loss of income. Isolation, loss of status and of course incidental degenerative diseases exert a chronic anxiety-producing stress in the aging individual and this leads to an increasing dependence on others at a time when the spouse or life-long friends have been lost. In addition, there is the anxiety of the younger generation regarding their own aging, which leads them to withdraw from the problems of the aged. This creates a vicious circle, whereby the anxiety of the aged becomes more intensified and its clinical expression in the neurotic symptomatology more severe and often incapacitating. (80)

Surprisingly, Canada's most esteemed somatically oriented dementia researcher was deeply concerned with psychological factors – a fact that has been forgotten. Moreover, in keeping with Rothschild, Kral posited a direct connection between how an individual copes with suffering and loss and the onset of dementia. Equally critical, both Rothschild and Kral were influenced by the prevailing theory of stress, championed by their Canadian colleague Hans Selye (at the University of Montreal). As I argued earlier, stress and anxiety remain the focus of Alzheimer's research (see Barton, "Anxiety May Speed Slide," *Globe and Mail*, 14 Nov. 2014, L7).

Kral's work also proved to be influential with respect to the contemporary constructions of Alzheimer's disease as a single disease category – a move that further consolidated Alzheimer's disease as a Gothic monster. In addition to linking benign and malignant forms of memory loss to stress, Kral viewed both forms of memory loss as being on a single continuum. Despite Kraepelin's initial decision to divide early and late-onset senility, and to give the former the status of a distinct disease process named after Alois Alzheimer, psychiatry had a tradition of "intellectual compactness, of lumping rather than splitting" (Shorter, *History* 303). The tendency toward lumping may have influenced Kral's position, cited below, on pathological memory loss:

One might speculate that the senile atrophic process, when it affects the brain only mildly … may be accompanied by the benign type of memory dysfunction. When, however, these structures are affected more severely, the malignant memory dysfunction may result. In favour of such a Unitarian pathogenic hypothesis would seem to be the fact that the neuropathological findings do not permit a strict differentiation between the brains of people who had died in possession of their mental capacities from those who had died from senile dementia. Cerebral atrophy, fibrillary degeneration and senile plaques are found in both groups, although they are somewhat more pronounced in the latter than in the former. (Kral 50)

Kral's tendency to side with the "lumpers" may also have led him to support like-minded clinicians in favour of revising Kraepelin's view of Alzheimer's disease as a rare, presenile illness. In keeping with the "lumpers," Kral wrote: "It is now generally accepted that the anatomical features of both conditions [senile dementia and Alzheimer's disease] are indistinguishable. The identical anatomical picture and the fact that both disorders have the amnestic syndrome as their symptomatological axis would support the hypothesis that only one nosological entity is being dealt with" (76). Although he revised Kraepelin's definition, Kral nevertheless insisted that the dementing process of the senium "remained a mystery" (51). In 1970, he also confessed that the therapeutic efforts directed towards the "chronic dementing process of the senium have not so far been successful" (81). To date, this situation has, unfortunately, remained unchanged.

Events in the US further consolidated Kral's decision to side with the lumpers and to collapse the division between Kraepelinian concepts of Alzheimer's and senile dementia. In 1976 Robert Katzman, neuroscientist and founder of the National Alzheimer's Association in the US, convincingly argued that these two forms of dementia were in fact a single disease; the irony of the situation lies in the fact that the distinct genetic basis of early onset dementia, which remains an extremely rare form of Alzheimer's disease, supports the original distinction made by Kraepelin. At the 1988 Ciba Foundation symposium on aging research, Katzman openly celebrated the success of his campaign to identify Alzheimer's as a disease: "I have spent a number of years trying to persuade people that AD is a disease, and not simply what used to be called 'senility' or 'senile dementia,'" and there has been marvellous progress in research. In my view this is because people now consider Alzheimer's as a disease" (in Ballenger, Self 110). The British geriatrician, J. Grimley Evans retorted: "this smacks of politics rather than science" (ibid.). Evans maintained that in the absence of a solid understanding of what exactly aging was, no conclusion should be reached regarding the issue of aging versus disease. Despite Evans's objections, which uncannily echoed those of Alois

Alzheimer himself when he objected to Kraepelin's desire to identify a new disease process, Katzman's position has prevailed – a position that has been extremely effective in drawing attention to the plight of elderly individuals coping with dementia and establishing dementia as a worthy cause for research funds, but, unfortunately, has also helped to consolidate the view of Alzheimer's as a Gothic monster.

Prior to Katzman's remaking of Alzheimer's disease, as noted earlier, physicians viewed it as a rare illness that struck people in their late fifties and early sixties. By linking Alzheimer's to what was then considered garden-variety manifestations of senility among elderly persons, Katzman increased the number of people experiencing a "disease" exponentially. Hordes of elderly individuals were suddenly labelled as contending with a disease and entire aging populations were viewed as being at risk of contracting it. In 2008 the eminent neurologist John Hardy stressed that the consolidation of the concept of Alzheimer's disease as a singular condition "was just a political maneuver to get funding, and some people then actually came to believe that this is the case" (in Lock 41). Similarly William Lishman, associated with the Institute of Psychiatry at the Maudsley Hospital in London insisted that the possibility must be entertained that Alzheimer's disease is, after all, "simply brain aging" (ibid.). He argues that until "a marker is found that is indisputably associated with the condition labeled as Alzheimer's alone, a marker never seen in healthy aging individuals," the idea that "Alzheimer's and neural aging are indistinguishable must not be dismissed" (ibid.). For the most part these cautionary views have been ignored in favour of sensationalist treatments of the illness. Katzman's reconceptualization of the nature and scope of the illness enabled him to bill Alzheimer's disease as the fourth or fifth leading cause of death in the United States. Prior to Katzman's Gothic refashioning of Alzheimer's into a "major killer" ("Prevalence" 217) – the phrase he used in his 1976 essay in the *Archives of Neurology* – the scientific community was not terribly interested in Alzheimer's. Before Katzman's 1976 article, for example, fewer than 150 articles had been published on Alzheimer's. From the time of that publication to Katzman's death in 2008, over 450,000 articles had been published (Lock 39–40).

Based on the conclusions drawn by the two British studies and the newly established view that Alzheimer's disease and senility were a single entity, four basic theories concerning the origins of Alzheimer's disease emerged in the 1970s. Since these theories served as the basis for virtually all of the discussions of senile dementia and have been analyzed at length in other studies, in what follows I will briefly summarize them. The first theory, which appeared in the Canadian media in 1988, posits that Alzheimer's is caused by the workings of a slow virus, such as those that cause scrapie in sheep, mad cow disease, or the rare brain disease in humans known as kuru. Initially Michael Kidd, a member of Roth's team, supported this view and proposed that Alzheimer's was transmissible (in Katzman and Bick 35). Some contemporary scientists such as Mira Katan, a neurologist with the Northern Manhattan Study at Columbia University Medical Center in New York City, likewise maintain that Alzheimer's is instigated by a form of the herpes virus.

The second theory, widely disseminated in the Canadian media through the 1980s and 1990s, holds that the disease stems from the toxic effects of aluminum. This view was briefly promoted by the Polish neuropathologist Henry Wisniewski. During his sabbatical, Wisniewski began working with Igor Klatzo at the National Institute of Health. Together they developed "an experimental model of aluminum encephalopathy thought to represent a form of cytoxic edema" (in Katzman and Bick 127). In the course of his research Wisniewski discerned a form of neurofibrillary tangles using light microscopy on rabbit brains, and this finding led to researchers probing whether aluminum toxicity plays a role in the etiology of Alzheimer's. In 1966, Wisniewski joined Robert Terry's lab, and introduced Terry to Klatzo's technique of inducing tangles. Soon after, however, they realized that their hypothesis was false: the fibrils in the rabbit tangles were "quite different than those in AD on electron microscopy" (ibid. 127–8). Although Terry and Wisniewski quickly abandoned the aluminum hypothesis, the Canadian researcher Donald Crapper McLachlan, who went on to help establish the Alzheimer Society of Canada and later served as the director for the Tanz Centre for Neurodegenerative Diseases, seized on this hypothesis and never ceased to champion the aluminum theory.[13]

The final two hypotheses, which remain the most powerful, link the origins of Alzheimer's to genetics and to deficits of the neurotransmitter acetycholine, respectively. Currently, scientists who accept these theories receive the lion's share of research funds (see Groopman). The genetic hypothesis has a solid foundation given the fact that in the 1950s and 1960s clinicians and scientists readily accepted and empirically demonstrated that some forms of mental illness were inherited.

In the 1970s, the recognition that children with Down syndrome succumbed to dementia further enhanced the genetic paradigm.[14] Later, in the 1990s, the identification of four genes that mediate the development of Alzheimer's firmly established the genetic approach as the cutting-edge scientific framework in Alzheimer's disease research. Peter St George Hyslop, a senior researcher at the University of Toronto's Centre for Research in Neurodegenerative Diseases, featured prominently in the Canadian media's treatment of the genetic origins of Alzheimer's disease. In keeping with the increasingly Gothic biomedical approach adopted in the 1980s and the concomitant view of diseases as puzzles to be solved by heroic individuals, one article describes Hyslop, who worked with McLachlan, as "a modern-day Sherlock Holmes."[15] In the 1980s both the Gothic model and the portrayal of scientists as "sleuths" became commonplace. In 1993, in an article with the Gothic title "On the Trail of the Mind Killer," Paul Taylor likewise refers to Hyslop's genetic research.

Of all the causal theories listed above, it is the idea of a deficit of the neurotransmitter acetycholine on brain functioning – the "cholinergic deficit" hypothesis – that has assumed pre-eminent status. This view was, in turn, based on the pioneering experiments that David Drachman published in 1974 (see Katzman and Bick ch. 5). In the 1980s researchers observed that the brains of patients who had died with Alzheimer-type dementia had a pronounced deficit of acetycholine (a neurotransmitter known to play an important role in memory and learning). This finding allowed researchers to construct a persuasive model of a proximal cause of dementia, known as the "cholinergic hypothesis."[16]

From the start, however, this theory suffered from several limitations. First, researchers recognized that there were other neurotransmitter systems involved in Alzheimer's disease. Second, the cholinergic hypothesis does not account for the other cognitive deficits characteristic of Alzheimer's – apraxia (the loss of the ability to execute or carry out learned purposeful movements), aphasia (the loss of the ability to speak, read, and write), and agnosia (the loss of the ability to recognize objects, persons, sounds, shapes, or smells), and disturbances of personality and affect (Ballenger, *Self* 93). Third, the focus on memory alone – "the elevation of memory loss as the primary symptom of dementia" – distorts Alois Alzheimer's original findings concerning the range of cognitive, behavioural, and affective symptoms characteristic of the illness (ibid. 98). Finally, and equally problematic, the hypothesis has nothing to say about the origins of the disease, namely, what causes the deterioration of this specific population of neurons in the first place (ibid. 93).

Neuroscientist Peter Whitehouse, whose research team was instrumental in generating the cholinergic hypothesis, publicly and repeatedly admits the limitations of this approach and insists that Alzheimer's is a multi-factorial disease that must be viewed in the context of both molecular and psychosocial factors. The evident limitations associated with the cholinergic hypothesis, in particular, and contemporary somatic theories, in general, have led to an increasingly visible and vigorous promotion of a public health approach to later life dementia. This approach targets the entire life course, rather than seeking a pill to cure symptoms of dementia in elderly persons. It addresses maternal health, education, exercise, nutrition, reducing environmental toxins, maintaining cognitive reserve, and preventing social isolation and depression among the elderly (see Whitehouse and George, "Myth" 219–63).

One of the striking features that emerges from a historical approach to Alzheimer's is the sea change that occurred after 2010 when, after a decade of failed drug trials, the media circled back to prior approaches and promoted changing people's lifestyles rather than waiting for science to discover the cure. An article from the *Vancouver Sun* raises a key question in its headline: "Alzheimer's: Should Prevention Rather than Cure Be the Focus?" (anon., 24 Nov. 2011, A14). In 2011, André Picard published an article in the *Globe and Mail* citing seven basic health risks including "low education, smoking, physical inactivity, depression, high blood pressure, diabetes, and obesity" (L6). Picard draws from a study that found that "half of Alzheimer's cases worldwide can be traced to seven common risk factors"; he argues further that the findings "also suggest that by tackling those underlying issues … the rising tide of dementia could be slowed considerably" (L6).[17]

From the Victorian era to the present, North American attitudes toward senile dementia have undergone a tremendous shift from an earlier reluctant acceptance of "dotage" to what has become an all-out "War on Alzheimer's" (see Whitehouse and George, "War"; see also Groopman). In its current approach to Alzheimer's disease, as in other cases – most notably, childbearing and menopause – science has planted its flag on what it deems the "pathological" aspects of the life course. Equally important, the rise of Gothic biomedical approaches to dementia have entailed a concomitant waning of religious and elegiac forms of consolation in the face of suffering and loss. Nowadays, as Thomas Cole observes, professional science offers "a secularized version of Calvinism's view of aging as unrelieved deterioration"; in place of "piety and divine grace, gerontology and geriatrics offered scientific knowledge and professional expertise as the path to salvation" (232).

Since the late 1960s researchers, clinicians, and drug companies have increasingly benefitted from society's panic in the face of the "menace" of the aging population, and, more specifically, the threat of this "dreaded disease." As I argue in the next section, the threat became vivid due to deinstitutionalization, which resulted in many more people with dementia and mental illness living on the streets. With respect to the mercantile facet of the pharmaceutical industry's response to this "threat," it is worth noting that in the 1980s the US Congress significantly loosened restrictions on the interaction between public and private research efforts; as a result, many academic researchers have taken personal investment stakes in their own research. As leading scientist Allen Roses, at Glaxo Welcome – one of the world's largest pharmaceutical companies – explains, the ability of academic researchers to benefit financially from their work has not always been good for science: "It brings out the worst in people. And there is no field as bad as Alzheimer's. I've been in several fields including muscular dystrophy and human genetics, which is known to be bad because things can be so easily stolen, but Alzheimer's disease is the epitome of this because there's so much money at stake" (in Shenk 187). For the most part, society eagerly attends to science's promise of "salvation" and supports researchers in their efforts to find a cure – a cure that is predicated on accepting the disease label and rallying behind it. Although people suffering from dementia and their caregivers find the disease label extremely reassuring and, at times, instrumentally useful, it remains questionable whether they have benefitted to the same extent as have researchers and clinicians.

In response to the recent G8 Summit on dementia, for example, and to the repeated vows "to find a cure for Alzheimer's disease," *Guardian* reporter Beth Britton, who had cared for her demented father, wrote: "Pledges to find new treatments and work towards a cure seem very far removed from the reality of day-to-day life with dementia and its stigma ... The argument about whether you look for short or long term improvements is an exceptionally difficult one. You have to be mindful of the 800,000 people (in the UK alone) who are living with a form of dementia, many of whom will be in the advanced stages and are unlikely to benefit from any future medical miracles. For them, improving their immediate quality of life and supporting those who are caring for them is vitally important" (Britton). As I have argued in the preceding chapters, historically, the needs of elderly individuals coping with dementia and those of their families have never been the predominant concern of the nation-state. In the next section I trace how in Canada the treatment of mentally vulnerable individuals in the 1950s reached a nadir, and led to the deinstitutionalization movement. In keeping with my effort to address the lived experience of people with dementia, in what follows I turn to the state of Canadian asylums and to the lives of their inhabitants from the 1930s to the 1960s.

SECTION V: THE EFFECT OF DEINSTITUTIONALIZATION ON PEOPLE WITH DEMENTIA, AND THE RISE OF SELF-HELP ORGANIZATIONS IN CANADA

During the Second World War, the overseas deployment of medical and health personnel to cope with the war resulted in a deprivation at home that was "little short of devastating" (Tyhurst et al. 3). Mental hospitals suffered in particular, and the effects were reflected in the "static if not deteriorating conditions of these services well into the late 1940s" (3). In 1947 J.V. McAree published an article entitled "Asylums of Canada Disgrace to Nation," which offered insight into the problem of overcrowding. As McAree explains, "there are 50,000 insane persons – or, as they are now called, mentally ill persons – in Canadian mental institutions, formerly called asylums. There is accommodation for perhaps two-thirds of this number" (6). At the end of his scathing review of the state of asylums across Canada, McAree mocks the notion that the mentally ill are receiving treatment: "Treatment, on the whole, is what the patients in Canadian mental institutions do not receive. Certainly they do not receive it adequately in any of them. One can imagine what treatment is possible when there is one doctor for three hundred patients or four hundred patients or even six hundred patients. What the patients get is custody" (6).

In response to these conditions, in 1948 the Canadian federal government established a system of mental health grants to the provinces to help "reinvigorate their programs"; over the next decade, tangible progress was made: "new buildings, new clinics, improved and increased staff, and the development of research programs all helped to establish a new professional interest in mental health and illness" (Tyhurst et al. 3). Between 1951 and 1956, the number of general hospitals that provided some psychiatric service increased by 78 per cent (85). Just when conditions were improving, however, the federal government ratified the Hospital Insurance and Diagnostic Services Act of 1957, which "specifically excluded mental hospital patients from the benefits offered to patients in general hospitals" (3). Both the patients with mental illness and the psychiatrists and staff who cared for them felt the effects of the act, which reflected the profound stigma against mental illness. As a result, people with dementia remained second-class citizens when it came to accessing health care. This structural discrimination persisted until the Canadian government, led by Lester B. Pearson, ratified the Canadian Health Care Act – which goes by the unofficial name of "medicare" – in 1966.

Since the opening of the first asylums in Upper Canada both the government and asylum superintendents promoted the view that asylums were not a suitable refuge for elderly individuals suffering from dementia. They repeatedly argued that the senile elderly should be cared for at home by their families. During the 1960s a concerted effort was made to rid asylums and hospitals of chronic and elderly patients. As Harvey Simmons explains, these patients became "pawns in a game intended to obtain federal cost-shared funds and were shunted aside into special residential units in hospitals. When this failed to attract federal funds, they were transferred to the Homes for Special Care Program, which then became an object of severe criticism" (xiv–xv). From 1961 to 1972, "hospitals discharged patients from mental hospitals and admitted them to residential units within the same hospital" (113). By March 1962, "nine residential units housing 3,466 residents had been established at the provincial psychiatric hospitals" (114). Substantial costs savings were achieved in this way thanks to the "economies [that] resulted from a lower level of care than that provided in the mental hospitals" (119). The Homes for Special Care Program of 1964 "established a second, lower tier of care for residents of psychiatric and mental retardation institutions, who, it was argued, could no longer benefit from active care" (ibid. 40).[18] From September of 1964 to February of 1973, a total of 11,500 people, most of them over sixty-five years of age, had been transferred from residential units to the Homes for Special

Care (119). Although many of the people discharged from the large mental institutions followed this route, others "were finding their way into municipal homes for the aged" (167). Due to overcrowding, Lawrence Crawford, the provincial director for homes for the aged, urged the municipal homes to "refuse admission to discharged patients"; he argued that the available beds should be reserved for people "actually living in the community who lack other necessary care facilities" (ibid.).

The rationale for these changes was partly inspired by an initiative undertaken in the late 1950s, when a group of psychiatrists – eight in total – was charged with the task of preparing a report that canvassed the attitudes and services currently available in Canada for the mentally ill. Published in 1963, the report, entitled *More for the Mind*, represented the culmination of five years of research and provided the philosophical foundation for Ontario's current approach to mental health services.[19] *More for the Mind* proposed radical changes to the system, including closing provincial hospitals for the mentally ill – veritable warehouses for people with mental illness, many of whom were elderly "chronic cases" – and establishing services in local, general hospitals. As the authors observed:

> Mental hospitals are often remote, isolated and far too big. Frequently patients are required to be transported long distances to hospitals, even from large cities. When these distances create delays, patients are lodged in jails and police cells in the interval. Professional opinion has been expressed with increasing emphasis over the last century or more that no mental hospital should be larger than 200 to 300 beds. Yet, for reasons which are often obscure, most provincial mental hospitals in Canada are attempting to care for 1,000 to 5,000 or more patients, often in buildings that are obsolete and inadequate even by minimum health standards. (Tyhurst et al. 27)

Cyril Greenwood, a social worker who left England to work at the Whitby asylum in Ontario in 1958, was appalled by what he saw. Worse, he found himself battling a corrupt system that not only tolerated but tacitly promoted patient abuse. "All our back wards," Greenland admitted, "including Whitby's pavilion 2B, represented extreme forms of abuse" (in Blom and Sussman 238). Mrs Holliday, a notorious staff member who was later sentenced and jailed for her crimes, had "a hundred or so patients working out in the community on farms and she was pocketing their wages" (212). She also regularly stole money by pretending to order new clothing for the inmates (212). If patients dared to complain, Holliday subjected them to electro-convulsive treatment, ECT (212). Shortly after he arrived, Greenland reported Holliday's crimes and embarked on a project known as "remotivation" that targeted the most desolate men's ward, 2B. This "Total Push" campaign took place over a period of three short months (220). I cite Greenland's experience because the infamous pavilion 2B was likely not too different from back wards at other similar institutions: an incredibly "bleak place" where patients, most of whom were naked, were either permanently in bed or pacing up and down and "pissing" in the corners (220). Many of the patients were "emaciated and looked like concentration camp victims" (220). Some were being starved simply "because the other patients were eating their food" (220).

In his reminiscences, Greenland emphasizes that the power imbalance between patients and physicians led to this horrific situation: "When I first arrived here in 1958 ... the patients weren't asked if they wanted E.C.T. or a leucotomy (brain surgery), we went ahead and did what we thought was best. This did a lot of damage, not only to the patients, but to our own self-respect and credibility. There were great abuses of power in those days ... The greatest abuse was our professional arrogance and paternalism" (in Blom and Sussman 237; see also 238). Under Greenland's supervision, many of the residents with senile dementia were transferred from 2B to old age homes.

Greenland wholeheartedly embraced the deinstitutionalization movement. Commenting in retrospect on the mistakes made by clinicians who, like himself, actively promoted the movement, Greenland confessed that he and other like-minded clinicians were under the mistaken impression that "chronic mental illness was a product of institutionalization" (ibid. 233; see also Shorter, *History* 272–81). He also admits that in their planning for deinstitutionalization, they failed to consider some of the strategic elements; "this is why no proper provisions were made for housing and community support systems. It was assumed, quite erroneously, that these resources would come from the community" (in Blom and Sussman 233).

Reports such as *More for the Mind* shared the prevailing optimism of the deinstitutionalization movement. And, in keeping with late-nineteenth-century asylum policy, the authors of the report expected families to bear the brunt of looking after elderly individuals with dementia. As the report states: "The possibility of keeping mentally ill patients out of mental hospitals altogether is becoming a reality with the development of community out-patient and day care services" (15). The report states that consultation services and acute hospital care must be readily available to the family "so that they do not feel they are going to be stuck with someone they cannot look after" (105). The report also insists that a major factor in "making domiciliary care possible may be provision of day centres, to which the aged may go for activity and socialization. This can provide a significant part of life for the aged person and may also be what is needed to enable the family or foster family to tolerate and care for him" (105). On the one hand, the report offers a far more realistic appraisal of the emotional and material burdens assumed by a family caring for someone with dementia. On the other hand, *More for the Mind*'s repeated bureaucratic references to "the aged person" continue to efface the lived experiences of elderly individuals incarcerated within the asylum or, following the deinstitutionalization movement, left to the mercy of what Shorter aptly terms "the rough care of the streets" (*History* 238).

In summary, this chapter analyzed the shift from psychosocial approaches to dementia to a decidedly somatic, biological approach. During this period the government oversaw the transfer of large numbers of elderly patients with dementia from psychiatric hospitals to residential units within these same hospitals, to nursing homes and to Homes for Special Care. At bottom, both transinstitutionalization and deinstitutionalization were effected to cut costs. To convey the effect of deinstitutionalization on the individual level, the next chapter turns from the material preoccupations of biomedicine, with its Gothic promise of a cure, to the psychological and elegiac concerns of fiction via an analysis of Alice Munro's short story "Powers." I chose this text because it addresses the impact of the deinstitutionalization movement on a woman with memory loss. In the process, "Powers" also explores the limitations of both the Gothic and the masculine elegy to accurately represent and console individuals coping with dementia.

A Narrative View of Deinstitutionalization: Alice Munro's "Powers"

The previous chapter examines the eclipse of psychological, stress-based theories concerning the etiology of late-onset dementia and the rise of somatic approaches – a shift that was accompanied by an increasing emphasis on the search for a pharmaceutical cure for age-related dementia in the late 1960s. The final section of chapter four analyzed the treatment of patients under these shifting conditions and the effect of the anti-asylum movement and deinstitutionalization in the late 1960s from the perspective of clinicians. In what follows, I offer a close reading of Munro's elegiac story "Powers" (2004) for several reasons. First, "Powers" shifts the perspective to literature and, as a result, offers new insight into challenges posed by deinstitutionalization. Second, the story explores a key issue raised in the previous chapters, namely the ramifications of the increasing dominance of biomedical approaches to mental illness and aging on Canadians from the perspective of patients and their caregivers. As we have seen, in an effort to locate pathological agents and mechanisms, what I term "Gothic" biomedical models rely on a metonymic[1] process of substitution of the person for increasingly smaller cellular and ultra-cellular units. One can think, for example, of the relentless focus on the brain of Auguste D. Yet, as "Powers" illustrates, literary genres engage in analogous processes of substitution and they, too, have limitations. In this chapter, I show how "Powers" highlights the drawbacks of the male elegy by calling into question the consolatory powers of the traditional English elegy triumphantly celebrated in Laurence's *The Stone Angel*. Whereas Laurence's novel celebrates the capacity of the imagination to console individuals in the face of loss, "Powers" repeatedly emphasizes the ethical limits of fictive consolation – by that I mean the consolation provided by fantasy and, by extension, literature.

Set in a small Ontario town after the First World War, "Powers" traces the lives of a group of young friends: Nancy, who has just finished high school; Wilf, the thirty-year-old town doctor; Wilf's younger cousin Ollie, who is Nancy's age; and Tessa, Nancy's childhood friend, who dropped out of school when she was fourteen due to an unnamed illness. Early on, Nancy cryptically explains that Tessa is "not in the world that the rest of us are in" (271). Readers soon learn that Tessa is a clairvoyant, and uses her psychic powers to help the townspeople locate hidden or lost individuals and objects. The first section traces Nancy's marriage to Wilf, and Ollie's less conventional relationship with Tessa, whom he later abandons in an asylum.

"Powers" addresses age-related dementia, institutionalization, and deinstitutionalization in several ways. First, toward the end of the story readers learn that Wilf succumbs to dementia later in life, and that Nancy faithfully serves as his caregiver. Second, the narrative reveals that Ollie, who was stricken with tuberculosis as a teenager, was treated in a sanatorium for three years. Third, after running off to the US with Tessa, and exploiting her psychic powers to further his career as a science journalist, Ollie has Tessa institutionalized. Like Wilf, Tessa also suffers from memory loss as an older woman. In the late 1960s, Nancy receives a call from the matron of the asylum where Tessa has been incarcerated for many years, because it is slated to close. Nancy must decide whether she is capable of looking after not one but two vulnerable elderly individuals. Already overburdened by Wilf, Nancy ultimately forsakes Tessa.

Told in fragments, the story spans approximately fifty years, beginning with Nancy's first-person diary entries in 1927 and closing with a third-person account of Nancy, as an elderly woman in the early 1970s, daydreaming about a happier resolution to Tessa's fate. In light of my book's overarching concern with the moral implications of biomedical and imaginative strategies for addressing the problem of age-related dementia, it is notable that "Powers" opens with Nancy's musing on the topic they used to discuss in the debating club: "Is Science or Literature more important in forming Human Character?" (272–3). As Nancy explains, however, the debating club was "scrapped after the War"; such serious subjects were no longer compelling after "everybody got cars to run around in and the movies to go to and started playing golf" (272). In an attempt to resist the times and again contend with weighty subjects, Nancy and her friends decide to read Dante Alighieri's *The Divine Comedy* together. Their plans are thwarted when Wilf proposes to Nancy because he convinces her to "give Dante a rest" (277). This phrase serves as the title of the first section, and suggests that the pleasures of modern society – "getting and spending" (300), to quote William Wordsworth's poem, "The World is Too Much with Us," (1807) which acts as the story's primary intertext – have made it difficult to ponder moral concerns. "Powers" repeatedly alludes to both Wordsworth's sonnet and to Dante's epic poem (composed between 1308–21), which likewise anatomizes good and evil in an effort to map the soul's journey toward God. Viewed in light of these poetic intertexts, Munro's sixty-five-page, multi-section short story, which charts Nancy's life, can be read as a secular response to both Dante's overtly religious and Wordsworth's spiritual portrayal of life's journey. In Nancy's case, the journey is fraught with ethical decisions that hinge on balancing self-interest with caring for others – specifically the frail elderly suffering from dementia.

Given Wordsworth's elegiac tone and my study's focus on the Gothic and its relation to the elegy – genres that both address how to cope with mutability, loss, and death – it is also significant that Tessa possesses the power to help people redress various forms of loss. As Nancy explains to Ollie, people drive to Tessa's house from miles away and line up to see her, "Mostly asking her about things that are lost" (293). "It isn't just things that people lose either," Nancy says. "She has located bodies" (294). The empirically minded Ollie immediately quizzes Nancy on the veracity of Tessa's abilities. "If that's true," Ollie replies, "why hasn't anybody investigated? I mean, scientifically" (294). Whereas Tessa's mysterious powers of consolation lie in recuperating what has been lost, Ollie's power seemingly lies in dissociating from his own vulnerability, and reducing women – most obviously Tessa – to scientific specimens. Ollie's strategy recalls late nineteenth and early twentieth century biomedical approaches to both hysteria and dementia, which entailed locating the disease processes in women's minds and bodies and using them as scientific material.

As noted earlier, readers learn that prior to visiting with Wilf and Nancy, Ollie spent three years in a TB sanatorium. As a patient he was subject to protracted, invasive treatments. Wilf, who is portrayed as an extremely dispassionate and detached physician, explains that doctors collapsed one of Ollie's lungs so that they could treat the infection (279). While Wilf calmly recounts Ollie's treatment, the latter puts his hands over his ears. As Ollie confesses, he prefers not to think about what was done to him. Instead, as he admits to Nancy, he "pretends to himself he is hollow like a celluloid doll" (279–80). Ollie's experience as a TB patient is relevant for several reasons. First, it recalls Sontag's discussion of the dread that attended TB – a dread that currently haunts Alzheimer's disease. Second, Ollie's traumatic experience may have motivated him to pass on this sense of dread. Ollie's response is significant because it offers insight into the predicament of the elegist, who, confronted with the death of the other, recognizes his own vulnerability and mortality. In the masculine elegy, the poet responds by deifying the deceased and, at the same time, celebrating his own survival. As we will see, Ollie's treatment of Tessa echoes this pattern.[2]

Ollie's mercenary, capitalist, and scientific bent also recalls chapter three's analysis of modernity's effect on the transformation of the meaning and experience of mental illness and dementia. In this regard, it is worth noting that the story's title "Powers" is cited in a letter Nancy writes to Tessa, in which Nancy directly quotes Wordsworth's sonnet, which rails against the negative facets of modernization, specifically society's obsession with commodification – "getting and spending" (300) – whereby "we lay waste our powers." In her letter to Tessa, written shortly after Nancy marries Wilf, Nancy expresses her fear that Ollie plans to take Tessa to the US, and she urges Tessa not to leave the small town to become the object of scientific research. "I do not know what kind of research he [Ollie] means," Nancy writes, "but I must say that when I read that part of his letter it made my blood run cold. I just feel in my heart it is not a good thing for you to leave here – if that is what you are thinking about – and go where nobody knows you or thinks of you as a friend or normal person" (301). Nancy's warning to Tessa not to leave the small town recalls the conclusion of Leacock's *Sunshine Sketches of a Little Town*. As noted in chapter three, Leacock's "L'Envoi" likewise warns the reader about the dangers of succumbing to the lure of the "unreal" city, a version of T.S. Eliot's wasteland.

In "Powers," Nancy's suspicions concerning Ollie's motivations spring from the fact that shortly after meeting Tessa, Ollie uses her to launch his career as a scientific journalist: he publishes his first article about Tessa's powers and the small town in *Saturday Night*. Nancy

shrewdly suspects that, far from caring for Tessa, Ollie plans to continue to use Tessa as lucrative research material. In a letter to Ollie
reprimanding him for publishing his article, Nancy – who may also
be jealous of Ollie's accomplishments and the attention he is paying to Tessa – bluntly asks Ollie if he obtained Tessa's permission to
exercise his "Scientific Curiosity": "Did you explain what you were
doing to her? Or did you just come and go and make use of us Prosaic
People here to embark on your Career as a Writer?" (298).

In effect Nancy is both angry and guilty, because she is the one who
first introduced Ollie to Tessa. At first, he suspects that Nancy is taking him to see a rural prostitute – a misunderstanding that horrifies
Nancy but also underscores Ollie's lifelong tendency to view women
as commodities. It is also Nancy who cajoles Tessa into displaying
her powers for Ollie because Nancy senses Ollie's condescension
toward her, the small town, and its inhabitants. As Nancy admits to
Ollie after their first visit to Tessa's home: "I took you out there on
purpose to show you we had something special here. Her. Tessa. I
mean, to show you Tessa. Because you don't think we have anything
here worth noticing. You think we're only worth making fun of. All
of us around here. So I was going to show her to you. Like a freak"
(295). Nancy's rash decision to make "use" of Tessa – a brief and
regrettable failure to care for Tessa as a friend – instigates further
lapses of compassion and humanity on Ollie's part.

The extent of Ollie's ill treatment of Tessa is only revealed in the
penultimate section, which takes place in the early 1970s. Nancy is
in her sixties, and she meets Ollie in Vancouver. Several years before
then, in the fall of 1968, Nancy receives a letter from the asylum
where Tessa has been a patient for many years, and she drives to see
her friend. After Nancy arrives, the matron explains that the hospital,
which had been "a catchall, literally, for those who were genuinely
mentally ill, or senile, or those who would never develop normally …
or people whose families could not or would not cope with them,"
is being closed down (304). Whereas many of the patients are being
transferred to alternative and, in some cases, specialized facilities,
there are some like Tessa, who, they hope, "could manage if they
were placed with relatives" (305). The Matron goes on to assure
Nancy that Tessa has been on "the mildest medication" (305) and
has also perhaps received some shock therapy (ECT). Her comments
recall those of the nineteenth-century superintendents who likewise
attempted to downplay the difficulties associated with caring for

mentally ill, elderly individuals – people in their "dotage" – in the hopes that their families and friends would look after them. As Nancy explains to the matron, however, caring for Tessa is beyond her; she is not Tessa's relative and she has her hands full looking after her husband, Wilf. "I have a husband," Nancy says, "who is – he would be in a place like this, I guess, but I am looking after him at home" (305). Although the matron offers Nancy the opportunity to leave without seeing Tessa, Nancy insists on visiting her friend. During their brief reunion, Tessa tells Nancy about her treatment in the asylum. "I had a hole in my head," Tessa explains, "I had it for a long time" (309). "They gave me the needles and the gas too," Tessa says. "It was to cure my head. And to make me not remember" (309). Toward the end of her visit, Nancy asks Tessa if she recalls her childhood powers. "Do you remember what you used to be able to do? You used to be able to – you used to know things. When people lost things, you used to be able to tell them where they were" (310). Tessa anxiously dismisses Nancy's comment. "Oh, no," Tessa says. "I just pretended ... It bothers my head to talk about it" (311). The terseness of her denial and her mundane explanation of her gift contrast with the earlier wonder that Nancy and Ollie and, by extension, readers experience when Tessa uses her power to magically itemize everything hidden in Ollie's pocket on his first visit.

In "Powers," the status of Tessa's clairvoyance remains indeterminate, which suggests that ethical consolation likewise occupies a similarly liminal space between truth and fiction. Moreover, Tessa's betrayal of her own powers – a denial that likely results from her protracted subjection to the biomedical model in the asylum – hauntingly mirrors Ollie's experience of himself as a hollow plaything. Tessa's disavowal of her gift also recalls that earlier question posed by the debating club: "Is Science or Literature more important in forming Human Character?" Munro's story prompts readers to wonder if Tessa is better off for having relinquished her belief in her imaginative powers. In effect, by juxtaposing Wilf's skill as a doctor with that of Tessa's power to heal and redress loss, "Powers" acknowledges the value of both arts, while demonstrating their respective limits.

In Munro's poetics, as Karen Smythe observes, empirical realism alone "is deemed an inaccurate method for representing the world and our experiences in it" (141). Smythe argues further that Munro's work "suggests that the quest for absolute precision may actually falsify reality, whereas artifice may serve to clarify or illuminate to a greater extent ... Pure fact is abandoned as an artistic dead-end in terms of elegiac consolation" (141). E.D. Blodgett maintains that the art that Munro strives for is "a mode of discourse that demonstrates that the problem of life, death, loss, and recuperation must pass into the telling" (in ibid.).

In "Powers," Nancy echoes the view that life's complexity is only comprehensible when transformed into a narrative when she explains why, as an older woman, she takes to reminiscing about her experiences. As she prepares herself for one of her imaginative adventures, she briefly considers her children's concern that she is increasingly forfeiting the chance to socialize in favour of sequestering herself in her house and "Living in the Past" (330). Yet as the narrator explains, "what she believes she is doing, what she wants to do if she can get the time to do it, is not so much to live in the past as to open it and get one good look at it" (330). In this passage, Nancy can be likened to a surgeon eager to "open" up and anatomize a patient. Looking, however, remains predicated on subjective elements – even within the supposedly objective realm of scientific research. As the controversies that attended the nineteenth- and early twentieth-century origins of the disease concept illustrate, Alzheimer's constituted – and remains – an enigma that serves as the site for powerful personal, familial, and national projections.

The look into the past Nancy obtains is self-consciously mediated by elegiac narrative patterns. Moreover as Kennedy admits, "a truthful elegy is an oxymoron, as the following lines from John Milton's "Lycidas" (1638) illustrate: "For so to interpose a little ease, / Let our frail thoughts dally with *false surmise*" (in Kennedy 69; my emphasis). In contrast to *The Stone Angel*, "Powers" self-consciously emphasizes that imaginative attempts to deal with mutability, loss, and death inevitably rely on various forms of "false surmise," and suggests, further, that both biomedical and imaginative accounts are, at times, treacherous constructs.

The overarching concern in "Powers" with how science and literature differently respond to loss is signalled early on by the narrative's treatment of Ollie's attempt to discover definitively whether Tessa's ability to find what has been lost is indeed magical or, conversely, artificial and fraudulent. Nancy raises similar concerns toward the story's conclusion when she meets Ollie in Vancouver, and asks him whether his public and clearly fraudulent performances of Tessa's powers, offered to audiences across North America for a fee, nevertheless relied on a code that might be considered "an art in itself" (325). "Powers" repeatedly acknowledges that "fiction itself might be a kind of fraud, a magic act and an act of faith that obscures a truth" (Blodgett in Smythe 141). Yet I would also suggest that Munro's stories rely equally on artifice to reveal, rather than merely "obscure a truth." Since, as I have suggested, all our ways of knowing are predicated on models that remain inherently partial and limited, literary narratives usefully supplement our understanding of the lived experience of dementia. With respect to both "The Peace of Utrecht" and "Powers," fiction reveals the burden on female caregivers who, due to the changes in governmental policy toward the mentally ill during the late nineteenth and twentieth centuries, were forced to cope on their own with loved ones suffering from dementing illness without support from the community.

The narrative suggests that Nancy has been extremely isolated while caring for Wilf. When she visits Tessa in the asylum, Nancy confesses that Wilf has "gone a bit round the bend" (307) and mentions the latter's habit of prowling around the room incessantly.[3] Tessa, a veteran of the mental hospital, replies knowingly: "Oh, there's some in here that do that" (307). Comforted by Tessa's compassion and insight into Wilf's illness, Nancy goes on to describe other behavioural changes in her husband – none of which, as it turns out, concern cognitive decline. Referring to Wilf's newfound dependency and paranoia, Nancy says: "It's 'Where's Nancy?' all the time. I'm the only one he trusts these days" (307). When Tessa asks Nancy pointedly if Wilf has become violent, Nancy assures her that although Wilf is suspicious and "mixed up," he is not physically abusive (308). Ironies abound in Munro's fiction. In this case, the self-sufficient, emotionally dispassionate doctor ends up suffering from dementia and is in need of constant care. Equally ironically, Nancy receives sage counsel and moral support from Tessa, a woman whom society has labelled mad and has institutionalized for decades.

When it becomes clear that Nancy will not look after Tessa after the institution closes, Tessa again demonstrates her *true* "powers" – her characteristic blend of insight, honesty, and compassion that Ollie, Wilf, and to an extent even Nancy herself lack. "I knew you hadn't come to take me away," Tessa tells Nancy candidly. "How could you?" (311). Nancy assures Tessa that it has nothing to do with her; it is just that she has to look after Wilf. "He deserves something," Nancy protests. "He's been a good husband to me, just as good as he could be. I made a vow to myself that he wouldn't have to go into an institution" (311). Tessa politely agrees that this would, indeed, have been a terrible fate. Only later does Nancy realize her tactlessness. Despite Tessa's dire predicament, she forgives her friend and thanks Nancy for making the trip: "You were good to come to see me, Nancy. You can see I've kept my health. That's something" (311).

As noted earlier, in Munro's fiction ironies proliferate. Despite having been repeatedly abandoned, incarcerated in an asylum, and subject to ECT as well as other medical interventions, Tessa – whose shoulders remain "square and stately" (306), and who cares not only for herself but for other patients in the asylum – gracefully assures Nancy that she is healthy. Moreover to Nancy's surprise, even after her tactless comment cited above "Tessa was smiling, and Nancy saw in that smile the same thing that had puzzled her years ago. Not exactly superiority, but an extraordinary, unwarranted benevolence" (311). In contrast to Rothschild's and Kral's valorization of the masculine traits of stoicism and detachment outlined in the previous chapter, Tessa's ability to withstand loss is predicated on her profound empathy and relationship with others, and on her seemingly magical – albeit potentially fraudulent – powers of the imagination.

Tessa graphically illustrates these powers and their fallibility when Nancy visits her in the asylum. Tessa is adamant that Ollie, whom she refers to as "That man," was murdered. "Oh, I saw him," Tessa insists, "he had his head wrapped up in a black coat. Tied with a cord around the neck. Somebody did it to him ... Somebody should have gone to the electric chair" (309). Nancy, who was never officially informed of Ollie's death let alone his murder, doubts Tessa's account, and gently suggests to Tessa that perhaps "that was a bad dream you had. You might have got your dream mixed up with what really happened" (309). It is possible that Tessa's delusion that Ollie was killed, and her sense of injustice – "Somebody should have gone to the electric chair" – serves as a screen for her own murderous sense of rage and betrayal. Before parting, the women return to the subject of Ollie's whereabouts. Using "a robust and reasonable tone," Tessa turns to Nancy, saying, if "he wasn't dead, why wouldn't he have come here and got me? He said he would" (312). These are the last words Tessa utters in the narrative, and to both Nancy and, by extension, readers they echo Auguste D.'s repeated utterance: "What do you want? My husband will come soon" (Perusini, "Histology" 84). The cry for the lost lover/husband also brings to mind the myth of

Orpheus and Eurydice. In "Powers," however, Tessa's plaint poignantly underscores Ollie's failure of care.

As noted above, a few years after visiting Tessa in the institution in 1968, Nancy bumps into Ollie – who, as it turns out, is alive and well strolling the streets of Vancouver. Nancy is returning from an Alaskan cruise that her friends urged her to take after Wilf's death. Footloose and fancy-free, Ollie is sojourning on Texeda Island. While conversing over dinner, Nancy discovers that her suspicions were correct. Ollie merely pretended to marry Tessa. He confesses that "it wasn't a thoroughly legal arrangement" (321). Far from regretting his deception, however, Ollie boasts that he was "ahead" of his time (321). Worse, he admits that after research funds dried up in the US during the Depression, he convinced Tessa to "go with the travelling shows" even though "that thing, too, was winding down" (324). Perhaps to assuage his guilty conscience for abandoning Tessa in an insane asylum, Ollie adopts a melancholy tone and tells Nancy an elaborate and entirely false story about Tessa's tragic death from leukemia, which, according to Ollie, occurred shortly after they were "married." As noted earlier with respect to Nancy's fate, and in accordance with the structure of the masculine elegy, "Powers" repeatedly draws implicit connections between marrying and burying wives.

Ollie's story about Tessa's supposed death also draws on one of elegy's characteristic topoi – the sea – introduced by Milton (Kennedy 6), echoed by Wordsworth, and, as noted, by *The Stone Angel*'s references to Shadow Point's proximity to the sea. As Ollie tells Nancy, Tessa asked to be cremated; "it was practically the last thing she had said to me, that ... she wanted to be scattered on the waves of the Pacific Ocean" (327). Unlike Matthew Arnold's poem "Dover Beach" (1867), which self-consciously undermines the consolatory powers of the English elegy, Ollie upholds the genre's fictive powers of consolation. He describes in realistic detail how he had "taken off his shoes and socks and rolled up his pant legs and waded in, and the gulls came after him to see if he had anything for them. But it was only Tessa he had" (327).

Even before he relates this elaborate falsehood, Nancy – who knows very well that Tessa did not die of leukemia, but was instead incarcerated in an asylum – is saddened by Ollie's "casual-sounding yet practiced speech in which it was said that life was indeed a bumpy road, but misfortunes had pointed the way to better things, lessons were learned, and without a doubt joy came in the morning" (319–20). It is Ollie's use of the elegiac structure to gloss over life's complexity *and* his moral failings – and not simply the latter – that galls Nancy.

For Nancy and for readers alike, in the light of Tessa's adamant claim that her husband was murdered, the fact that Ollie is *alive* comes as a terrible surprise, and his lies concerning Tessa's poetic death are equally if not more shocking. Both revelations constitute epiphanic moments in the narrative. As critics observe, Munro's fictions are frequently studded with epiphanies. Traditionally, an epiphany draws attention to the role of the subject that perceives and thinks, rather than the object that is perceived. In accordance with the Kantian sublime, the perceiver of the epiphany typically receives consolation from an awareness of his capacity to use his reason to derive insight. In "Powers," however, epiphanies do not produce this kind of self-assurance and knowledge. Instead they point to glaring gaps in the perceiver's understanding – gaps that remain unresolved. Put somewhat differently, Munro constructs her story so that readers share Tessa's experience of having "a hole" in their heads (309). The epiphanies in "Powers" thus function more akin to shocks than to opportunities for gaining insight.

As Smythe argues, Munrovian epiphanies recall the notion of the shock put forward by German philosopher Walter Benjamin (1892–1940): "Where thinking suddenly stops in a configuration pregnant with tensions, it gives that configuration a shock" (Benjamin 262). By relying on these shocking epiphanies, "Powers" functions as a counter-discourse to the traditional masculine elegy, and specifically to its false forms of imaginative consolation and mastery. Instead Nancy is subjected to what might best be described as Munrovian "shock therapy," which entails experiencing the double impact of the reifying powers of the masculine elegy and the biomedical model.

Munro's reliance on the aesthetics of shock recalls the Surrealist's dedication to this technique and its intended effect. As noted in the introduction, André Breton famously asserted: "It must never be said that we did not do everything within our power to annihilate this ridiculous illusion of happiness and *understanding*" (*Manifestoes* 152). In light of Munro's evocation of the asylum, it is also worth noting that the Surrealists deployed shock tactics in the service of re-creating a "state which can only be fairly compared to that of madness" (175). Of all the Surrealists, Antonin Artaud was perhaps the most devoted to the aesthetics of shock. As Sontag asserts, it is one of the great ironies that "the man who was to be devastated by repeated electric-shock treatments during the last three of nine consecutive years in mental hospitals proposed that theatre administer to culture a kind of shock therapy" ("Essay" xxviii). For Artaud, to improve and edify individuals, art must be "brutal – and also an experience suffered, and charged with extreme emotions" (xxix). In a similar fashion, readers of "Powers" are shocked to discover that within the asylum and in Ollie's story, Tessa is similarly objectified and stripped of her healing gifts. As Munro's narrative deftly illustrates, both discourses compromise the agency of vulnerable individuals.

In contrast to Hagar's celebration of falsehood at the end of *The Stone Angel*, Ollie's deceitful story of Tessa's death self-consciously highlights the dangers of substituting the writer's consoling story – be it an imaginative or a biomedical artifact – for the lost individual. Put differently, whereas Tessa seemingly possesses the magical ability to recover lost bodies, Ollie, a natural-born charmer who exploits other people, possesses the opposite power: his false elegies bury the living.[4] I would argue further that in "Powers," Ollie's version of the traditional masculine elegy – with its emphasis on detachment and substitution – hides a Gothic crime. In this case, the crime is not, as in Mary Shelley's *Frankenstein*, that people fall ill and die. Instead, the crime is linked to failures of empathy and compassion that doom women and the frail elderly to experience a dreadful form of death-in-life.

In keeping with Hagar's erasure of John's experience in *The Stone Angel*, "Powers" likewise demonstrates that our loss of empathy is encoded in how we represent people who suffer from mental illness and dementia. For instance, when Tessa and Nancy discuss Ollie's supposed death Tessa says: "I thought you would've known. *Didn't* Wilf know?" (308; emphasis added). However Nancy corrects Tessa, saying: "*Doesn't* Wilf know," speaking in an "automatic way, defending her husband by placing him amongst the living" (310). Nancy's determination to place her husband among the living contrasts with Ollie's decision to narrate Tessa's death. In this way "Powers" repeatedly emphasizes the potentially corrosive and, at times, murderous relationship between language and its referent, particularly when the referent lacks agency due to a dementing illness. Ultimately, "Powers" argues for using language and the imagination to secure and maintain empathetic bonds and, within limits, to promote recuperation in the face of loss.

Both the tendency to rely on the imagination to secure consolation for the living, and the limits of this practice are strikingly evident in the concluding episode. Sitting in Wilf's old recliner in the sunroom of her house, Nancy begins to daydream; in accordance with their contrasting approach to language outlined above, Nancy's dream challenges Ollie's fantasy. In her daydream Nancy finds herself entering another room where she finds Ollie and Tessa, moments before he makes the decision to have her committed. Contemplating Ollie's nefarious actions, Nancy presumes that his faith in Tessa's "extraordinary powers" likely waned. She imagines Ollie siding with the empirical, biomedical assessment of Tessa's powers, and deciding that they were not a gift but rather an index of "a threatening imbalance in her mind and nature" (334). Nancy surmises further that Ollie retained the services of a doctor and convinced him that living with a "unique" person was "a strain, in fact perhaps more of a strain than a normal man can stand" (334). In Nancy's fantasy, Ollie has already secured the papers he needs to commit Tessa but they remain hidden in his coat pocket. Recalling how Tessa sensed what was in Ollie's pocket when they first met, in Nancy's fantasy Tessa likewise knows what lies hidden. In Nancy's consoling revision of history, however, Ollie reconsiders his decision: "He says to himself that he will get rid of the papers as soon as he can, he will forget the whole idea, he too is capable of hope and honor" (334). Equally important, in Nancy's fantasy Tessa recovers her lost powers. After finding a pile of dead flies behind a curtain – a reference perhaps to Emily Dickinson's elegiac sonnet "I heard a fly buzz" (1863) – Tessa is ecstatic because she *"knew they were there"* (333). In Nancy's imaginative revision of events long past, in the face of loss and death, rejuvenation (repair) prevails over dehumanization (waste). Nancy relies on familiar pastoral and religious imagery to describe Tessa's face after the revelation that her powers have returned: "Now her eyes are shining as if she has had the dirt rinsed out of them, and her voice sounds as if her throat has been freshened with sweet water" (333). Ultimately, however, the narrative undermines Nancy's reliance on imagination, which, in keeping with the masculine elegy, sanctions the shift from helpless participant to detached, masterful observer. In contrast to Ollie who clings to "false surmise," the narrative suggests that Nancy unconsciously chooses the ethical yet far less consoling option of recognizing the limits of fantasy.

In interviews, Munro has spoken candidly about the allure of the imagination and its utility in getting out of a messy situation.

Referring to her story "An Ounce of Cure" (1968), Munro explains that when the protagonist's circumstances become hopelessly messy, when nothing is going to go right for her, "she gets out of it by looking at the way things happen – by changing from a participant to an observer. This ... is what a writer does ... I made the glorious leap from being a victim of my own ineptness and self-conscious miseries to being a godlike arranger of patterns and destinies, even if they were all in my head" (in Smythe 111–12). As this statement suggests, Munro understands the temptation to enjoy fantasies of mastery. "Powers" illustrates both the allure of fictive consolation and the necessity of relinquishing it in favour of a more expansive narrative that also conveys an engagement with one's "own ineptness" and life's "miseries." Like Prospero – the magician in Shakespeare's *The Tempest* (1623) who relinquishes his powers and famously tells the audience, "Now my charms are all o'erthrown, / what strength I have's mine own" (5.1.2405–06) – Nancy ultimately relinquishes her fantasy. As I have argued, in the case of the elegy the notion of control is precisely what is at issue; in Nancy's case, it is more accurate to say that the fantasy itself gives way when confronted by the immutable fact of death. Readers are told that "deep in that moment [Nancy's daydream] some instability is waiting" (335). Although she is determined to ignore it, Nancy "is aware already of being removed, drawn out of those two people and back into herself" (335). In keeping with the allusions to Dante throughout "Powers," the conclusion recalls Virgil's role in *The Divine Comedy* as a spectral guide who leads the narrator from hell to paradise. As Nancy explains, she feels as if "some calm and decisive person – could it be Wilf? – has taken on the task of leading her out of that room ... Gently, inexorably leading her away from what begins to crumble behind her, to crumble and darken tenderly into something like soot and soft ash" (335). In Munro's rewriting of *The Divine Comedy*, the figure who leads Nancy out of her daydream and thus limits the powers of imaginative consolation is, quite fittingly, the empirically minded physician Wilf, who initially urged her to "give Dante a rest." Whereas Ollie refuses to recognize that his wife is alive and imaginatively reduces her to cremated ash, on some level Nancy grapples with the fact that her husband is dead, using the same image of "ash." On the one hand, Nancy's reliance in her daydream on pastoral imagery with respect to Tessa's rebirth and its final reference to Wilf leading Nancy back to the world of the living reinstall two of the central elements of the traditional English elegy. On the other hand, due to its references to the abject "soot and soft ash," the conclusion inverts the elegy's tran-scendent impulse to elevate the subject to a god-like stature. Nancy's reluctant waking from her reverie thus effectively contrasts with both Ollie's embrace of falsehood and *The Stone Angel*'s unequivocal cele-bration of the imagination, signaling the story's challenge to both the biomedical model and the masculine elegy.

To summarize, "Powers" offers insight into the lived experience of deinstitutionalization and the fate of cognitively impaired, elderly individuals who were released from asylums. Equally important, Munro's narrative highlights the fact that both biomedical and lit-erary require "material" that is inevitably subjected to reductive processes of selection and substitution. Put differently, "Powers" explores the limits and the ethical dangers associated with attempts to singlehandedly capture life's complexity – a complexity that is inextricably bound to transience, loss, and death. In keeping with the story's ultimate refusal of elegiac forms of consolation, readers learn that Nancy neither looks after Tessa nor writes to her. As she confesses, she had meant to write, but "Wilf became such a care as soon as she got home, and the whole visit … became so disturbing, and yet unreal, in her mind, that she never did" (312). After bump-ing into Ollie Nancy tries to track Tessa down, but her efforts prove futile. Her letter is returned unopened: "Apparently no such hospital existed anymore" (332). Even her letter to Ollie is returned to her "with one word written on the envelope. Moved" (332). In "Powers" transience and loss remain absolute and without redress.

The next two paired chapters continue to explore the challen-ges associated with caring for a loved with dementia in Canada. Chapters six and seven trace the experience of two Canadian broth-ers, Michael and Andrew Ignatieff, who adopted very different approaches toward their mother Alison's dementia, which resulted in her death in 1992. Andrew's response – which I align with both a historical, religious elegiac approach and a turn toward "ordin-ary ethics" – entails exploring the founding of the Alzheimer Society, a worldwide organization founded in Toronto. Influenced by the increasingly Gothic, biomedical view of dementia promoted by the media, Michael's response entailed writing *Scar Tissue*, a Gothic and melancholy fictionalized account of his brother's experience of car-ing for their mother.

A Tale of Two Brothers:
Andrew Ignatieff and the Rise of the
Alzheimer Society of Canada

In keeping with the previous chapter's focus on literature – specifically Munro's short story "Powers," which traces the effect of deinstitutionalization from the perspective of patients and caregivers – both this chapter and the next examine the responses of two Canadian brothers, Michael and Andrew Ignatieff, to the dementing illness that took the life of their mother Alison in 1992. I have chosen to focus on their experiences in order to probe the broader social ramifications, from the late 1970s to the early 1990s, of the remaking of Alzheimer's disease in Canada. When Alison Ignatieff's symptoms became evident in the early 1980s, medical researchers had only recently begun to assert that Alzheimer's disease was the primary cause of senile dementia and that the stereotypical cognitive changes associated with aging were not inevitable. In 1974, US President Richard Nixon signed the Research on Aging Act that established the National Institute on Aging (NIA) within the National Institutes of Health. The latter organization already had a thriving life processes institute, the National Institute of Child Health and Human Development (NICHD). The newly fledged NIA thus urgently needed to establish a socially cohesive group that could advocate for increased funding. But as medical historian Patrick Fox explains, rallying such a group would require "a disease the new institute could call its own" (213–14).

The same year that NIA was formed, neurologist Robert Katzman, at the Albert Einstein Medical Center in New York, co-wrote his now famous paper with Tokoz Karas that eliminated the separation between Alzheimer's disease and senile dementia. Due to the effects of the deinstitutionalization movement of the 1960s, the remaking of

Alzheimer's disease gained widespread public recognition. No longer
hidden by asylum walls, cognitively impaired individuals were now
living in urban communities, providing visible proof of the influence
of dementia on elderly people, a burden that was increasingly being
shouldered by family members.

From the late 1970s to the 1990s across North America, a host
of researchers began positing that cognitive decline was the manifestation of specific disease processes, most notably Alzheimer's
disease, which could be identified, analyzed, and, ideally, cured. As
Fox writes: "The reconstitution of senility cum Alzheimer's disease
signaled the transformation in the public mind of the meaning of
brain impairment associated with age from an inevitability to a possibility" (224). In the United States, Katzman and psychiatrist Robert
Butler successfully championed the disease model and went on to
spearhead the Alzheimer's movement. As NIA's first director, Butler's
goal was profoundly humanitarian, and lay in countering one of the
most feared connotations associated with growing old – epitomized
by the pernicious stereotype of elderly people as "forgetful, unable
to manage their everyday affairs, and totally dependent on others
for survival because of cognitive impairment" (ibid.). In his role as
director and as a practicing psychiatrist, he strove to emphasize that
many conditions that lead to dementing disorders or memory loss
were neither natural aspects of aging nor irreversible.

Generally speaking, although the fundamental aim of medical science in regards to Alzheimer's represents "one of the noblest forms
of human endeavor – to treat and cure disease – it is also a business"
(ibid. 228). As such, it involves powerful economic interests invested
in "the marketplace of disease diagnosis and treatment" (228). For
one, the acceptance of the definitional transformation was politically
crucial for neurologists such as Katzman and other bench scientists
because it conferred power on medical professionals as "arbiters of
normal versus diseased elderly people" (224).

This reconstitution of senility as Alzheimer's disease instigated an
even more profound "crisis mentality," in which old people and old
age itself were cast as major contributors to an ongoing, global
healthcare crisis. Alzheimer's disease may have effectively constructed "new subjectivities for later life," including "Alzheimer's victims," but it also gave the concerned "much more to worry about"
(Gubrium 200). In the late 1970s, with the help of the media – which
drew on the metaphors previously used in the first half of the twentieth

century to describe the category of the "feeble-minded" – Alzheimer's created new identities in the public imagination such as the "grey tsunami," which portrayed the elderly as burdens on the younger generation. In the US, largely due to the efforts of NIA and the Alzheimer's Association, the introduction of the disease paradigm also ensured that the interests of "an elite group of biomedical researchers emerged as the primary focus of federal AD policy" – a policy that, by and large, has failed to develop programs to meet the needs of caregivers (Fox 220). Although medical historians have documented the effect of this paradigm shift in the United States, which saw "dotage" and "senility" recast as "disease," to date little is known about Canadian responses and the rise of the Alzheimer Society of Canada.

I have opted to write two chapters focusing on the Ignatieff family's experience because Michael's and Andrew's responses to their mother's illness highlight the tensions between elegiac and Gothic views of Alzheimer's disease. Although Michael was no doubt intimately involved with and emotionally affected by his mother's condition, he ultimately opted for a more public, literary, and philosophical perspective. By contrast, Andrew adopted a faith-driven, practical response. Both of their approaches attest to the range of social responses generated by the scientific paradigm shift in Canada.

In the foregoing chapters I outlined the strengths and limitations of both the biomedical and the literary models of dementia. In this chapter I address an alternative response to dementia formulated by some of the founding members of the Alzheimer Society of Canada such as Andrew Ignatieff and Lori Dessau. The former worked on the board of the Alzheimer Society for Metropolitan Toronto (ASMT), and the latter on the board of the Alzheimer Society on the national level. I argue that their participation in these voluntary groups represents a more mundane, yet immensely powerful popular response to the challenges posed by Alzheimer's disease – in essence a shift from cure to care.[1] Andrew's involvement with the ASMT reflects today's more secular context that calls for what might best be described as "ordinary ethics." Rather than rely on a traditional narrative structure such as the Gothic or the elegy or offer a prescribed set of rules or codes of conduct, practitioners of ordinary ethics spontaneously attempt in "every day practice and thought to inhabit and persevere in light of uncertainty, suffering, injustice, incompleteness, inconsistency, the unsayable, the unforgivable, the irresolvable, and the limits of voice and reason" (Lambek, *Ordinary* 4). Put differently, individuals who practice ordinary ethics inhabit the ironic space of illness and indeterminacy.

In the early 1980s Andrew left his job in Peru, where he worked for the Canadian arm of Save the Children, to return to Toronto and care for both his parents. His role as caregiver became increasingly demanding after his father's death in 1989. Throughout this tumultuous period, Michael remained in Europe with his wife and young family. "I was the absent brother," Michael told *The Guardian* (in Valpy). Whereas Michael's essays and novel *Scar Tissue* (1993) about his mother's illness speak clearly and eloquently for his position, Andrew left little written trace of his experience either as a caregiver or as a board member of the Toronto branch of the Alzheimer Society. The dearth of information about Andrew's experience as a caregiver prompted me to engage in two formal interviews and a series of email conversations to address specific queries that emerged from our face-to-face interviews.[2]

Faced with the challenges associated with caring for Alison, Andrew derived comfort from religious observance and the support of his church congregation. Andrew's father George was a deeply believing Russian Orthodox Christian, and Andrew followed in his footsteps. Andrew's connection to the church enabled him to draw on prior elegiac approaches to illness and death, and provided him with both consolation and a communal approach to the challenges posed by dementia. Although his mother was a thoughtful lifelong agnostic, who rejected traditional organized religion of every sort, she happily accompanied George and Andrew to church. As Andrew explains, by the time he returned to Canada to care for his parents, who were both struggling with very different age-related illnesses, his mother had entered a particularly difficult phase in the evolution of her dementia. She had become fearful – a complete alteration in her character. She suddenly became afraid of abandonment, of making a fool of herself in public, of getting lost and not knowing the way home. Perhaps the greatest of her fears was that her husband was leaving her. This last fear made any outing stressful for them both as she would clutch at George, argue with him, and accuse him of plotting to leave her. Whenever he was out of sight, she demanded to know where he was and what he was doing.[3]

After Andrew returned to care for his ailing parents, he began accompanying them to church on Sundays. As he explains, he trailed along "mostly to keep an eye on Alison so that George could have

some freedom to devote himself to the worship and social interactions with his fellow parishioners." Once inside the church, Alison
was apparently a different person. She was instantly calmed and
entranced by all the goings on – the singing, the incense, the icons, the
embroidered brocade vestments, the gleaming gilt candlesticks and
lecterns – which Andrew fondly refers to as "the smells and bells,"
the more theatrical aspects of traditional Orthodox liturgy. Soon
Andrew began to attend other services in the week, and increasingly
saw his caregiving responsibilities in the framework of an emerging
awareness of faith. This drift in his thinking was not new. In Peru,
for example, immersed in development programming, he frequently
partnered with religiously observant individuals and Christian-based
communities who were inspired by the liberation theology of the time.

In keeping with his experience abroad, when he returned to Toronto
to look after his parents Andrew found consolation in religion, and
joined forces with a group of care providers – the nascent ASMT
that, unbeknownst to many, was instigated by clinicians. In the early
1990s Andrew became a member of the ASMT and, later, served on
the board. In the second half of the chapter I turn to Andrew's engagement with the ASMT, using his experience with the local branch as a
point of departure to chart the rise of the little known, yet immensely
important, history of this Canadian national organization.

In Canada, as in the United States, the biomedical characterizations
of Alzheimer's disease provided the foundation for the emergence
of a social movement dedicated to the eradication of the disease. In
the wake of the deinstitutionalization movement, sufferers and care
providers in Canada primarily relied on each other to formulate ethical strategies for coping with cognitive impairment. The Alzheimer
Society of Canada sprang from this endeavour; as the Society's website proudly declaims, "It was the first organization of its kind in the
world" ("Milestones"). Although the ASC's more practical approach
to Alzheimer's conceived of the illness as an unequivocal evil, the
organization, particularly in its early days, put less emphasis on finding a cure and more on the care afforded to people struggling with
cognitive decline.

SECTION I: ORDINARY ETHICS

When he was in his mid-thirties Andrew received a letter from his
ailing father, asking him to come home. After he returned from Peru,

his father suddenly died from a heart attack. The stricken family was tasked with coming up with a plan for Alison since there was no prior care arrangement for her. Initially, as a care provider, Andrew was often out of his depth. At night, he had taken to sleeping on his father's side of the bed so as to reassure his mother that she was not alone. By sleeping beside her, he could calm her restlessness and prevent her from getting up and wandering away in the night.

His mother had always been a good sleeper, but she snored. One night, she fell asleep but her snoring kept Andrew awake. At a certain point he reached over and put his hand over her mouth to quiet her, but the snoring continued. He tried turning her over, first to on one side, then the other. He even pinched her nose shut. Each time, she would cough lightly, take one or two breaths, only to resume snoring loudly a moment later. Finally, sleep deprived and unable to stand the noise any longer, Andrew pulled his mother's pillow out from under her head and placed it firmly over her open mouth. It worked: she stopped snoring. But he pulled back in horror, thinking: "I have just tried to kill my mother." Jumping out of bed, he raced out of her room, locked the door, and went to sleep in another room. When he tiptoed into her bedroom the next morning, she was sleeping soundly. After he roused her and started their daily routine, it dawned on him that her illness had progressed far beyond his capacity to care for her.

After breakfast, he looked up the number for the Alzheimer Society of Canada and called them. As soon as he heard the woman from their telephone counseling service ask, "How can I help you?" Andrew blurted: "I think that I tried to kill my mother last night! I need help!" There was a pause before she gently enquired, "Is your Mom OK now?" When he responded in the affirmative, she invited him to outline his predicament. After hearing his story, she reassured him: "Your Mom is just fine. You're doing the very best you can. You're just stressed out." She went on to explain what he could do for himself and for his mother. As Andrew recalls, all it took was a single phone call, and he felt able to resume his role as a caregiver.[4] Whereas in conversation Andrew tends to recount these and other instances as darkly comical events, we will see that in his fictional adaptation Michael portrays these same events as unequivocally Gothic trials. As their diverse perspectives illustrate, the use of different narrative genres changes the meaning and the affective nature of one's experience of dementia.

Far from minimizing the challenges involved in caring for his mother, Andrew repeatedly admitted his fear that as her illness progressed he would not be able to go where it threatened to lead them. When Alison received the definitive diagnosis of Alzheimer's, it dawned on Andrew how much of his persona was wrapped up in her identity and their relationship. He thought to himself: "When she can't remember my name, or doesn't recognize me, I'll just die; when she becomes incontinent, I will die of shame." Though she always recognized Andrew, she soon forgot his name and lost any understanding of their relationship, a fact of life that receded in importance in the day-to-day effort of caring for his mother. As for incontinence, it passed almost unperceived by either of them. As Andrew recalls: "We were out for our afternoon walk when Alison let out a soft squeak. We stopped and we both looked down at the sidewalk where her urine fell and a stain began to spread. 'Well,' I said, 'I think that we've had enough walking for today. Let's go home.' As we hastened back home, I said, 'Guess, what, mom? For a treat when we get home, I'm going to give you a nice hot shower, towel you down, and then we get to choose a whole new outfit.' It wasn't till much later, when I was lying in bed wide awake, mulling over the day, that it dawned on me my mother had just passed a major milestone on the downward road of AD. We had passed it together."[5] As this episode suggests, in caring for his mother Andrew strove to view her illness "as a part of daily life," to borrow his words, and to maintain a sense of her "personhood" at all times. Maintaining this perspective was hard because, as Andrew admitted, "as a caregiver, you're obsessed with what's been lost."

When we first met, Andrew recounted the story of a transformative visit from an old family friend, who for privacy's sake he referred to as Uncle Jack. Alison and Jack were friends of long standing, their bond forged by a shared grief from wartime London. Over the years, their friendship had grown to include respective spouses and children. Shortly before Alison's death, Jack called to say he was determined to see her one last time. Andrew tried to dissuade him, telling him to hold on to his memories of her rather than visit, as she was now infirm, unable to speak coherently, and seemingly had no memory of anyone or anything. But Jack was determined to make the journey and to see her at all costs. As Andrew dressed his mother, combed her hair, and put on her makeup in preparation for their reunion, she was completely unresponsive. She was equally impassive listening to Andrew's cheerful monologue concerning their visitor: the mention of Jack's name, the anecdotes concerning Jack and his family, and even Andrew's own excitement at the prospect of seeing their dear friend had no impact. The moment Andrew escorted Alison through the door, however, her eyes shone with recognition. She made her way across the room as fast as her legs could carry her and fell into his arms. They sat on the couch, side by side, with their hands on each other's knee or with their arms draped over each other's shoulder. Alison smiled, laughed, and burbled incomprehensibly while Jack shouted – he was stone deaf – the latest news of his family and recounted episodes from the long years of friendship. Afterwards, Andrew escorted Alison back to her room. Before departing, Jack turned to Andrew, saying, "You're far too pessimistic about your mother, you know. Ali was as marvelous as ever. And she's still as beautiful as she was when I first met her forty years ago." Despite everything Alison had lost, Jack still saw *her*. His parting words reassured Andrew that crucial aspects of his mother had, indeed, endured.

At my request, Andrew repeated this story in an email in June 2014. In thinking about how, in Munro's words, his mother's illness passed into "the telling," I am struck now by the complexity of the position of the narrator/witness in the story, a position in which, as listener, I was also implicated. As arts and age studies scholar Anne Basting observes, in the story of dementia conveyed in Hollywood movies such as *The Notebook* (2004), there is likewise "a sharp contrast between who the person *was then*, and who the person *is now*" (*Forget* 40). Basting explains further that these narratives typically climax "in a moment when the two worlds (then and now) come together to reach some sort of harmony" (40). More precisely, and in keeping with Andrew's story, the climax "is commonly a moment of sudden lucidity – in which a woman suddenly recognizes her husband" (40). Basting goes on to explain that this "can also be a "moment of clarity for the caregiver about his or her perspective on the disease" (40). In his story of his mother's reunion with Uncle Jack, Andrew implicitly portrayed himself as the one who was in doubt as to whether his mother's illness had irrevocably transformed her beyond recognition. It was Uncle Jack who assumed the authoritative position and insisted that Alison remained unchanged. In telling and repeating the story later via email, Andrew remained silent as to whether he wholeheartedly agreed with Uncle Jack. Simply put, it was Jack, rather than Andrew, who adopted the position of certainty. In contrast to the Hollywood script, Andrew and the listener (in this case, myself) were left in an indeterminate position – the uneasy, doubtful space of ordinary ethics.

In his conversations with me, Andrew frankly discussed the ethical complexities of caring for his mother. As he explained: "A caregiver must make all the decisions based on a deep sense of the other's need. You really need to know them. In caring for my mother, I was the custodian of her memory."[6] In addition to championing what scholars now term "patient-centered care," Andrew also vociferously resists the medical view of people with Alzheimer's as "victims." Instead he sees them as "heroes." When I asked "Why heroes?," he explained that Alzheimer's "is the absolutely worst thing that can happen to a person and her family. The person doesn't know you're there." His perspective here, like that of the narrator in *Scar Tissue*, reflects the Gothic view of the disease. Wiping out a loved one's memories and sense of connection to kith and kin, Alzheimer's gives the lie to John Donne's famous injunction, "No man is an island." For Andrew, caregivers and sufferers alike are heroes because together they must work tirelessly to rebuild interpersonal bridges.

In his role as the custodian of his mother's memory, Andrew drew particular strength from evening prayer, which in the services that he attended, included the *Nunc Demittis*, The Orthodox Prayer of St Simeon:

> Lord, now lettest thou thy servant depart in peace according
>   to thy word.
> For mine eyes have seen thy salvation,
> Which thou hast prepared before the face of all people;
> To be a light to lighten the Gentiles and to be the glory of thy
>   people, Israel.[7]

This prayer resonated deeply because it evoked personal and communal experience. On the one hand, it consoled Andrew as a caregiver with parents preparing to leave the world. On the other hand, it also spoke to communal memory because it was given particular mention in the story of his father's family's flight from Russia during the revolution. In reciting this prayer, Andrew explained that he felt part of a community: "I was no longer alone, no longer isolated in caring for my mother." Ultimately, although there were "no fully satisfactory answers to many of the questions posed" by his parents' lives and deaths, Andrew's growing faith provided him with a framework for coming to terms with their illness and making decisions on their behalf.

In Andrew's case, deriving consolation from religion and teaming up with the Alzheimer Society of Canada were essential to his ability to care for his mother; he was on the board of the ASMT from 1990–95. As he wrote: "When I got involved in the Toronto Chapter of the Alzheimer Society in 1990, I had the feeling that we were close to ground zero, that we were making it up as we went along, that the moment of creation was within the volunteer commitment of many of the people around the table, like me – family members who had survived the Alzheimer experience and knew what was necessary to support the person and their family and caregivers as they made their way through this unknown land."[8] Surprisingly, no one has written the history of this remarkable organization, making it yet another chapter in the story of Alzheimer's disease that has been forgotten. To remedy this oversight, in the following sections of this chapter, I offer an overview of the development of the Alzheimer Society of Canada. Unfortunately, like many grassroots organizations, there is no official archive. What follows is thus not a scholarly medical history, but instead an account based on a series of interviews conducted via email and in person with Andrew Ignatieff and Lori Dessau, two of the founding members.

SECTION II: ORDINARY HEROES: THE FOUNDING OF THE ALZHEIMER SOCIETY OF CANADA
PART I: THE HEARTBREAKING NEWS

In 1977, Lori Dessau, a young social worker with a BA in Sociology, was hired as a research assistant on a three-month contract for Dr Arthur Dalton, a psychologist doing research on people with Down syndrome. Dalton's research partner, the neurologist Dr Don McLachlan, was investigating Alzheimer's disease. Both Dalton and McLachlan worked at Surrey Place, a community clinic established by the University of Toronto's Department of Psychiatry for people with developmental disabilities. They recognized that adults with Down syndrome who came to autopsy after the age of forty showed all the signs of suffering from what was then a little-known illness – Alzheimer's disease. More precisely, the characteristic tangles and plaques of Alzheimer's disease marked the brains of adults with Down syndrome. "They were the only group," Lori explains, "that we knew for sure – 90% sure – if they lived long enough would show the signs of AD. But we didn't know why."[9]

In effect, it was predominantly the study of Alzheimer's disease in individuals with Down syndrome in the late 1970s that led to the development of a key hypothesis concerning the role played by amyloid – the protein responsible for the formation of unhealthy plaques in the brain (Dalton and Wallace 2). For people with Down syndrome, "cognitive decline – in the form of pre-senile dementia such as Alzheimer's – features commonly" (Wright 8). Dalton's and McLachlan's clinical research at Surrey Place confirmed what caregivers in the L'Arche communities had been observing for several years.[10] In L'Arche communities, adults with developmental disabilities live and work together with their caregivers. As Lori explained, before institutions like Surrey Place and L'Arche communities existed, "people with Down syndrome didn't used to live that long. Typically, they would die of other diseases." Workers at L'Arche saw that when their patients reached approximately forty years old, "they didn't recognize their workers. They didn't remember what they were supposed to be doing." No one wholly understood what was happening, but as Dalton's and McLachlan's research confirmed, they were showing signs of Alzheimer's disease.

The 1950s and 1960s saw the birth of clinical genetics – a paradigm shift that transformed how medical conditions were viewed and understood. Trisomy 21 (the addition of an extra chromosome) was discovered in 1959 as the genetic cause of Down syndrome (Dalton and Wallace 3). But the connection between Down syndrome and Alzheimer's could only have happened in the 1970s. As Dalton observes, thanks to the deinstitutionalization movement, starting in the 1960s people with intellectual disabilities were "increasingly more visible as they moved from institutional to supported community group homes" (3). With the general improvement in living and social conditions associated with places such as L'Arche and others, "life expectancy improved" (3). By the late 1980s the lifespan of people with Down syndrome increased "from nine years at the middle of the last century to at least middle age and older" (3). At bottom, the connection between Down syndrome and Alzheimer's is based on the fact that people with Down syndrome inherit a third copy of chromosome 21, giving them an extra helping of a gene that makes amyloid precursor protein, or APP, which is linked to the production of plaques in the brains of Alzheimer's patients. Nowadays scientists understand that virtually all individuals with Down syndrome "develop Alzheimer's disease neuropathology by the 4th decade of life" (Geller and Potter 167).

In the post-Second World War era, associations advocating on behalf of children and adults with Down syndrome sprang up at the grassroots level, "most often the result of small groups of parents who sought out other families in similar situations for peer support" (Wright 147–8). As Dalton's and MacLachlan's work at Surrey Place attests, however, organizations sometimes partnered with universities to support research (ibid. 149). Although researchers and caregivers in L'Arche communities were making the connection between Down syndrome and Alzheimer's disease, it was Lori's job to break the news to the parents. "Here I was," Lori explained, "talking to parents of young children who were in infant stimulation programs, and parents who had fought forever to get their kid into a group home or a workshop or a work situation." Just when these beleaguered crusaders thought they could relax, Lori had to tell them that, if their child lived past forty or forty-five, it was likely they were going to start showing the symptoms of this illness called Alzheimer's disease. Their kids were going to start to lose their short-term memory and judgment. Although they had been fighting for group homes and work situations, these same parents now had to think about later in life, when they would not be there to care for their children. Who would look after them as adults when they had Down syndrome and dementia? "Imagine how difficult it was for treatment," Lori said. "How would you put someone who is 55 and has Down syndrome *and* Alzheimer's in a nursing home? I had to tell the parents that they were going to have to think of placing their kids elsewhere. It was crucial to give them the heartbreaking news because they had to start advocating immediately."[11]

Lori's job became even more challenging when McLachlan asked her to consider working with families of adults who did not have Down syndrome – people in their fifties and upwards who were showing signs of dementia. She recalled McLachlan saying, "There's nothing out there to help them … Absolutely nothing." McLachlan was concerned that he was offering families a diagnosis of a little-known disease at a time when it was still being labelled "presenile" or "senile" dementia, and viewed as a part of normal aging.[12] As David Shenk wrote:

> Medical schools in early and mid-twentieth century taught as gospel that there were two clearly distinct types of dementia, easily separated by the age of onset:
>
> *A disease* –
>
> A very rare disease afflicting people in their forties and fifties, characterized by plaques and tangles. Cause unknown.
>
> *Senile dementia* –
>
> A relatively common condition affecting the elderly (sixties and older), caused by cerebral arteriosclerosis.
>
> Senile dementia was not regarded as a disease, just an unfortunate side effect of getting old. (73–4)

As noted in previous chapters, during this period dementia among the aged was not considered a Gothic crime instigated by an evil disease. Instead it was understood as a given, and the elderly as a group were dismissed for their general weakness and moral failure to maintain health and well-being. Although in previous chapters I have outlined the limitations of the biomedical model, there were also important benefits. As Robert Katzman clearly understood, labelling age-related dementia a disease and folding it into the same disease that afflicted younger people – people who deserved attention, compassion, and medical help and resources – was a politically and economically empowering narrative move.

Given the prevailing view in North America in 1977, Art McLachlan was on the vanguard by labelling the cognitive and behavioural changes associated with dementia as distinct from normal aging – a separate set of syndromes and a disease called Alzheimer's. Although he was making the diagnosis, the general public and many physicians had never heard of the disease. The families McLachlan spoke with had lots of questions, but there was no support program in place for them. As well, McLachlan and Dalton urgently needed brain tissue donations for their own research; families had to agree to donate their loved ones' brains because the only sure way to diagnose Alzheimer's disease was post-mortem. That is why they asked Lori for her help.

PART II: "THIS IS TO HELP YOU WITH YOUR WORK"

At the time, Dalton and McLachlan were not entirely sure if care-givers would be interested in forming an organization. When Lori put out a notice for their first family meeting, as she explained, "we expected maybe 20 people, but 60 people showed up. We didn't have enough chairs." Every time they called a meeting, the attendance was overwhelming. That kept happening as more people spread the word. At the initial gatherings, Lori offered information about the symptoms and canvassed people to see if they would be interested in starting an organization. They knew they could not create anything viable unless they had family members involved.

One of the first people who came to the meetings and joined the initial steering committee was Marni Besser, whose father had Alzheimer's but had not been clearly diagnosed.[13] Besser later became the first president of the society after it was incorporated. Another key player was Dr Walter Lyons, head of social work at Baycrest Centre. His wife suffered from dementia. "They were an amazing couple," Lori recalled, "very dedicated to each other." Lyons generously offered to donate his expertise and lead family support groups, if Lori could get them organized. Lori recalled him saying, "When people call up to get information from you, ask them if they are interested. If you get ten people, we'll start a group. You just give me the time and the place and I'll show up." Lyons capably led the first family support groups, and later joined the Board of Directors.

Around the time of these initial meetings, award-winning journal-ist Hana Gartner, host of CBC's *Take 30*, interviewed Lori. Their brief interview galvanized people across Canada and the US. "I had five minutes," Lori recalled breathlessly, "probably less, to talk about this new disease that we were discovering, and what we were try-ing to do with this organization." After the show aired, Lori was inundated with letters from concerned listeners. "These were not information letters," Lori explained. "They were heartfelt ten page letters that read 'my husband has been ill, but everyone thought I was crazy.'" The letters were voicing the fundamental, everyday problems associated with coping with dementia, and mental illness in general.

Unlike physical ailments such as the flu or a broken leg, mental illness is most often invisible. In the case of Alzheimer's, the disease is what "doctors call a disease of 'insidious onset,' by which they mean that it has no definitive starting point. The plaques and tangles proliferate so slowly – over decades, perhaps – and silently that their damage can be nearly impossible to detect until they have made considerable progress" (Shenk 32). It drifts from "one stage to the next in a slow-motion haze" (34). As a result, it is notoriously difficult for people not directly affected (and, even in some cases, those who are) to grasp and accept its existence. On the outside, people coping with Alzheimer's look much the same. Although the changes occur gradually, these people's cognitive abilities decline and their judgment and behaviour can change profoundly. The average interval from diagnosis to death in Alzheimer's disease is currently eight years (40). Under these circumstances, the name "Alzheimer's disease" consolidated people's experience. The diagnostic language provided a powerful symbol that allowed formerly isolated individuals – men and women who had become islands unto themselves – to form a community whose members could support each other.

Since few people had heard of Alzheimer's disease in the 1970s, most were suspicious if someone suggested that their husband or wife needed to be put into a home. As one woman told Lori, "my husband's family thinks I'm brutal because I'm considering a nursing home for him and he's only 55 years old." Caregivers, who were making agonizing decisions with little or no support, were routinely treated with skepticism and distrust. People wondered if they were just trying to get their spouses out of the way. Were they after money? In many cases, when they went to their doctors they could not identify the problem, either.

As Lori explained, "I was giving credibility to all of these caregivers, when I told them on the radio, 'We've identified that you need to take your spouse to a neurologist because they could be suffering from Alzheimer's disease.'" Caregivers were immensely grateful. They could put a name to something that they knew was happening to their loved one. As David Shenk writes: "The disease name is public recognition of a shared affliction. The name says, THIS *is what you are suffering from. You are not alone. Others are suffering from the same thing.* The name also says, *We're going to fight this thing*" (79). For caregivers, the name Alzheimer's disease was profoundly reassuring. Naming a disease, Shenk asserts, "is tantamount to launching an assault against that disease" (ibid.; emphasis in original).

But, as I repeatedly noted in the previous chapters, naming does not merely bring caregivers together. In his discussion of the effect of the label "Down syndrome," David Wright offers insights applicable to the refashioning of Alzheimer's disease: "The very label of a disorder threatens to obscure our view of the individual and, indeed, most insidiously, affects the self-identity and behaviour of the persons themselves. In these situations, the danger is that individuals disappear in the powerful shadow of the medical syndrome" (15). Although many scholars, including Anne Basting, have addressed the stigma associated with Alzheimer's and dementia (*Forget* 25–30), historically, the label played and continues to play a very complex role.

For Lori and her team, the disease label in conjunction with her five minutes on air instigated the beginnings of what Shenk, cited above, described as an assault. More and more letters kept arriving. Some people had slipped a twenty-dollar bill into the envelope, saying, "This is to help you with your work." Within a brief period, there were over two hundred letters. Overwhelmed by the response, Lori asked herself, "What am I doing?" She finally took the correspondence and the money to Dalton and McLachlan. It was time to make a decision. "Here's the thing," she told them. "People are sending us cash and cheques. We either have to deposit them and set up an account and start an organization, or we have to send the money back."

From the start, Lori, Dalton, and McLachlan knew that whatever happened, "it was going to be big." The two researchers did not hesitate; they asked Lori to find out how to get a charitable organization incorporated. From their clinical practice and the responses that Lori was receiving from across Canada, they also knew that it was going to be "bigger than Toronto." From the beginning, the Steering Committee envisioned provincial chapters sprouting across the country. They wanted to make it easy for people in every province to access information and find support. Rather than force each chapter to apply for incorporation, they simplified the process by incorporating nationally. As Lori laughingly recalled: "I researched how to start a national charitable organization as though I were reading a recipe to bake apple pie." She interviewed people from other organizations such as Huntington's and ALS, and developed a model for what, in 1978, became federally incorporated as the Societé Alzheimer Society – a name chosen to accommodate both French and English potential members. As luck would have it, they were able to incorporate quickly; "it was easy back then." Shortly after the organization was formed in Canada – the first of its kind in the world – the US and Britain followed suit. As Mary Ann Chang, the President of the Alzheimer Society of Metropolitan Toronto (1982–85) wrote: "It is an exciting historical fact that all Alzheimer Societies in the Western world owe their beginning to an important event that took place in Toronto in 1977" (1).

Although incorporating was easy, Lori was still working out of "a little corner" in Dalton's office. After the Alzheimer Society incorporated, they opened a bank account with an initial deposit of one hundred dollars (Alzheimer Society of Canada, "Milestones"). When people called asking for information, Dalton, McLachlan, and Lori quickly made up information packages, stuffed them into envelopes, and mailed them out. As well, they urged people to start chapters in their own communities. Researchers from across Canada also heard about the society and were calling to get information packages and find out how they could access funds for their research. Lori fielded calls from scientists at Baycrest and McGill. They were asking "if we had a million dollars to support their research. Art [Dalton] and I would just look at each other. People thought as soon as we started that we were big. But we were basically a group of family members who formed a committee." "They gave me a title, Vice President," Lori said, "so I could be part of a burgeoning new organization." And it was an organization that was being pulled in different directions: patients and caregivers needed practical help and advice; researchers and clinicians wanted money to support basic research.

PART III: THE LOSS OF THE ORDINARY LIFE

From Dalton and McLachlan's initial recognition that children with Down syndrome were vulnerable to Alzheimer's disease to the formation of the national Alzheimer Society of Canada, families and caregivers provided the central raison d'être of the organization. It was in the initial meetings and through consultation with families that the Society developed its four key goals: education, support for families, research, and advocacy. "We were passionate about making support for families as important as research," Lori insisted, "so that resources would be in place while researchers sought for a cause and a cure."

The major challenge for the new organization was lack of awareness and information associated with dementia. Moreover, until Alzheimer's disease was recognized, it made no sense to list it as a cause of death. Thus at the time, when doctors stated the cause of death they listed the secondary causes, such as bronchial pneumonia, instead. Due to lack of public awareness, fundraising was very difficult. "It was a struggle," Lori recalled, "to get our first donations for an office and the infrastructure needed to help start chapters and spread the word. We made presentations to the Ministry of Health as well as to corporate funders and the general public." Indeed the disease was so little recognized that the letters they received were frequently "addressed to the 'Old Timers' Association."

In the 1970s, if dementia struck people under the age of sixty-five, it was typically misdiagnosed. When Rita Hayworth showed signs of forgetfulness at midlife, no one suspected she suffered from dementia. Given the negative view of aging, it was difficult if not impossible to believe that an old person's illness could afflict the young. Yet Hayworth began having trouble remembering her lines during the 1960s, while in her forties. The fact that Hayworth drank heavily at times complicated matters: "her fellow actors largely suspected alcohol as the cause. So did her doctors" (Learner). Like many families and victims coping with dementia, the overriding concern for the people in Hayworth's life was avoiding embarrassment and shame. As a result, her family, colleagues, and friends engaged in "extensive denial, continuing to book her for appearances and take her to parties" (ibid.). In the 1970s, Hayworth's mental status worsened considerably: "She experienced several distressing public spectacles. The worst was in 1976, when she became agitated on a plane trip to London, and photos of the disheveled actress were broadcast worldwide" (ibid.). In 1979, the cause of her illness was finally named: "The New York psychiatrist Ronald Fieve made a diagnosis of Alzheimer's … Two years later, the diagnosis was made public" (ibid.).

When the media cited Hayworth's cause of death as Alzheimer's, it was a watershed event. In May of 1987, her death made the headlines in the Montreal *Gazette* and the *Toronto Star*: "Rita Hayworth Dies at 68; 'Love Goddess' of '40s a Victim of Alzheimer's" (*Gazette*, 16 May 1987, H1). Journalists who wrote about her death followed up their stories with explanations of Alzheimer's disease and how people could obtain more information. Suddenly the public had an image in their mind of what the disease looked like – they had a face, and it belonged to Rita Hayworth, the beautiful and beloved pinup girl from the Second World War. Here was a figure who was as far from the typical vision of an abject "hag" as one could get. Hayworth was the first of many public figures, including Ronald Reagan, who shaped public awareness of dementia.

Four years after Hayworth's death in 1987, researchers unlocked the molecular structure of beta-amyloid, "the main component of plaques" (Shenk 143–4). On 15 September, 1983, the US House of Representatives passed a resolution declaring November national Alzheimer's disease month (Ballenger, *Self* 113). Three years later, in 1986, the tangles were also decoded (Shenk 144–5). In the early 1990s, much of the work "had shifted to molecular genetics," as researchers began to uncover the precise genetic links to Alzheimer's on the human genome (ibid. 150–1). Ultimately, they learned that "only 5 percent of Alzheimer's cases – most of them involving onset in middle age – are caused directly by a single gene" (ibid. 151). The causes of the other 95 per cent of cases are not as clear. Researchers now understand that Alzheimer's is a profoundly complex and multifactorial illness. Biomedicine's promise of salvation, which seemed imminent, has repeatedly proved highly elusive.

Prior to these paradigm-shifting discoveries in the late 1970s, the newly fledged Alzheimer Society of Canada and its supporters were doing the crucial work of disseminating information. People needed to understand the symptoms and the progression of the illness so that they could properly plan for patient care, treatment, and support. To create a workable, effective strategy to deal with an illness, families need to know what is happening and, equally important, what lies ahead. The support groups facilitated by Walter Lyons reflected the need for this type of basic, practical information about dementia. In the US Jaber F. Gubrium studied Alzheimer's groups and, as he explains, Alzheimer's disease only became "a widely shared framework for assigning personal meaning to the cognitive experiences of later life in the 1970s ... Narratively, what became a disease experience – as opposed to one of the natural facts of old age – provided a new framework for formulating stories about the experience in question" (196). It was also "the period in which the future of Alzheimer's disease was being formed at the level of everyday life" (182). The initial meetings in Toronto brought together people living with a spouse or a family member who had Alzheimer's disease. For the first time, they were all in the same place, and they were asking each other questions that inevitably began, as Lori recalled, "So what do you do when" and "how do you handle it if. " As Lori explained, total strangers soon became "emotional and social backups for each other." At these meetings, someone would typically share a problem: "What do you do when your husband helps you to prepare supper, eats the meal with you, helps you with the dishes, puts them away, then ten minutes later says, 'I'm hungry. When are we having supper?' How do you deal with the fact that he doesn't remember eating?" Another person would respond: "Oh, when my husband does that I just give him carrots and celery because if I say we just ate, he says, 'No, we didn't,' and we get into an argument, and he just gets angry, and feelings get hurt, and then I have to deal with that, too. So I give him carrots and celery, and he's not hungry anymore." Everyone listening to these exchanges was busily writing things down.

In the support groups Gubrium studied, there was also talk of recent and possible breakthroughs in research and treatment: "Facilitators and savvy participants made it a point to convey new information. Oddly enough, such new information might be combined with, or followed by, self-help discussions aimed at encouraging people to 'go it alone' – that is without the well-meant but useless interference of researchers and professionals. It was occasionally said that professionals knew little about the ordinary character of an affliction that had no cure. Pessimism was expressed about the possibility of a cure for what otherwise sounded much like the condition of the aging mind which was once simply called 'senility'" (183). In Lori's groups, another key topic was whether to keep loved ones at home or put them in nursing homes. "There aren't any rules," Lori explained during our interview, and "it's a mistake to think that you should keep the person at home." As she told me: "Sometimes I thought it was a disservice to make it seem as if the best thing were to keep them at home as long as possible, because it depended on what kind of network of support the person had at home. If you lived in a community or if you had family or if you had such strong support networks that you could have other people come in, then that was one thing. But that wasn't always the case." She recalled people saying to her: "As soon as he is incontinent, that's the turning point ... I can't deal with that."

Lori learned that everyone has a different turning point. For some people, it has to do with matters of safety; for instance, if their loved one starts wandering, they might not be able to cope with them at home any more. For others, it is when the illness progresses to the point that the person with dementia no longer recognizes them. Speaking of her husband, one woman confessed: "As long as he knows who I am, I can't put him in a home. But when he doesn't know who I am." Ultimately Lori discovered that it was not the number of supports that made the difference for caregivers, but how normal their lives could remain. She recalled reading a powerful study affirming that it was not the number of services at your disposal, but how ordinary your life could still feel that made it easier to cope with dementia. As Lori explained, in the late 1970s a lot of women were looking after their husbands, and they were crying and saying: "If I could only get out, go shopping, get to the hairdresser, get my nails done, then I could deal with this." For people caring for someone with dementia, normal life disappears. "Imagine you're going out shopping," Lori said, "and you tell your husband you're going, you'll be back soon. Five minutes later, he forgets what you've told him. You've already left, and he starts panicking: 'Where is she?' When you get back, he's upset, shouting: 'You didn't tell me you were going out.' You can't do it that way, so you try leaving him with someone else. But he doesn't know that person as well as he knows you, so he panics again." When you live with someone suffering from dementia, "everything has to be meticulously planned."

In addition to losing the daily routines that keep life familiar, the care provider's social life also begins to fray. "Maybe you used to play bridge with other couples," Lori explained, "but you can't play anymore because he can't remember the game. And other folks you know are threatened by mental illness, so they don't come to the house any longer." Lori recalls meeting the wife of a minister. He was a mild-mannered fellow, but due to the effects of dementia, he started cursing all the time. His wife was so embarrassed by the change in his personality that she stopped inviting company over. Sometimes the opposite shift happens: someone who was dominant and confident suddenly "trails behind you all the time, meekly following you everywhere you go." "What do you do," Lori asked, "when you have company over for dinner, and your husband appears at the top of the stairs stark naked. He forgot that he was supposed to put clothes on; he forgot what 'clothes' meant."

Taken together, Lori's experience with families dealing with Alzheimer's taught her two central lessons: first, more than anything else, people want to feel ordinary – an impulse that may well run counter to the increasing biomedical testing at memory clinics and technical nomenclature such as mild cognitive disorder (MCI) involved in tracing the progress of Alzheimer's disease. Second, coping is easier if one has a sense of humour. Referring to the previous scenario, for example, Lori insisted that the story does not have to end in embarrassment and shame. "You can educate people, prepare them, and then invite them over. If they understand and they're good friends, then when your husband shows up naked, everyone laughs, and you help him back to his room and put on some clothes. And the evening goes on." Humour and a sense of acceptance may well be at odds with viewing people suffering from Alzheimer's as victims of a dread disease.

Reflecting on the role she played in the formation of the Alzheimer Society of Canada, Lori recognized that she was part of a larger, over-arching set of social movements that shaped the 1960s and 1970s. Fuelled by the energy of civil rights activists and second-wave feminists – young people who fought the government and held consciousness-raising meetings – she believed they could change the world. It was an especially euphoric time for youth in Toronto, a period in which it surpassed Montreal as the nation's largest city and the centre for commerce and (arguably) culture (see G. Stewart). Toronto was also home to the infamous Rochdale College: the experimental, student-run, alternative educational institution and co-operative. Located at the southwest corner of Bloor and St George, Rochdale housed 840 people. In keeping with the spirit of L'Arche communities, Rochdale was a free university where students and teachers lived together and exchanged knowledge.

As a university student, Lori marched in front of the American consulate to protest against racism in southern Alabama and the war in Vietnam. "You had the feeling then," Lori mused, "that you could do incredible things and that you could really make a difference." In hindsight, it is clear that the activists associated with the Alzheimer Society felt that they were contributing to an organization whose mission was to help sufferers and caregivers. They had the heady sense that their voices and their desires were shaping the direction of the society.

As the foregoing account attests, Lori worked for a grassroots organization that placed an emphasis on care and maintaining daily life, and that relied on a non-hierarchical, non-professional support group for guidance. The balance between care and cure has now shifted, and research has emerged as a priority. In 2012, the Alzheimer Society of Canada awarded $3.4 million in research grants ("Highlights"). According to the mission statement, their current vision "is a world without Alzheimer's disease and other dementias" ("Vision").

On the surface these accomplishments and goals seem admirable. Yet as David Shenk and many others have observed, biomedical research for Alzheimer's disease, which has "no cure and not much in the way of treatment" (39), has become extremely lucrative. As a result, it is essential to consider carefully who actually benefits from the "war." Since the 1980s, for example, changes to US laws have enabled scientists to function as entrepreneurs. Many researchers work for, and profit from, multinational pharmaceutical companies. At a recent conference, one scientist explained: "An important subtext of these battles ... is that all of these scientists have patents on their discoveries. There's a lot of money at stake" (Shenk 157). As noted in the previous chapter, Glaxo Wellcome's researcher, Allen Roses, believes that the for-profit nature of current research "brings out the worst in some people ... And there is no field as bad as Alzheimer's" (in ibid. 187). Roses also accepts the fact that "information is withheld," however, and believes that the "ends justified the means" because he has faith that "the market" will "sort things out" (189). Reflecting on the role of the pharmaceutical industry, Anne Basting observes that it has played a profound role in influencing the media in the US, which due to its well-funded public relations department, portrays Alzheimer's as a "tragic story, in which science is the white knight" (*Forget* 38, 39).

To date, medical progress has provided the foundation for what Jay Olshansky describes as "unprecedented rates of survival into older age." Yet clinicians worry that with no cure in sight for Alzheimer's, biomedicine has merely extended "frailty time" – what epidemiologists refer to as a "prolongation of morbidity," in essence, the end stage of dementia. Reflecting on the changes affecting Canadians from the 1970s to the present, I have become increasingly concerned that the incredibly lucrative biomedical focus on Alzheimer's disease is potentially eclipsing the perspective and needs of families and caregivers. At the end of his brilliant and compassionate account of Alzheimer's disease in the US, which traces the biomedical debates with fascination and respect, David Shenk argues that senile dementia is "a condition specific to humans and as old as humanity that, like nothing else, acquaints us with life's richness by ever so gradually drawing down the curtains. Only through modern science has this poignancy been reduced to a plain horror, an utterly unhuman circumstance" (252) – a Gothic horror story. In the next chapter, I turn to Michael Ignatieff's novel *Scar Tissue* to trace the implications of viewing cognitive decline solely as a narrative of horror and despair.

7

Gothic and Apocalyptic Horror:
Michael Ignatieff's *Scar Tissue*

SECTION I: THE FAILURE OF DOCTRINES
AND DOCTORS: *SCAR TISSUE'S* MELANCHOLY BABY

As I argued in the previous chapters, the construction of Alzheimer's as a disease concept instigated a profound crisis mentality. In the late 1970s, the public was informed that rather than succumbing to dotage in their later years, their loved ones were being stalked by a mysterious disease. Crucially, the disease paradigm legitimized the interests of a group of elite researchers. As the analysis of Michael Ignatieff's novel *Scar Tissue* (1993) in this chapter demonstrates, however, the disease model often failed to provide solace to both sufferers of dementia and their caregivers. In Canada, government agencies began directing substantial funds to Alzheimer's in the early 1980s. From the 1980s to the 1990s, the Canadian media tracked research findings and the results of drug trials. From the 1980s onward, newspapers alerted the public about supposedly pathological substances associated with Alzheimer's, ranging from aluminum pots to tea to DDT.[1] The media also broadcast information about potential curatives, ranging from nicotine, to ginseng, to ginkgo, to Gila monster spit.[2] Likely because a cure has not been discovered the language used by reporters from 1980 to 2010 seems mind-numbingly repetitive: "scientists find," "researchers develop," "new hope for patients," "hope in Alzheimer's battle," "drug offers hope," "drug approved for clinical trials." Without fail, the media's optimistic pronouncements are followed by acknowledgements of failure: "hopes dim," "study fails to show," "test drug fails to slow," "vaccine removes plaque but not dementia," "ginkgo fails," "doubt cast on effectiveness and safety of drug," "drug a waste of money." In 2012, after two pharmaceutical companies, Pfizer and Johnson and Johnson, pulled the plug on intravenous drug treatment, calling it a failure, Gary Rotstein stated: "it has been a frustrating year – a depressing decade, in fact – for people hoping for breakthroughs in Alzheimer's research and treatment (E2). In contrast to its staccato account of the rise and fall of potential pharmaceutical cures, the media also published a stream of articles about the impact of Alzheimer's on families, caregivers, and the unceasing efforts of charitable organizations to raise money for research. Police alerts also regularly appeared about missing persons, followed several days later by news of the outcome: "Alzheimer victim found wandering the streets" or, in the worst case, "victim found dead."[3]

Set in this historical context, *Scar Tissue* offers the first-person account of a middle-aged philosophy professor who cares for his mother with Alzheimer's, and whose brother, a neurologist, remains physically and emotionally detached from her plight. As Marsha Lederman observed, "it is easy to assume that Michael Ignatieff was his mother's primary care provider"[4] when, as noted in the previous chapter, it was his younger brother, Andrew, who returned home to care for both his father and his mother until her death. The confusion is understandable because to a great extent, the narrator's experience follows that of Andrew rather than Michael.

For the purposes of my book, it is significant that *Scar Tissue* poignantly illustrates that when Alzheimer's emerged as a *disease* experience – as opposed to one of the natural facts of old age – it provided new confusing and frightening diagnostic identities for those concerned. As *Scar Tissue* illustrates, these new identities emerged within an overarching Gothic framework. In his fictional response to his mother's death, Michael incorporates fragments from religious, scientific, and classical narratives – most obviously, the myth of Oedipus – to create a Gothic novel that articulates the fear and rage generated by the "disease." In *Scar Tissue*, the narrator views the dementia that runs through his family as a curse akin to the one that plagued Oedipus and his descendants. As we will see, *Scar Tissue* highlights the ethical and existential dilemmas associated with a protracted historical moment in which Canadians found themselves caught between a waning faith in religious consolation and an as-yet-unrealized promise of a biomedical cure for dementia.

During the 1990s and in the decades that followed, a number of Canadian writers expressed this tension in their works. In Anne

Carson's essay "The Anthropology of Water" in *Plainwater* (1995), the narrator blends biomedical and religious narratives as she ponders her father's experience of dementia.[5] Similar tensions between science and religion are also apparent in Sandra Sabatini's short story collection *The One with the News* (2000). The final stories in the collection briefly address the limitations of both religious and biomedical narratives, as well as the pain that attends waiting helplessly for a cure for Alzheimer's.[6] Dreams of finding a cure for Alzheimer's are likewise central to Jeffrey Moore's *The Memory Artists* (2001).[7] In contrast to *The Memory Artists*, which ends with the discovery of a cure, *Scar Tissue*, like *The One with the News*, treats this desperately sought outcome as a deferred promise and emphasizes the longing for religious consolation.[8]

In *Scar Tissue* science is waging war against dementia but the narrator despairs that he will live to see a victory. Confounded by a disease he cannot master, he succumbs to depression. Leaving his wife and children, he ends up isolated and overcome by his obsession with the illness, which he perceives as a curse that threatens to claim him. Although the narrator draws on fragments of classical literature, religious rituals, and empirical, scientific research to assuage his fear of Alzheimer's disease, *Scar Tissue* portrays the devastating subjective and interpersonal impact of the shift from senility to Alzheimer's disease, and the failure of all the narratives cited above to offer consolation for the losses instigated by the emergence of Alzheimer's disease – a newly baptized, seemingly insurmountable force of evil.

On one level, Michael's account of his mother's struggle recalls Laurence's novel *The Stone Angel*, since both works graphically illustrate the characters' waning faith in religious consolation. But *Scar Tissue* portrays the additional existential anguish associated with the contemporary historical moment, which has pinned its hopes on science and, more precisely, on an as-yet-unrealized biomedical cure for dementia. As noted in the previous chapter, my aim in tracing the brothers' response to their mother's dementia lies in emphasizing their differing approaches: whereas Andrew, supported by religious faith, adopted an elegiac perspective and grappled with the impact of dementia on the level of everyday life, Michael adopted an imaginative, philosophical, and literary approach to explore the painful existential questions raised by Alzheimer's disease, which he categorized in no uncertain terms as an evil akin to original sin.

While working as a journalist in Europe, Michael Ignatieff published two autobiographical essays and one fictional account – *Scar Tissue* – dealing with his mother's battle with Alzheimer's. The essays appeared in the prestigious literary journal *Granta* – the first, "August in My Father's House," in 1984; the second, "Deficits," in 1989. In "August in My Father's House," Michael characterizes his mother as an outlier in a distinguished family: "a Toronto schoolmaster's daughter, squint-eyed and agile, next-to-youngest of four … the tomboy in a family of intellectuals" (39). Early on, the essay recounts an episode when his mother, at seven years old, sat at the dinner table, surrounded by her erudite, well-educated family. "Who remembers the opening of the Aeneid?" asked her father, the principal of Upper Canada College. Even though her brothers and sisters, Margaret, Charity, and George – who later achieved fame as a philosophy professor and the author of *Lament for a Nation* (1965) – were "all better scholars," Alison was the one who proudly and correctly recited the opening words to the poem in Latin (40).

In 1944, beautiful and independent-minded, Alison married George Ignatieff, the youngest of five sons from a noble Russian family. George's mother was Princess Natalia Nikolayevna Mescherskaya and his father was Count Paul Ignatieff, a close advisor to Tsar Nicholas II. In the early days, Alison pursued her love of painting, while George engaged in a successful career as a diplomat. Then the boys arrived: Michael was born in 1947, and Andrew in 1950. As a young man, Michael was fiercely devoted to his mother. In his early writings, Michael cast himself as the protector of his mother's precocious intellect and creative spirit – attributes that were already under threat by her patriarchal family long before she was diagnosed with Alzheimer's disease. At one point, Michael accused his father of allowing his career to take precedence and thwarting his mother's aspirations for herself: "I said to him, You have crushed her. She used to paint. Not any more. She has wishes for you and for me, but none for herself. Not anymore" ("August" 46). Although Michael raged at his father, an even greater tragedy struck the family when Alison's battle with dementia became evident in the early 1980s.

Speaking to journalist Sandra Martin about his decision to go public about her struggle with the disease, Michael said he felt "compelled to honour his mother's suffering in the best way he knew – by writing about it" (in Valpy). But what many viewed as a bold and courageous decision did not sit well with members of his mother's family, a family whose cardinal rule was "Never make a fuss" ("August" 40). Alison's sister Charity and her brother George, as well as his wife Sheila, reportedly "could never bring themselves to forgive Michael for having publicly exposed his intensely private mother" (Valpy). Alison died in 1992 and despite – or perhaps because of – the family's umbrage at Michael's violation of his mother's privacy, the following year he published *Scar Tissue*, his critically acclaimed *fictional* account of her illness. In effect, in writing about his mother's experience, Michael was renouncing the silence that typically shadows mental illness, and attempting to say "the unsayable" (Lambek, *Ordinary* 8).

In the novel, the narrator maintains that a new and confusing world order was instantiated by the medicalization of Alzheimer's disease. The following passage is worth citing in full because it clarifies the palpable confusion associated with the remaking of Alzheimer's disease at that time:

What in my childhood had been called "hardening of the arteries of the brain" was now called "premature senile dementia." The one was as absurd as the other. My mother was disturbed but she was anything but senile. Then the doctors took to calling her condition a disease. This at least had the merit of conferring clinical interest upon what, until then, had simply been regarded as the demented confusion of the elderly. When post-mortem examinations of the patients revealed a characteristic pattern of scar tissues in the neural fibers, doctors suddenly believed they had a clinical mystery to unravel.

However, the more that doctors discovered, the more puzzling the disease became. While the tangles and plaques – the scar tissue – did obstruct the neurochemical transmission of electrical messages in the brain, they showed up in alert people whose symptoms were confined to mild memory loss associated with normal ageing. Some experts weren't even sure whether the scars were a cause or a consequence of the forgetting. (54)

As noted in the introduction, the disease model instigated a shift away from elegiac modes of consolation and provided the foundation for a Gothic plot, installing a "clinical mystery," but one with no clear perpetrator or cause and effect. In this liminal space, Michael's narrator argues, the boundary between public and private is no longer clear: "No one knows any more what should be said and unsaid, what should be respected and kept in silence. No one knows any more what proprieties should attend a person's dying" (168). I argue further that this shift in public perception and etiquette was accompanied by a transformation in genre from elegy to Gothic. On every level, then, there were changes in the rules.

The confusion surrounding the disease also gave rise to powerful emotions that Michael chose to fictionalize, although he retained many of the autobiographical elements from the previous essays. As he explained, the novel was written in "a three-month burst" in the early 1990s, as he struggled with his mother's Alzheimer's and the death of his father in 1989: "It's one of the few times I've written something where I just had to get something out of my system ... One of the difficult aspects of this, and it's difficult even to talk about, is in its advanced stages, Alzheimer's feels like a kind of living death. Death is kind of in the room. It's present; you can feel its power. So a lot of what you write is a kind of struggle with the fear and anxiety that that presence creates in a family, and creates in your life" (in Lederman). In keeping with my book's aim of tracing the shift from elegy to the Gothic, it is significant that *Scar Tissue* is predicated on Michael's belief that he was engaged in a battle with a disease that felt, to him, like a literal embodiment of death. Equally important, and in keeping with the shift from elegy to Gothic, although *Scar Tissue*'s narrator turns to science, religious ritual, and even classical literature for consolation, he cannot ultimately allay the terror aroused by the disease.

In addition to installing Alzheimer's as a Gothic story, *Scar Tissue* underscores the failure of both religious and scientific narratives to console victims of this newly baptized dread disease. The novel signals its debt to religious and literary narratives with its opening epigraph: "So by this infirmity may I be perfected / by this completed. So in this darkness, / may I be clothed in light." Taken from John Milton's "Second Defence of the English People" (1653), the passage speaks of the Christian poet's blindness and desire for insight. In *Scar Tissue*, the epigraph likewise highlights the overarching desire to understand and be redeemed by suffering since it prefaces the narrator's opening account of an elderly woman's final, agonized moments of life; only later does he reveal that the woman is his mother. From the start, the nameless narrator informs readers that "the banal heartlessness" of his mother's death and his lack of insight into its deeper meaning instigated his quest for redemption – to find "some way back to the unscarred beginnings" (1).

On the one hand, the task he sets for himself to redeem her death and return to a more Edenic state recalls Milton's attempt to explain the ways of God to Man, a feat the latter undertook in his epic poem *Paradise Lost* (1667). In his poem, Milton offers a Christian account of the evil that "brought death into the World, and all our woe" (l.3). On the other hand, *Scar Tissue*'s narrator's task also echoes the Gothic quest of Victor Frankenstein, an infamous literary son who responds to maternal death by attempting to transcend mortality. Like Mary Shelley's hero, Ignatieff's protagonist turns to science in the hopes of achieving revelation and insight. In *Scar Tissue*, returning to the "unscarred beginnings" before death marred human existence paradoxically calls for an apocalyptic form of redemption through destruction – the evil must be exorcised and destroyed. At bottom, the narrator's goal, like that of Victor Frankenstein, lies in mastering rather than reconciling himself to his mother's dementing illness – the harbinger of her death and, potentially, his own. Taken together, the quotation from Milton along with more explicit references to Christianity and the novel's reliance on philosophical and biomedical accounts signal the narrator's pervasive, yet ultimately futile attempt to rely on literature, religion, and biomedicine for consolation. Even classical literature and the act of writing itself fail to allay the narrator's fear and rage at the losses he incurs.

In what might best be compared to a wasteland of broken master narratives that circulate in the novel, fragments of religious rituals repeatedly inform his obsession with mastering dementia. In an effort to console the narrator, who is clearly distraught with grief, his neurologist brother introduces the narrator to Moe, one of his patients afflicted with ALS who is a devout Christian and finds comfort in God's love. After listening to Moe's perspective, however, the narrator responds by confessing that he is "more of a rage rage type," alluding to Dylan Thomas's famous elegy for his father, "Do Not Go Gentle into that Good Night" (139). Later, he asserts that "it became obvious to me that I was one of those unfortunate people who happen to have a religious temperament without having a scintilla of religious belief" (174). In the narrator's case, his rage fuels a desire for a divine weapon powerful enough to defeat the threat, rather than an authentic belief in religious salvation. Although he ostensibly eschews religious doctrines, he admits that the extremes of religious life continue to draw him "like a magnet," particularly the rituals of "fasting, mortification and cleaning which all religions require of believers before they submit to god" (175).

Similarly, although he also claims not to benefit from science and the long-distance, dehumanizing gaze of biomedicine, the latter approach dovetails with his philosophical attempt to unveil the mystery of dementia. Refusing to live with the complexity of Alzheimer's, the narrator understandably seeks clarity. He finds modern science particularly seductive because it promises to render the body and, more precisely, the brain, transparent. As the narrator confesses, the "dream of the transparent body, of seeing inside yourself, has always been the fantastic underside of the official history" of the modern self (193). Toward the novel's conclusion, the narrator recalls the dizzying sense of power he experienced when, during an operation on his kidney, he first saw the insides of his own body projected on a TV screen: "this was who I really was, just this urging pulse, this shape of bones, and the particular fate that had made my kidney fail. All this and on live TV! This was narcissism with a capital N. I had become the Visible Man" (194). Although he recognizes both the artifice and the narcissism inherent in such an interpretation of this technological projection of his image, he confesses that he yearns for the same knowledge concerning Alzheimer's disease and the fate of his brain: "I long to know, to be certain, to be face to face with the thing itself. I long to see the pathways of my own brain. My brother is right. No antidote to fear compares with knowledge" (194).

Yet just as religion fails to eradicate the threat, science also cannot deliver on its promise to solve the mystery at the heart of Alzheimer's disease. As the narrator explains, he distrusts biomedicine both due to its dehumanizing paternalism and because, to date, science lacks the power to resolve the mystery of dementia and thereby alter his family's fate. Unlike his brother, who gains comfort from the belief that the answers "will surrender themselves eventually," and that science will ultimately find a cure, the narrator cannot sustain himself with deferred hope. Citing Kafka, he states: "there is hope, but not for us. It will come too late for me" (194). The narrator's inability to find consolation in either religious or scientific narratives is exacerbated by his fear of his own supposedly tainted genetics. He clings to this fear despite rational reasons to believe that he is not fated to succumb to dementia. Far from an idiosyncratic response, the narrator's preoccupation with the genetic basis of Alzheimer's disease – a basis which, as his brother insists, is highly complex and not a factor in the majority of cases (6) – petrifies him and narrows his sense of himself to that of a diseased body to the exclusion of all of his other social roles. In the end he views himself solely as the progeny of a diseased mother, and the next target of the familial curse.

The narrator concludes his memoir with a melancholy show of embracing his fate as the next victim of Alzheimer's disease – a tactic that strikes me as a vestige of his earlier reliance on fragments of religious discourse to offer a framework for understanding evil. Echoing the biblical Fall, which places the blame squarely on Eve, the narrator traces the illness along the maternal line. In keeping with his earlier allusion to Milton, the narrator recalls the structure of the book of Genesis when he maps the genealogy of his mother's dementing illness. As he explains, according to family legend, dementia was passed from his great grandmother, Annie MacDonald, to his grandmother, Nettie, to his mother. He concludes his genealogy by positioning himself as the nth Adam – the bearer of Eve's sin – and by confessing his fear that he will be Alzheimer's next target. Surprisingly, in his first autobiographical account, he reputedly told his mother that he does not "believe these things run in the family" ("August" 48). Clearly, he changes his mind. As noted, however, the novel is characterized by a melancholy oscillation that bears witness to the narrator's incomplete faith in both religion and biomedicine.

Rather than wholly accept the illness as God's will and thus part of the divine plan, the narrator turns away from religion toward science. Again, this shift is in keeping with broader social trends. In the case of Ignatieff's narrator, the turn toward science enables him to conceive of his mother's fate as a violation of normal aging and thus a Gothic crime that he personally must resolve. From the start, both the classical image of fate and the Judeo-Christian notion of a loving but inscrutable God are juxtaposed to a secular and mechanistic model of biological inheritance that highlights the criminal nature of Alzheimer's disease.

For the narrator, fate is a gun, and the villain – genetics – pulls the trigger (6). Contemplating the bullet's trajectory toward his own vulnerable flesh, the narrator links his current terror to the fear and dread he experienced as a child at his maternal grandmother Nettie's funeral. As he says, "I've always thought of that moment at Nettie's funeral as the instant my childhood ended. It was as if I discovered, in my innocence, that there was such a thing as fate and that it could take a life and dismember it" (5). Later, he explicitly cites Sontag's views concerning illness and fear to probe the basis of his own terror. Drawing on Sontag, he observes that diseases "whose cures have been found become mere diseases; those we do not yet understand become metaphorical carriers of everything we fear and loathe" (66–7). For the narrator, the disease is not simply a source of terror. In this respect it differs from earlier scourges such as tuberculosis and polio. The terror of his mother's dementing illness springs from his dreadful anticipation that the disease will affect him directly. His response attests to the fact that, as noted in the previous chapter, the disease paradigm instigated a profound "crisis mentality," which gave the concerned "much more to worry about" (Gubrium 200).

SECTION II: SCIENCE AND THE DEHUMANIZING GAZE

As noted above, the narrator critiques science's tendency to infantilize patients as well as its inability to overcome its habit of finding cures only after diseases have taken the lives of scores of innocent victims. Yet, by participating in the scientific narrative that views Alzheimer's as a disease – a threat and a problem to be solved – *Scar Tissue* both illustrates and remains complicit with the ramifications of this shift, namely, a seemingly inescapable tendency to reduce human beings to objects of scientific scrutiny. In addition to relying on humanists such as Sontag in an effort to master his fear, the narrator ponders his tendency to adopt a dissociated, scientific approach to Alzheimer's. Again recalling his response to his grandmother Nettie, he muses: "I can remember wondering even then why I felt merely distant and curious. This must have been the first time I turned something I at first found fearful into something interesting" (5). Far from an idio-syncratic response to the newly coined Alzheimer's disease, his trans-formation of a dreadful mystery into an object of scientific scrutiny characterizes the socially pervasive shift in North America from the late 1970s to the early 1990s. To a great extent, North American society has become tremendously "interested" in brain health and in diseases of the brain.

Scar Tissue's value as a cultural document lies in the fact that it does not suggest that we can discover the "right" way to face the truth of mortality and loss. As the narrator realizes, scientific models have pitfalls, but so do literary and religious models. Equally important,

every approach depends on imagination and storytelling, and none
is patently superior as a mode of experiencing reality or dealing with
our mortality. Equally crucial, rather than merely highlight the shift
toward the Gothic, the narrative also reveals elided aspects of the
disease paradigm. For example, the novel repeatedly portrays physicians who scrutinize the mother's brain while effacing her humanity.
When the family first gathers in the doctor's office for a diagnosis,
the narrator reports that the doctor, a "big specialist in the city" (54),
looks at "Mother's PET scans and sees a disease of memory function,
with a stable name and a clear prognosis. I see an illness of selfhood,
without a name or even a clear cause" (56). The narrator is horrified
when the doctor softly utters the prognosis, telling his father: "Your
wife will be dead in three years" (57). Before the family leaves, the
doctor explains to the father that she wants to include his wife in
her study: "The clinical picture she presents will be of great interest
to us" (61). Touching a form with "a red fingernail," she asks him
to sign the consent form. When he asks, "Consent for what?" she
replied, "To allow us to remove her brain following autopsy for special study here at the clinic" (61). The chapter ends with the father's
wordless gesture: "He picks the paper off the desk and flicks it back
at her with a brisk gesture of contempt. Then he strides out of the
room" (61). Whereas the doctor's interest lies in "the clinical picture," which rests on obtaining a brain sample after the patient dies,
the narrator's father remains aligned with his wife, as a living person
deserving of respect.

   Despite their best efforts to maintain a sense of the mother's unique,
human identity and their kinship roles, even the narrator's brother,
a neuropathologist, admits that in his eyes, his mother is "like a lab
experiment" (125). After his marriage breaks down, the narrator visits his brother, who runs a lab at a US teaching hospital. Standing side
by side, the narrator and his brother take turns looking down the eye-
piece of an electron microscope at cells on a glass slide from "the temporal lobe of a patient in her late sixties" (129). Afterwards, they gaze
at the same patient's DNA scan. Pointing to row six, his brother identifies "the defect on the middle arm of chromosome 21" (130). The
narrator remarks on his brother's methodical, neutral voice, which
makes him sound like a stranger. Touching the DNA scan, his brother
comments that "being a neuropathologist is like joining a pool game
in the middle" (130). His final comment, "This is how we find the first
shot" (310), recalls the narrator's initial metaphor of fate as a bullet

fired by genetics. Equally important and in keeping with the novel's emphasis on detachment, the narrator withholds the fact that the patient whose images and DNA are being scrutinized is their mother. What begins, then, as his attempt to redeem his mother's senseless death and tell her story, inevitably also includes the partial erasure of her subjectivity instigated by the disease model. As the passages above indicate, in *Scar Tissue*, the narrator's difficulty in maintaining a sense of his mother's humanity is exacerbated by the scientific protocols and institutions that deny her a proper name and a respectful death. As he explains: "Certainly no proprieties were observed in the place where she died. Nurses at the end of their shift walked to and fro, smoking cigarettes. In the next bed, behind the green curtain, another person coughed and sighed. There was even comedy of a sort, when a keen young intern entered the room and asked whether we thought some morphine might be appropriate, and my brother managed a dry, wise laugh and said, 'I think my mother has just died'" (169). Although the narrator protests against the dehumanizing facets of her treatment in the institution, like so many frightened and grieving individuals in his position, he, too, is frequently unable to see his mother for the disease. As noted earlier, he repeatedly conflates his mother and, indeed, all of the matriarchal figures in his family, with the dreaded illness itself. The Gothic repercussions of this type of reductive thinking are strikingly apparent when the narrator lies in bed with his mother to prevent her from wandering at night. This scene was drawn from his brother Andrew's experience, cited in the previous chapter. While she sleeps, he muses that fragments of his infantile, pre-verbal identity are locked within the cells of her deteriorating brain. "She is the silent custodian of the shadow zone of my own life. She is the only one who can tell me what I was like before I began to remember, the only one who can decipher those first senseless scenes when memory begins" (50). When she falls asleep, however, a murderous impulse threatens to overtake him: "How easily, how mercifully, how quickly it could all be done. One pillow held over her face for long enough. There is no one to stop me, no one to know. Two minutes is all, and enough pressure. No one would blame me. I am sure I could manage it if I did not have to see her eyes staring up into mine. I lie there debating whether I have the right to save her, whether I have what it takes ... Then I realize she is not sleeping but awake beside me, as if she had been listening to my innermost thoughts. Her face against the pillow is like Nettie's now" (51). In his eyes, his mother is losing the battle against the disease, which he views as a living death. To borrow Michael Ignatieff's earlier comment, Death "is in the room" (in Lederman). He views actual death, what he calls "saving her," as more merciful than what he imagines she is experiencing.

Although in this instance, the narrator resists his violent impulse, his ambivalence toward his mother – who in his mind is simultaneously a beloved individual and both a transmitter and a victim of disease – continues to haunt him. At one point, the narrator considers telling his brother about the night when he imagined taking his mother's life: "I wanted to confess the shame of that to someone, to unburden myself of that memory and the rage it contained. Then, just as quickly as those feelings came over me again, I found myself thinking how absurd they were. Why had I ever wanted to do such a thing? Her awareness, that fragile and damaged thing, suddenly seemed infinitely precious to me, like a painted egg I might have crushed in my hands and now saw for the thing that it was" (144). Although he aims to protect his mother, in the wake of his refashioning of Alzheimer's as a heritable illness, the mother's identity has already irrevocably fractured into a someone "infinitely precious" and the transmitter of an evil disease.

Due perhaps to the magnitude of his panic about inheriting the disease, we never gain a clear sense of what the illness means to her. Early on, the narrator signals his overarching tendency to view his mother as his mirror – the keeper of his memories and hence his own identity and fate, rather than her own. Readers learn, for example, that when he was fourteen, his mother painted his portrait: "We had struck a bargain ... I would have her all to myself for a week. In return, I had to surrender to her scrutiny. I had to give myself to her without reserve. That was the deal. And of what she had seen, she would reveal only what she chose to depict" (14). After two weeks, she produces an image that offers him profound insight into his character – insight that remains valuable to him throughout his life: "In her picture, I get to see myself through her eyes, and I think that it takes me about as deep into myself as I am ever likely to go ... I find it strange that forty years on I have changed so little. All the cells in my body have been replaced a number of times, and I have had a life. Nevertheless I remain what I was when she painted me" (17).[9] In contrast to the mother's portrait of him, his memoir charting her illness – which likewise requires her to surrender to his scrutiny – paradoxically reveals very little about her. Instead *Scar Tissue* powerfully demonstrates how the mysterious, Gothic disease leaves him petrified and trapped in the role of a traumatized son.

To convey the power of his rage, fear, and survivor's guilt, the narrator repeatedly invokes the story of Oedipus, the mythical King of Thebes. In the classical story, Oedipus unwittingly murders his father and marries his mother, inflicting a curse upon the entire city. The curse is only lifted when Oedipus recognizes his crimes and blinds himself. Michael Ignatieff first drew on the Oedipus myth in "August in My Father's House," which opens and closes with both implicit and explicit allusions to the tragic story. The essay begins with an account of the tempestuous origins of his parents' home in Provence that highlights the seemingly universal battle between fathers and sons. As Michael explains, his parents' farmhouse once belonged to a "retarded" shepherd boy and his abusive father. One night, "crazed by his father's beatings," the son rose behind his father and smashed in his skull. Afterwards, the horrified townspeople took the boy away and buried the father, but the house "fell into ruin, marked in the village memory by the stain of parricide" (39). In this way, the essay foregrounds the devastating impact of both cognitive impairment, portrayed as a patricidal "feeble-minded" child – a figure which, as I explain in subsequent chapters, haunted the social imaginary during the first half of the twentieth century – and Oedipal rage in its opening paragraphs. But the conclusion offers an even more explicit reference to the myth of the tragic King of Thebes. In the closing paragraphs Michael relates how he and his wife drove to the next village where a theatre troupe was staging *Oedipus* on a tiny stage built into the sandstone cliffs at the foot of the village: "Oedipus and Jocasta circle each other slowly against the towering folds of sandstone: the eternal story unfolds in the night air. Oedipus turns his bleeding eyes upon us: 'Remember me, and you will never lose your happiness.'" Hearing these words, Michael recounts how a five-year-old boy, seated between his father and mother in the audience, rocked "backward and forwards on his seat" and said to himself "in a small voice, 'Now I understand everything'" (48).

Michael Ignatieff's ongoing reliance on the myth reinforces his desire to understand suffering using age-old tools – the power of myths to offer understanding and consolation. Over the ages myths have provided a narrative armature that can bear the weight of profoundly devastating emotions. But Michael's invocation of the Oedipus myth also belies a desire to universalize and elevate suffering by aligning it with a divine curse in a royal family. The narrative may also offer a means to justify the narrator's inability to move beyond the role of his parents' immensely gifted, yet cursed son.

In *Scar Tissue*, the Oedipal nature of the familial conflict is underscored by the fact that many of the scenes are drawn from the original autobiographical essay. Moreover with few exceptions all of the central characters, including the narrator, are referred to in terms of their kinship roles rather than their first names, enhancing the reader's tendency to conflate the author with the narrator. Readers also never learn the given names of the narrator, his father, his mother, his brother, or the narrator's wife.

In keeping with the emotional palate of "August in my Father's House," in *Scar Tissue* the narrator's desire for his mother and hatred for the father colour the entire novel. Early on, the narrator admits that all his life, he vied for his mother's attention. From the start he confesses to the ongoing rivalry between himself, his father, and his brother – "three men all competing, mostly for her [his mother's] favour" (25). He maintains that fighting with his father gave him proof that he was something "more than a son. Yet a son I have remained" (25). Even though after his father dies the narrator realizes it is time he fully embraced his role as a parent of two children, his mother's illness triggers both his separation anxiety and regression. At one point, prior to his divorce, the narrator accuses his wife of secretly condemning him for having "never grown up," for being forty-five years old, yet "still tied hand and foot to the pair of them ... Even though one is dead and the other might as well be" (106). In this enraged monologue, he continues to betray his Oedipal obsession. "Ever since I can remember you've been thinking, 'Why the hell doesn't he stand up to them? Why does he let them walk all over him? Why does he clean up after every goddamned one of them?'" (107). As these passages illustrate, the narrator berates himself for never moving beyond the role of "a son" and fully embracing additional adult roles.

The destruction of his identity is perhaps best illustrated when his mother's disease clearly takes hold and makes it impossible for her to communicate verbally. At one point, the narrator again encourages her to draw his portrait. Initially, she complies and he fantasizes again that he can see himself within her: "It was as if she were suddenly a transparent figure and I could see within her to the secret chemistry of art, to the neurological impulses that had made her able to paint, as no one else ever had, the true likeness of myself" (152).

On this occasion, however, his mother fails to complete his portrait, and he comments on the rupture of their mutually constitutive identities: "There was no way to tell that the person depicted was a son and the artist his mother. There was a disconnection between her and me and between her hand and herself" (152). For the narrator, the break in the intersubjective bond instigates powerful Oedipal fantasies of a return to dyadic oneness – fantasies predicated on the collapse of the difference between self and other.

SECTION III: ALZHEIMER'S, DEPRESSION, AND MELANCHOLIC DESTRUCTION

The narrator's fantasies of oneness are linked to his depression – a depression triggered, in part, by the "spoiling" of their mutual identities exacerbated by the introduction of a Gothic disease model (see Goffman). To this disease, figured as a mythic curse, the narrator attributes a host of ongoing losses that he and his family endure – losses for which he can find no lasting consolation in religious, scientific, or literary narratives. I invoke the terms "oneness" and "depression" and link them to the "disconnection" between the narrator and his mother because he self-consciously ponders his drive toward oneness and links it to psychoanalyst Melanie Klein's writings on the subject: "Melanie Klein would have us think of depression as a longing for the lost oneness with the maternal breast. The individual of adult life is thus haunted by a preconscious memory of a time when we had no selves at all. The self may not be natural, may not be naturally at home with itself; in depression, some rejection by the world, some success or failure, triggers a more essential disappointment with the project of individuation itself, in the form of longing for return to the beginning. The depressive is a kind of mystic and depression is a meditation on a lost paradise beyond the prison of selfhood" (179). For the narrator, however, selfhood only becomes a prison when it is aligned with an inescapable, intergenerational disease.

The negative repercussions associated with the narrator's tendency to repeatedly conflate his destiny with his mother's identity and fate and to escape into fantasy are vividly illustrated in the episode in which he gives his mother, who is now institutionalized and very ill, a photograph of himself, taken when he was six years old. He pins it up on the bulletin board beside her bed. This time, rather than merely fail to function as his mirror, she responds to his gesture with seemingly irrational violence – a gesture that once again highlights the mutual destruction of their identities: "I had already laid the pin in the centre of the top margin of the picture, when I placed the photo in my mother's hand. She held it there for a second and stared carefully at this image of a child who was once her son. Then with sudden savage deliberation, she removed the pin and jabbed at the picture, puncturing both of my eyes. There was not a shadow of a doubt as to what she intended. It had been a blinding" (196). By viewing her gesture in the light of the blinding in the Oedipus myth, the narrator signals guilt for his obsession with his mother.

Yet after his mother dies the narrator dramatically revises his interpretation of this wounding gesture in order to support a fantasy of attaining mastery over her illness and regaining a sense of oneness with her: "Now, of course, I understand," he says. "If you hold the picture up to the light, radiant illumination streams through the eyes. It is the light streaming from the terrain beyond the gates of truth" (196). Rather than accept her loss, he embraces his supposedly imminent reunion with her "beyond the gates of truth." Despite the claims of his wife, children, and even his mistress (he briefly has an affair with his mother's caregiver), the narrator imaginatively pursues his mother into and beyond the disease.

Taken together, the narrator's distraught behaviour raises a fundamental question that speaks to our own angst-ridden historical moment: Why is he unable to mourn and resign himself to loss? To answer this question, it might be helpful to distinguish between what Freud termed "mourning" versus "melancholia." According to Freud, the work of mourning allows one to come to terms with the loss of a loved one by withdrawing one's attachment to the object and incorporating it within the ego. By accomplishing this labour the ego succeeds in freeing its libido from the lost object and, in time, another object can be substituted for the one that is lost. In contrast to supposedly healthy grief, the inability to free the libido from the lost object and move on, a central aspect of melancholia, appears to Freud as the mark of a morbid "pathological disposition" (252). As I noted in the introduction, Freud's model of mourning has been criticized for substituting the lost object too rapidly – a limitation feminist critics have also found in the male elegy. In fact, both mourning and melancholia have been deemed inadequate to the task of resolving the evils associated with illness, loss, and death – evils that are only exacerbated by the current mysterious aura surrounding dementia.

In the case of *Scar Tissue*'s narrator, loss cannot be legitimately relegated to memory since the family illness of dementia, which instigates his "pathological disposition," threatens him as well as his young son, and thus cannot be relegated to memory and put to rest. As the narrator's opening account of his genealogy and the image of the gun fired by genetics suggest, in the cultural imagination Alzheimer's disease, as it was refashioned in the late 1970s, was transformed into a speeding bullet whose flight never ceases; to use another metaphor, it represents an ineradicable taint in the gene pool. As such it inflicts an irreparable wound on the narrator's psyche and, by extension, on the collective unconscious – precisely because it exceeds the individual and results in potentially endless intergenerational trauma. As *Scar Tissue*'s narrator remarks: "It does seem ironic that we have just enough knowledge to know our fate but not enough to do anything to avert it. Genetics now routinely predicts outcomes which medicine can do nothing to prevent. We can identify the children in a particular family who will inherit certain forms of as yet incurable disease. Geneticists call this form of knowledge the new clairvoyance" (7). This is a melancholy condition, indeed. The narrator attests to his melancholic plight when he confesses that his rage and inability to separate from his parents spring from what he terms a "wound" and a "primal attachment" (113, 114).

His choice of the term "wound" is especially apt because it is the basis of the word trauma (from the Greek meaning a "wound"). As he explains, his difficulty lies in the fact that he is not simply mourning the death of his mother, but the fall of his entire household: "Since my father's death, I had been mourning something larger than one life. It had been our whole existence at the farm, that whole world of mine now destroyed by illness. Why my wife couldn't let me mourn that, I didn't understand. If she wouldn't, I had no choice but to do it somewhere else" (114). Although the narrator speaks of mourning, his behaviour more closely resembles what Freud viewed as mourning's pathological double, melancholia.

The intergenerational, traumatic source of the narrator's melancholia and his reference to the destruction of his entire house – which recalls Edgar Allan Poe's Gothic tale "The Fall of the House of Usher" (1839) – is illustrated in an episode that takes place shortly before the narrator's mother completely succumbs to dementia. Dancing with the narrator's son, she croons into the little boy's ear: "Come to me, my melancholy baby" (40). Abruptly, the mother stops dancing with her grandson and, addressing her two grown sons, she announces prophetically: "I'm sure I will make a cheerful old nut. Don't you think so? In any case … it'll be much worse for you" (40). This scene also features prominently in Ignatieff's first autobiographical essay concerning Alison Ignatieff's illness, attesting to its haunting significance ("August" 47). I offer this detailed account of the narrator's melancholy predicament because it highlights the potential implications for the paradigm shift associated with biomedicine's insistence that Alzheimer's is now a disease. As *Scar Tissue* illustrates, the outcome of this shift for some individuals may entail a dangerous combination of rage and paralysis.[10] Although compelled to rescue their loved one from the disease, they may conclude that their only option lies in waiting for the experts – researchers and other trained professionals – to discover the cure. Worse, as the narrator's account of his mother's treatment emphasizes, the shift toward the disease model potentially exacerbates the tendency to dehumanize people suffering from cognitive decline.

Although the narrator does not find consolation in either scientific or religious narratives, he nevertheless turns to religious rituals in an effort to usher in apocalyptic destruction. For instance he engages in a related, quasi-religious urge to exorcise his parents' home that culminates in the sale of the family home and the eradication of all traces of his parents' existence. The narrator's urge to destroy the family house is instigated by his father's death. Worn out from looking after his wife, the father suffers a heart attack and dies beside the front porch. The narrator's brother, who frequently checked his father's health, insists that his father's "heart was fine" (86). This information lends credence to the narrator's covert belief that his mother's illness murdered his father: "He had enslaved himself to it and when it had finished with him, it had thrown him away" (83). This language of slavery further conveys the narrator's overarching sense of powerlessness that triggers his enraged fits of destruction. As he says after selling the house: "If I could have, I would have ripped the pictures off the hooks, the hooks out of the walls, the carpets off the floors, the covers off the sofas. I could have torched the place. As if to say: you took him, so take the rest, so take everything. As if to say, I don't want to remember anything … I wanted to lose it all. I felt flames roaring in my head and my heart was full of savage joy. Then twenty black garbage bags were full and it was a new day … This house, I believed, had been inhabited by illness and I had purified it.

This place had been possessed. I had cleansed it" (95). This passage invokes familiar apocalyptic rhetoric: images of purification, fire, and cleansing in anticipation of "a new day." In light of his mother's vocation as a painter, it is also significant that he begins by imagining ripping "pictures off the hooks." It is perhaps not a coincidence that the narrator's house cleaning and sale of the family farm is followed by his confession to his brother about the role he played in destroying his mother's paintings. After their mutual participation in "cleansing" the farmhouse, as he says: "It was no longer a betrayal to tell him our secret" (164).

He proceeds to relate how, with his brother away at college and his father away at a convention, while he was alone at the farm with his mother she ordered him to mix all of her paints until the colours bled together, "losing themselves in a viscous, oily paste, the colour of despair" (165). She then demanded that he paint over all of her canvases while she walked out into the orchard leaving him alone. Relating this episode, the narrator insists he had "no choice" and that in half an hour he covered over "her life's work" (196). Again, the narrator frames his cleansing in terms of a spiritual rite: "I had assisted at a scene of mutilation, like the mourning rituals of countries where widows cut and daub their own garments and beat their temples in sorrow" (166). He equates her gesture with a general "surrender to the dying that is in all our cells from the beginning" (167). He imagines further that she "chose to make her peace with it early, given that she knew, not merely how she would die, but that she would lose the memory that she had ever painted any pictures at all" (167).[11] Unable to take ownership of his own enraged, melancholic "compulsion to destroy" (108), as the passage cited above suggests – the paintings painted over in the colours of *his* despair – he stubbornly maintains that destruction was passed down to him from his mother in the form of a family curse. Moreover he symbolically passes the legacy of this compulsion to destroy when he bequeaths his gun to his son. Knowing that the little boy is reluctant to bring the weapon home to his mother's house, the narrator tells him: "I know what your mother thinks, but I want you to have this. It was mine, and now it's yours" (116). Although literally he is referring to his gun, previously he figuratively connected the weapon to the supposedly predetermined genetic nature of the family disease. Thus symbolically the gesture suggests that he is passing down "Death and all our Woe."

Despite the narrator's repeated attempts at purifying the family home, he remains haunted by a disastrous future he cannot prevent and by the dead he cannot mourn. Although his physician assures him that all the tests demonstrate that his brain remains unscarred, he insists he is gradually succumbing to dementia: "The cells are too small to see. But I know. I feel them inside me. My fate has come to meet me. My voyage has begun" (198). Not only does he cling to the belief that he and his mother share the same fate, he also believes his commitment to apocalyptic revelation and destruction will be rewarded. In this respect, his behaviour recalls Julia Kristeva's comments concerning the depressed individual's identification with the abject: "One can understand that [the abject] is experienced at the peak of its strength when the subject, weary of fruitless attempts to identify with something on the outside, finds the impossible within, when it finds that the impossible constitutes its very *being*, that it *is* none other than the abject" (*Powers* 5; emphasis in original). In his fantasies, the narrator follows his mother, escorted by an angel, through the "gates of truth" (181). For the narrator and, indeed, for virtually every adult in Canada in the twenty-first century, death and its harbinger Alzheimer's lurk in every room. Incited by the panic instigated by the refashioned disease, and unable to win the war in his lifetime, *Scar Tissue*'s narrator responds by idolizing the abject and elevating himself to one of Alzheimer's elect.

The protagonist's Oedipal obsession with his mother and father recalls Kathleen Woodward's account of the limitations of Freud's Oedipal model in her essay "Inventing Generational Models" which, as Woodward explains, is twofold:

> The constitution of male and female sexuality, established within the nuclear family, is understood to be achieved simultaneously with the rigid separation of the two generations, the generation of the parent from the generation of the child. Both the two sexes and the two generations are ever after to remain unequal in power. The triangular geometry of this nuclear family is established through the threat of force, which entails for the child the emotions of guilt over the desire for the parent of the opposite sex, fear of punishment, and jealousy of the parent of the same sex. Classically the father is cast as the third term that intervenes in the mother-child dyad. (*Figuring* 150–1).

Woodward argues, however, that the longevity of older people in the twenty-first century offers society an unprecedented opportunity to rethink the implications of Freud's binary, agonistic model. Simply put, more older women are alive and recording their own experiences of aging into old age. Focusing on the import of this transformation for women in later life, Woodward explains: "Historically we have not before had what I call generational consciousness of older women, which is being shaped for us today by what I have referred to, following Bollas, as "evocative objects," cultural texts that are helping us to imagine our possible futures. Thus we necessarily cannot reproduce the Freudian model of revolting against the previous generation" (*Figuring* 163). Ultimately, drawing on her reading of Margaret Drabble's novel *A Natural Curiosity* (1989) Woodward argues for the possibility of leaving the future "open-ended" and linked "not through the trope of familial identification but rather through a curiosity akin to affection" (ibid. 161). Whereas *Scar Tissue* frames dementia as an uncanny familial secret, Woodward's insights remind us that people with dementia and their caregivers exceed the Oedipal configuration and its structure of intergenerational warfare.

In the remaining two chapters I explore two novels, Caroline Adderson's *The History of Forgetting* (chapter eight) and Jane Rule's *Memory Board* (chapter nine), that link homosexuality and Alzheimer's disease. Recalling the discussion of Sontag's work on AIDS in the introduction, these novels prompt readers to analyze the similarities and differences between society's rejection, fear, and reductive view of these two marginalized groups – old people and homosexuals. As Adderson's and Rule's novels clarify, both groups arouse similar fears of degeneration. As Sontag reminds us, and as I noted in the introduction, the most dreaded illnesses "are those that seem like mutations into animality ... What counts ... is that it reflects underlying, ongoing changes, the dissolution of the person" (*AIDS* 41). In contrast to *Scar Tissue*, however, Adderson's and Rule's texts offer intergeneration models of care that deconstruct societal fears of degeneration and Freud's two-generational Oedipal model. Rather than uphold heteronormative modes of reproduction and caregiving as the norm, *The History of Forgetting* and *Memory Board* both promote practices of caregiving based on affiliation rather than filiation, on friendship rather than kinship bonds. Such caregiving practices are energized, in Woodward's terms, by "a curiosity akin to affection."

8

A *History of Forgetting*: Cognitive Decline and Historical Cycles of Degeneration

This chapter extends my investigation of Gothic metaphors currently associated with Alzheimer's disease by addressing Caroline Adderson's *A History of Forgetting* (1999), which depicts a long-term, homosexual relationship in which one partner suffers from Alzheimer's. *A History of Forgetting* is significant for several reasons. First, it offers an alternative to the Oedipal model of intergenerational rivalry and promotes a model of care based on friendship rather than filiation. Second, through its repeated allusions to the Second World War, Adderson's text draws attention to the casualties of our current war against dementia. Third, it resists the myth of progress by emphasizing how both individuals and nations experience episodes of repetition, decline, and loss. Fourth, and perhaps most important, *A History of Forgetting* rejects a strictly biomedical account of dementia in favour of an imaginative and socio-historical contemplation of the origins of human evil, which it unequivocally locates in the repeated failure of individuals, families, and nations to recognize the Other as represented in the novel by the homosexual, the Jew, and the animal. In its evocation of the Second World War, the narrative offers a historical foundation for contemporary society's obsession with cognitive decline and fascist promises of perfection. At its core, *A History of Forgetting* draws parallels between the first half of the twentieth century and the international eugenics movement. Adderson's novel focuses, in particular, on the movement's unjust treatment of cognitively and physically "defective" individuals and other so-called undesirables. The gruesome history of the eugenics movement is mirrored by Western society's current approach to elderly citizens suffering from dementia.[1] The final chapters, set in

Auschwitz, drive home the novel's overarching fear that Western culture's contemporary desires for cognitive perfection are the secret sharers of Nazi Germany's state-sanctioned policies. This uncanny connection is based on the shared bureaucratic approach to and normative standards of mental and physical health, and the desire to perfect society by purging the nation of its "defective" citizens.

Set in Vancouver during the 1980s, *A History of Forgetting* traces the experience of a group of young hairdressers working at "Vitae," an avant-garde hair salon. Decked out as a parody of a Roman temple – "fourth-century laurel-wreathed emperors hang in profile on platter-sized medallions" (75) – the salon's décor recalls the fall of the Roman Empire and introduces readers to the novel's overarching themes of degeneration and decline. As critics observe, the word degeneration "was itself a curious compound. First of all, it meant to lose the properties of the genus, to decline to a lower type … to dust, for instance, or to the behaviour of the beasts of the barnyard. It also meant to lose the generative force" (Chamberlain and Gilman ix). The dictionary definition likewise conveys the sense of a profoundly negative physical and moral transformation: "The process of degenerating or becoming degenerate; the falling off from ancestral or earlier excellence; declining to a lower or worse stage of being; degradation of nature" (*OED*). It is worth noting in regard to ethics that the first recorded use of the term in 1607 links "degeneration" to the biblical Fall (*OED*).

In the late nineteenth century, degeneration enjoyed a "respectable scientific pedigree" (Goodey 367). In 1857, for example, French psychiatrist Bénédict-Augustin Morel defined degeneracy as "a marked departure from the original type tending more or less rapidly to the extinction of it" (in ibid.).[2] Although some scientists regarded degeneration objectively, as Edgar Miller observes the concept was also used to pathologize individuals, families, and supposedly inferior races: "At its crudest, the notion of degeneration implies that a mild abnormality such as a cleft palate or an over-anxious personality may appear in one generation, to be followed in the next by something rather more far reaching like madness or scrofula, and with complete idiocy, or some other equally dreadful affliction emerging in the third" (367). Dr Alfred Tredgold (1870–1952), one of the most influential Edwardian medical commentators on the problem of dementia and a strong proponent of eugenics, explained the process of degeneration and its purported links to cognitive decline: "At first the mental change which results is slight and shows itself as migraine, hysteria, and the milder forms of epilepsy. Later, and in subsequent generations, it becomes more pronounced and gives rise to insanity and early dementia; whilst at a still later stage we see the conditions with which we are now concerned, namely, actual defect of the mind structure – amentia or mental deficiency" (in Jackson 99). I cite these views because they remain central to Adderson's narrative interrogation of their legacy. By linking late-onset dementia to earlier periods in history when society was equally concerned with the "burden" posed by the "feeble-minded," *A History of Forgetting* invites readers to remember the violence that can attend efforts to delineate two levels of existence – the fully civilized, healthy human, on the one hand, and the diseased or defective subhuman, on the other.

In *A History of Forgetting*, although the AIDS crisis has taken its toll (one of the stylist's lovers is dying) the hairdressers insist they are untouched by violence and remain "apolitical." Their lives are tragically altered, however, when one of their beloved colleagues, Christian – a diminutive, young gay man, born with unusual facial features – is brutally murdered by a gang of homophobic neo-Nazis during the Christmas holidays. The novel focuses predominantly on two of Christian's colleagues, Malcolm and Alison, and their responses to the tragedy. Taken together, their respective experiences at work and at home constitute the central narrative. Ultimately, their interpretation of Christian's death as a continuation of Nazi ideology reinforces how the violence in the present is informed by the past. In keeping with the work's titular emphasis on forgetting, the narrative suggests, however, that Western society forgets or, more precisely, represses its capacity for moral decline and aggression.

In theorizing repression Freud observed that individuals repeat in lieu of remembering – an opposition often characterized as a tendency toward acting out rather than working through. Freud noted, for example, that his patients did not have certain memories at their disposition: "it was a question of things which the patient wished to forget, and therefore intentionally repressed from his conscious thought and inhibited and suppressed" (in Laplanche and Pontalis 392). In Adderson's novel the compulsion to repeat on the microcosmic (individual) level provides both the content and, equally important, the logic for what plays out on the macrocosmic level of history. As analyst Hans Loewald famously insisted, the cure for the potentially eternal return of the repressed entails turning ghosts into ancestors, a process that relies on narrative. Viewed in this light, the title of the novel, *A History of Forgetting*, recalls the ancient symbol of the ouroboros (the tail-devouring snake) since both individual and national history require memory, but the repression of things we wish to forget eats holes in the linearity and order of the historical understanding that we so desperately seek to establish and maintain as individuals and nations. Yet in the act of telling repression remains at work, and so the process is marred by falsification and breaks down, instigating another narrative cycle.

In the first section of this chapter, I briefly review how the plot of *A History of Forgetting* highlights its central preoccupation with individual and national forms of degeneration. In section two, I offer a historical context for Western society's concern with the relationship between idiocy, personhood, and citizenship beginning with the late eighteenth century. Based, in part, on distinctions carved out during the Enlightenment, Western nations established the concepts of idiocy and degeneration, thereby laying the foundation for later and more pernicious articulations of the elusive goal of ensuring the health of the larger social body by means of ridding the nation of nature's supposed flaws. In the late nineteenth and early twentieth centuries, European and North American nations, including Canada, pursued this goal by means of enforced sterilization, euthanasia, and, during the Second World War in Germany, mass extermination. In section three, I offer a close reading of *A History of Forgetting* to illustrate how the text's rhetorical features – the image of the mirror, the allegorical treatment of Christian as a Christ figure, and the portrayals of animals as figures of abjection – forge connections between distinct marginalized groups – homosexuals, Jews, and dogs – and, in the process, emphasize the similarities between past and present apocalyptic solutions to the problem posed by the Other.

SECTION I: A HISTORY OF DECLINE

From the start, the novel's protagonist, Malcolm, finds himself surrounded by degeneration and decline at work and at home. In his late fifties, Malcolm is decades older than his new colleagues and has no rapport with his fellow hairdressers, who sport a variety of tattoos and piercings. Pondering his youthful co-workers' aesthetic sense, Malcolm muses: "Something had gone grotesquely wrong from the start" (85). He wonders if they can sense his disapproving view "that they were flowers of degeneration," and he concludes that, for them, "freakishness and mutilation had replaced beauty as a standard. Theirs was a torture chamber aesthetic" (85). Although Adderson's novel may lack the familiar trappings of the Gothic, including ancient castles, evil counts, and kidnapped maidens, its ongoing meditation on beauty and its loss within a Goth-inspired youth culture recalls early Gothic writers' concern with humanity's primitive roots and capacity for violence.

In *A History of Forgetting*, individual and cultural forms of degeneration are juxtaposed and repeatedly mirror one another. Malcolm's preoccupation with degeneration as it is reflected in the culture of his younger coworkers, for example, is echoed and amplified by his domestic circumstances. His long-time companion, Denis – a Frenchman whom Malcolm met in 1959 when Denis was opening a salon in Paris, and with whom he worked and lived for over thirty years – suffers from advanced dementia. With respect to national degeneration, Malcolm repeatedly emphasizes that despite its reputation for beauty and civility, Paris oppresses him because he can never forget its violent history. By contrast, Malcolm thinks of Canada as a place where nothing "ever happened" and he sees that "as idyllic" (152). As he tells Christian, speaking of his life with Denis in Paris: "In our own neighbourhood, heretics had been burned during the Inquisition, the Bastille stormed, guillotines erected in hotel court-yards; Jews had been rounded up there during the war and, in the eighties, bombed in delicatessens" (152). Although Malcolm never feels at home in Paris, he continues to reside there until Denis becomes too ill for him to care for by himself (24). Eventually, Malcolm takes Denis to Vancouver and, ultimately, puts him into long-term care.

The novel opens after Malcolm brings Denis to Vancouver. During the day Malcolm works happily at "Faye's of Kerrisdale," a humble establishment that caters primarily to elderly women, while Denis is looked after in their home by Yvette, a French-speaking caregiver. But Faye soon retires. Before selling her business, she legally ensures that Malcolm can still continue to look after his elderly clients at the salon's new incarnation. Amanda, "Vitae's" twenty-something owner, is dismayed at this prospect, however, as she does not "want a bunch of old ladies tottering around spoiling the concept" (84). Initially, as the passage cited above suggests, it seems as if the only prejudice tainting the paradise of Vancouver is ageism. Yet traces of the Old World's violent past begin to erupt in Malcolm's domestic life. As Denis's illness progresses, Malcolm witnesses his erstwhile kind and gentle companion become physically violent and shout anti-Semitic invectives. Rather than view Denis's behaviour solely as the result of a neurodegenerative disease, Malcolm attributes it to cultural factors. In keeping with the theme of national degeneration he blames Denis's upbringing in France, where anti-Semitism was both widespread and condoned, for corrupting his lover (see 153, 290). Past and present continue to intersect in the novel as Denis's increasingly violent and abusive behaviour uncannily echoes Christian's murder. Both are predicated on a lack of recognition of other people's humanity and culminate in bloodshed. Gradually Malcolm, and by extension the reader, recognize that Denis's illness and Christian's death exist on a continuum (211).

The novel links Christian's tragic fate to a set of archetypal religious and historical narratives including the story of Christ, the extermination of the Jews during the Holocaust, and Dante's *Inferno*. These intertexts serve to emphasize, and in fact universalize, social degeneration and its tragic outcomes. Owing to its reliance on these well-known intertexts, as noted above *A History of Forgetting* offers a socio-historical analysis of the origins of human evil. According to the narrative, evil inheres in the failure to recognize the Other. The repercussions of these failures of recognition are graphically illustrated through Christian's murder by young men who do not recognize homosexuals and disabled persons as fully human. This lack of recognition is evidenced both by the deadly beating they inflict on a helpless young man and by its aftermath.

Due to the savagery of their aggression, Christian's face is unrecognizable after the attack. The police escort Malcolm to the morgue to identify the body, but when the sheet is drawn back, Malcolm is at a loss for a response. Rather than admit to the police, "I don't know this person," Malcolm asks a far more basic and morally loaded question instead: "Is this a person?" (194). He goes on to reflect that this question also relates to Denis's illness and the fate of other caregivers who likewise visit friends and family members in the long-term care facility only to be confronted by people whom they no longer recognize: "All of them had seen their loved ones become different people. Denis had become demanding and unlikeable, hate-filled ... It tormented Malcolm wondering which Denis was real, the gentle man he had seemed to be up until his illness, or how he was now. Yet his situation was hardly unique" (194). The juxtaposition between the violence of Christian's murderers and Alzheimer's disease suggests that the latter potentially effects a similar destruction of personhood and a foreclosing of recognition on both sides. For instance, it torments Malcolm that Denis's transformation might actually be a revelation of a pre-existing truth about Denis and who he is (and is not). This breakdown in the process of recognition implicates both characters and, by extension, readers. In the scene at the morgue, although he remains unable to identify Christian visually, Malcolm overcomes his estrangement by opting for touch.[3] He easily finds the telltale callous on the forefinger and thumb that identifies Christian as a kindred hairdresser. Unlike the thugs who violently inscribe their denial of personhood onto the body of the Other, throughout the text, in his relations with Christian, Malcolm insists on the latter's humanity.

Although Christian's murder leaves Malcolm utterly bereft, it brings him closer to his colleague Alison, a naive girl in her early twenties who started working at "Vitae" a few months prior to Christian's death. Like Malcolm, Alison has also been befriended by Christian. Whereas Malcolm is familiar with both anti-Semitism and homophobia, Alison has not personally grappled with either prejudice. When she becomes depressed in the wake of Christian's murder, her live-in boyfriend Billy counsels her to take anti-depressants and forget the gruesome episode. In this way the narrative pits Billy's intellectual and scientific approach to life against Alison's visceral compassion. A bright and ambitious university student, Billy researches the behaviour of rats and sleeps beneath a poster of a giant rat on his ceiling. As he explains to Alison, he finds the image comforting. "It's sort of like believing there's a God" (130). Alison, by contrast, comes from a family of caregivers – with a mother who ran herself ragged for charity and a Shriner father (91). Rather than accept Billy's view of a universe as governed by a rat-God and acquiesce to the banality of human violence, Alison is determined to remedy her ignorance of human history, specifically the history of the Third Reich that inspired Christian's killers. To Billy's dismay, his formerly uneducated, happy-go-lucky girlfriend, who was once content to have sex with him whenever he wanted and whom he playfully called "Shit-for-Brains," begins reading books about Nazi ideology and the Holocaust. After learning about the extermination camps, Alison recognizes that Christian embodied everything European and North American societies in the 1930s and 1940s deemed defective; as a "small, deformed" gay man, he was "marked for death" (221). Whereas Billy views Christian's murder as the outcome of a set of predictable, animal behaviours, Alison interprets it in the context of Western history's repeated episodes of moral degeneration.

As a result, she becomes even more determined to learn from history and to treat others with kindness rather than embrace forgetting. Ultimately, she determines that "it was possible to care, even for a total stranger" (226). In the end, Alison breaks up with her boyfriend and persuades Malcolm to travel with her to Auschwitz. The narrative concludes with Malcolm and Alison's tour of the concentration camp. Their visit culminates when the two hairdressers enter a room filled with hair shorn from the heads of countless victims. As the narrator explains, "They had come just in time, before it turned to dust" (344).

Rather than focus solely on the contemporary plight of cognitively impaired elderly individuals within the biomedical disease model, *A History of Forgetting* contextualizes society's fears and stigmatization of a set of marginalized groups within the overarching framework of twentieth-century responses to supposed threats to the health of the nation. One the one hand, *A History of Forgetting*'s portrayal of Denis's degenerative illness ultimately reinstalls a Gothic view of dementia due to its repeated use of spectral tropes and images of monstrous transformations to describe his experience. On the other hand, the narrative underscores that the most pernicious disease of forgetting, which is unequivocally identified as evil, does not lie in an individual's brain cells. Instead evil constitutes a far more pervasive cultural disease, whose characteristic symptom involves adopting violent, apocalyptic solutions to living with people who are deemed imperfect and thereby mirror our disavowed imperfections. In effect, the novel's transposition of the terror-inducing flaw of forgetting to a broader social context implicates both individuals and nations. While it may be tempting to see those afflicted with dementia as absolved from the corrosive effects of repression, the novel's treatment of Denis – specifically, the emergence of his seemingly latent anti-Semitism – intimates that everyone's hold on his or her present (conscious, civilized, recognizable) self is tenuous and, to borrow Sontag's words concerning Artaud's dark insight, "the purest contingency" ("Essay" xxi).

SECTION II: THE LEGACY
OF ENLIGHTENMENT VIEWS OF IDIOCY

As medical historian David Wright observes, prior to the Enlightenment in the eighteenth century, profound dementia, whether from birth – "Amentia (congenita)" – or due to senility later in life – "Amentia (senilus)"[4] – was termed "idiocy," and did not draw much medical attention. "It was considered a regrettable and incurable condition about which medical practitioners, both orthodox and unorthodox, could do little" (28). By the time of the French Revolution in 1789, however, the situation had reversed: "idiots ceased to be a mere footnote in medical texts and occupied a surprisingly important role in the emerging ideas of Enlightenment philosophy and scientific medicine" (28). As Alan Bewell asserts: "It is probably not too great an exaggeration to say that the philosophical discovery of the idiot took place in the eighteenth century" (57). During the Enlightenment the definition of "an idiot" from Anthony Fitzherbert's *Natura Brevium* (1652) was cited repeatedly: "Such a person who cannot count or number twenty, and tell who was his father or mother, nor how old he is, so that it may appear that he hath no understanding or reason, what shall be for his forfeit, or what for his loss" (in Andrews 82). Although the criteria might seem to be empirically based, as C.F. Goodey observes, the social meanings associated with mental handicap were in fact "sheer invention" (215) – an "invention" that historians largely credit to the English philosopher and physician John Locke.

Early modern notions of idiocy merged from several "previously distinct schemata including the imbecility of women, children, and old people" (Goodey 224). Locke, however, relied on the concept of the idiot to shape the modern, psychological concept of the self.[5] Locke's *Essay Concerning Human Understanding*, which is "very much a treatise on memory," relied on idiocy to show that all memory is "a product of education and culture" and humans are not, in contrast to René Descartes's theory, born with innate impressions (Bewell 57). For the purposes of my analysis of *A History of Forgetting*, it is important to appreciate, in particular, Locke's use of the phenomena of mental disability to define the nature of consciousness, will, and citizenship (Wright 18). Critically, Locke contributed to the contemporary view of idiocy as a mental state that lies "beyond what is human" (Goodey 227). He based his view that idiots were not men on the fact that they lacked the capacity for abstraction (ibid. 234). The central importance of the idiot for Locke, according to Bewell, was that, in standing "outside language" and exhibiting "only a rudimentary power of memory, the idiot occupies the threshold between nature and man, and could be seen as linking the two states" (57).

Memory, or rather the inability to remember, was vital to Enlightenment definitions of idiocy. Relying heavily on Locke's theories, in 1798 the English physician and medical writer John Haslam wrote: "Memory is the first power which decays ... how treacherous the memory is without reinforcement. The necessity of a constant recruit [sic] and frequent review of our ideas, satisfactorily explains why a number of patients lapse nearly into idiotism ... Mr. Locke well observes, 'that there seems to be a constant decay of all our ideas ... so that if they be not sometimes renewed ... the print wears out'" (in Andrews 94). For Locke and his many supporters, both a flawed memory and an inability to draw conclusions from sensory perceptions placed idiots "on par with beasts" (Wright 30).

These distinctions were of tremendous practical import because eighteenth-century English law identified criminal intent based on an individual's ability to distinguish good and evil. English judge and lawyer Sir Matthew Hale's *History of the Pleas of the Crown* (1736), for example, devotes an entire chapter to the discussion of individuals with mental impairments (see ibid. 22). According to Hale, whereas men of reason were subject to criminal punishment, idiots, "if totally deprived of the use of reason, could not be guilty ordinarily of capital offenses, for they have not the use or understanding, and act not as reasonable creatures, but their actions are in effect in the condition of brutes" (in ibid. 22–3). Rationality and freedom were inextricably connected for Locke; in his view, both idiots and children were "beyond the law" (Goodey 240). As Locke states, "There is no reason that we should deal with the case of children and idiots (fatuis). For although the law is binding on all those to whom it is given, it does not, however, bind those to whom it is not given, and it is not given to those who are unable to understand it" (in ibid.). As I noted in the previous chapter, the figure of the deranged, idiot child, which appears in Michael Ignatieff's fiction, haunted the social imaginary from the Enlightenment to the Second World War.

In *A History of Forgetting* the intelligence of animals and human animals is a central concern, as evidenced for example by Billy's research on rats. As well, the pivotal courtroom scene establishes the fact that Christian's murderer Vorst is not an imbecile but, instead, a highly intelligent individual who is thus morally responsible for his actions. The fact that Vorst is not "feeble-minded" is crucial to the narrative since it suggests that people who are mentally disabled do not necessarily represent a threat to society as the eugenics movement insisted. Instead the threat inheres in those who believe themselves to be endowed with the responsibility to cleanse the world of so-called undesirables. As I note in my book *DisPossession*, the concept of degeneration was built into imperialism and colonialism: "it was formed and functioned within [these] institutional arrangements ... which reflected and furthered the needs of ... European culture to reify its own power and to institutionalize the powerlessness over which it exercised its dominion. This dominion was both literal and figurative and included the real world of the European colonies" (Chamberlain and Gilman viii).

Equally significant to the novel's debate concerning animal versus human intelligence, Malcolm buys Denis a dog named Grace and the narrative repeatedly emphasizes dogs' inferior intelligence yet superior capacity to offer unconditional love to their frail, elderly companions. Viewed in this light, in the novel dogs serve as a device to underscore the presence of a crucial attribute that cannot be measured through an IQ test, namely the capacity for empathy that prohibits people from treating others as waste matter. I use the term "waste" because – in addition to recalling the Victorian theory of waste and repair cited in chapter three – as Mark Jackson observes, in the 1930s eugenicists repeatedly associated "imbecility with waste" or the "residuum" of society to argue that the "feeble-minded" were a "bestial" lot who led "a parasitic existence at the expense of society" (139).

A History of Forgetting's repeated pairing of animals and dementia recalls the historical connections drawn during the Enlightenment between cognitive impairment and animality – connections that were bolstered by scientific research in the early twentieth century. Reginald Langdon-Down (whose name is now associated with Down syndrome), for example, identified the characteristic "single transverse palmar crease" (Wright 83) – an unbroken line running across the palm – in individuals diagnosed with what was at that time termed "Mongolism." For him, this finding was significant because a similar crease is often found in primates, which explains why he dubbed it the "simian crease" (ibid.). In the early decades of the twentieth century, the preoccupation with degenerative traces of animality among humans was fuelled by Darwin's paradigm-shifting theories of evolution. Public intellectuals repeatedly expressed the anxiety that due to the taint of brutishness among certain individuals, races, and classes, if left to their own devices human beings would slide down the rungs of the evolutionary ladder and degenerate to the level of their ape-like ancestors rather than achieve their divine potential. These concerns were particularly prevalent during the first decade of the twentieth century, when "the optimism of the mid-Victorian period had given way to darker speculations about racial degeneration, as eugenic ideas had taken hold across a vast swath of the educated middle class in Britain and elsewhere" (Wright 83). In 1910, for example, the year after Langdon-Down identified the "simian crease," Winston Churchill, then British Home Secretary in the Liberal Asquith government, circulated a document to his cabinet that warned of "120,000 or 130,000 feeble-minded persons at large in our midst" (in ibid.). In July of that same year, Churchill spoke in the House of Commons, stating his belief "that there is no aspect more important than the prevention of the multiplication and perpetuation of this great evil" (84). I offer this information to demonstrate that the current panic concerning dementia and Alzheimer's is not the first time that Western nations have anxiously debated questions of national efficiency and the social costs of disability. It is also helpful to recognize that the international eugenics movement had supporters across Europe and North America. Although *A History of Forgetting* adopts the familiar eugenics storyline, which "leads from Nazi Germany to the death camps" (Brave and Slyva 37), it is a mistake to attribute these attitudes solely to Nazi Germany. In the 1930s, German eugenicists looked to and roundly praised the United States and particularly the state of California for leading the charge in sterilizing the "feeble minded" (see Kühl).

By the early twentieth century, anxieties about "the social impact of mental deficiency were driven by pervasive beliefs that the number of defectives was increasing" (Jackson 34). Statistics gleaned from asylums, prisons, workhouses, and from expansive surveys of school children "combined to inspire fears that the proportion of the population that could be considered defective was rapidly expanding" (Jackson 34). In his 1910 House of Commons speech, Churchill flatly stated: "If by any arrangement ... we are able to segregate these people under proper conditions, so that their curse died with them, and was not transmitted to future generations, we should have taken upon our shoulders in our own lifetime a work for which those who came after us would owe us a debt of gratitude" (in Wright 114).[6] Although by no means the sole or original source of our current panic, our contemporary anxieties concerning dementia can be traced to changes in the nineteenth century when, owing to the advent of

compulsory education and the testing of IQ, a new class was created
– the class of "the feeble minded" (114). The growing awareness of,
and estimates about, "mental backwardness" in children paralleled
a broader trend that became pronounced at the turn of the twentieth
century: a desire for state authorities to establish quantitative estimates of mental deficiency in the general population (90). During
the early twentieth century, the Victorian-era's preoccupation with
the health of children and, by extension, the fitness of the nation,
was transformed into a concern with the social costs of disability. As
eugenicists across the Western world slowly realized their inability
to augment fertility amongst the most valuable members of society,
Wright explains, "they became preoccupied with the potential danger of the feeble-minded. Everyone seemed to believe that in calling for the eradication of the disabled, they were acting urgently on
behalf of future generations" (114).

Viewed in this light, the Nazi leadership's policy in Germany of
"euthanizing" individuals held in long-term care in mental hospitals – which began in 1939, but had a long genesis prior to being
made official – constituted part of an overarching trend among
Western nations. Ordered by Hitler himself in a memorandum dated
1 September 1939, the policy, known as the Aktion T-4 Program,
began in October of 1939 and ended in August 1941, killing
between 70,000 and 95,000 mentally and physically disabled adults
and another 5,000 children (104). In 1941, when the program was
officially cancelled, most of the medical personnel involved were
"quickly transferred east to implement the Final Solution to the
Jewish Question" (107).

While historians have demonstrated the profound connections
between the Nazis' eugenics policy and that of the United States
(see Kühl), it is equally important to recognize that many Canadians
embraced the eugenicist ideology. Angus McLaren observes, for
example, that during the first decades of the twentieth century, "a
preoccupation with the feeble-minded" swept Canada (41). Activists
made their case for intervention by quantifying the costs of "mental
defectives," who were thought to have large, illegitimate families that
"burdened the tax roles and clogged the hospitals, industrial schools,
and reformatories" (McLaren 30). Eugenicist speakers regularly pro-
pounded their ideas at the Canadian Club in Toronto (see Kühl 35).

In Canada, Dr Helen MacMurchy, a leading Ontario public health
activist, was "probably the most outspoken medical eugenicist"

(Comacchio 19). MacMurchy was a founding member of the Toronto-based eugenicist Canadian National Committee on Mental Hygiene, established in 1918 (McLaren 59). As the first "Inspector of the Feebleminded" for Ontario, she issued annual reports that, as one official stated, "did much to impress upon medical and political leaders the extent of mental deficiency" and its threat to the Canadian nation-state (in ibid. 39). MacMurchy strongly advocated for segregation and sterilization of the "feeble-minded" (Comacchio 19). She continued to "call for the forcible control of the reproduction of the feebleminded" through sterilization into the 1930s (McLaren 37–47).

Echoes of late-nineteenth and early twentieth-century eugenicist anxieties concerning the menace of the "feeble-minded" can be discerned in the use of the same phrases to describe people coping with mental disability in the twenty-first century. At the dawn of the twentieth century, "mental defectives" were repeatedly and publicly decried as a "burden to society"; moreover, the narrative of the "burden" played a crucial part "in the eugenic calculus" up to and during the Second World War (Brave and Slyva 41; Jackson 2). As noted in the introduction, these same Gothic tropes and threats concerning "the economic 'burden' of the unfit" (Brave and Syla 41) are now being deployed in the repeated images of the "rising tide" or "tsunami" of demented, aged individuals threatening the nation.[7] I cite these parallels because *A History of Forgetting*'s juxtaposition of the Holocaust and contemporary approaches to dementia alerted me to the fact that the use of Gothic literary tropes and animal imagery to describe the "feeble-minded" is not new; the target may have shifted from the cognitively challenged to children to elderly individuals, but the language and intent remain similar.

SECTION III: DEMENTIA AS METAPHOR – "THE PROBLEM IN THE MIRROR"

These historical associations help to explain why *A History of Forgetting* repeatedly juxtaposes the Nazis' extermination program with contemporary attitudes toward mental and physical disability. From the start, the prologue to the first section, "Its Image in the Mirror," illustrates how throughout the narrative, the past is repeatedly mirrored in the present. Early on, the narrator describes a pair of mirrored sunglasses worn by the taxi driver who escorts visitors to Auschwitz. We are told that the driver's glasses "reflect back in miniature and reverse the entrance to the Muzeum" (9). This seemingly insignificant image graphically hints at how microcosmic ("miniature") isolated events in the New World, such as Christian's murder and Denis's protracted decline in the long-term care facility in Vancouver, mirror past ("reverse") events in the Old World. Ultimately, the characters and readers alike recognize that Christian's death at the hands of his homophobic, skinhead executioners beside the train tracks was motivated by the same logic that rationalized the concentration camps in Europe, where a host of people with mental and physical challenges, and other undesirables including Jews, Gypsies, Jehovah's Witnesses, political dissidents, and homosexuals were likewise transported by trains to the gas chambers and executed en masse.

To emphasize the connections between the death of defective individuals in the present and during the Holocaust, each of the novel's four sections set in the present begins with a brief italicized prologue set in Auschwitz. The final three prologues cite (in English, French, and German, respectively) the words printed on the sign that greets visitors to the concentration camp, warning them of the horrors that await them: "You are entering a place of exceptional horror and tragedy. Please show your respect for those who suffered and died here by behaving in a manner suitable to the dignity of their memory" (75; see also 182, 271). Within the narrative, the sign refers both to Christian's brutal murder in a washroom in a Vancouver park and to the horrors perpetrated at Auschwitz. As noted above, in the final section Alison and Malcolm travel to Poland to visit the concentration camp, thereby providing a rationale for the appearance of the signs throughout the text. Until they embark on their trip, however, the repeated oscillations between the cryptic, italicized prologues and the events set in Vancouver are profoundly disorienting.

Rather than align the experience of disorientation with disease, the novel suggests instead that making sense of one's existential position is a difficult task for everyone, irrespective of one's cognitive capacity. Again the novel shifts the locus of "impairment" to humanity as a whole, and effects this both formally and thematically to implicate readers. For individuals and nations, the past constantly intrudes on and disrupts one's experience in the present. As Malcolm tells Alison: "History does not belong exclusively to the place in which it occurred. It is borne along currents of air and on the Internet" (266). Readers are also told that the first thing Alison learned working at "Vitae" was about history: "that the present rests upon layers of the past, but is a stratum so unstable, so shot with fault lines, that now and then the *then* rears up and knocks down the *now*" (111; emphasis in original). As Malcolm asserts, past and present are abstractions that inhere in the air we inhabit (the spaces, objects, bodily gestures, institutions, and languages we have inherited) and the Internet – as insubstantial and permeating as human consciousness. In Ingram's words: "The immaterial, like words and thoughts, can reach across the gap and make material changes in the brain" (255).

Perhaps because the inherently unstable relationship between past and present is so terrifying, we project it onto people suffering from Alzheimer's disease. Yet, as Malcolm observes, the blurring of past and present is in fact ontological and global rather than, as Ingram posits, merely individual and biological. Viewed in this light, the novel illustrates how disease simply amplifies or makes visible what is known but disavowed, namely, that we are all corrupted by and implicated in the sins of history. Ordinary consciousness and our everyday amnesia concerning our past just allow most people to deny it.

In the narrative, Christian's murder constitutes the most overt and uncanny return of the past. When Malcolm and Alison attend the court proceedings, they come face to face with their friend's killers. Vorst is the leader, a teenager who sports a swastika tattoo on his skull. As Malcolm observes, in his "long career he had seen his share of scalp afflictions ... but here, on this teenager's square skull, was a disease of an entirely different magnitude marked out in right angles with a razor. The last time he'd seen a swastika was on a wall in the Paris Metro" (206). Returning to the salon, Alison informs the other stylists at "Vitae" about the trial and explains that the neo-Nazis came from Surrey. As soon as she says this, however, she realizes "they had come straight out of the past" (216). By virtue of its repeated, self-conscious allusions to the Shoah, *A History of Forgetting* emphasizes that neither an individual's history nor that of a nation-state can ever be accurately described as a story of unmitigated progress. Instead, the novel formally and thematically insists that history includes episodes of repetition and degeneration. Both the novel's oscillating structure and the ambiguous identity of Christian's killers reveal that, as noted above, the most pernicious and potentially ineradicable disease is not dementia per se. Instead, it is the refusal to recognize that we are inextricably bound to facets of our past, an existential predicament that makes it possible for all of us, and not merely people coping with dementia, to become strangers to ourselves and estranged from others. In the novel, dementia merely amplifies the perils of reaching the limits of recognition of both the self and the Other as fully human and deserving of respect.

In *A History of Forgetting*, the image of the mirror serves as a governing metaphor that underscores both the necessity and difficulty of reflecting on one's existential and historical context, and, by extension, of affirming the humanity of self and other. The failure of this type of ontological recognition and the concomitant experience of disorientation are foregrounded in the novel's first chapter. Wakened in the middle of the night by a strange noise, Malcolm imagines that he understands how Denis feels not knowing what city he is waking in – or what room, for that matter. Whereas Malcolm's disorientation is momentary, however, for Denis, "it just went on and on" (13). Investigating the noise, Malcolm discovers that it was caused when Denis, wandering in the dark, "slight and spectral," toppled the Christmas tree. When Denis turns and faces Malcolm, readers are told that it was as if Malcolm "had seen a ghost and now the ghost saw him" (14). Later, escorting Denis back to bed, Malcolm observes that Denis had adopted a "vaguely simian posture, arms heavy in their sockets ... 'Come on, King Kong,'" Malcolm says, as he leads Denis back down the hall to the bedroom (15). In accordance with the previous section's analysis of de-humanizing perceptions of cognitively challenged individuals, in this episode, the references to ghosts and simians/apes offer a portrait of Denis as the Gothic victim of a monstrous, degenerative transformation. Later, Denis mistakes a shop girl's solicitous behaviour toward him for idiocy. Denis chatters to her in his native tongue, unaware that she does not understand a word. When Malcolm urges her to respond, she blurts out, "*Je t'aime beaucoup*" (I love you very much). When Malcolm compliments Denis for collecting admirers everywhere they go, Denis smiles but insists that she is mad: "*Elle est bête*" (49). Throughout the novel, the use of French highlights the potential for misinterpretation. In this episode, however, the word "*bête*," which is etymologically related to the word "beast," recalls the historical links forced by Locke and others between idiocy and brutishness – which placed both "outside language" (Bewell 57) – and the concomitant exclusion of both brutes and idiots from the category of human, with all its rights, privileges, and protections afforded by the law. The narrative's treatment of Denis recalls Loewald's assertion that the psychoanalytic task entails turning ghosts into ancestors, remembering instead of repeating. In short, as Allison's determination to learn from documents on the Holocaust suggests, the answer to the Gothic is history.

Owing to its Gothic treatment of Denis's illness, the novel both articulates and enacts the challenges associated with recognizing individuals coping with dementing illness as persons rather than portraying them as spectres or brutes. Gothic doubling – recalling infamous doubles such as Victor Frankenstein and his monster as well as Dr Jekyll and Mr Hyde – pervades the text. For example, in chapter one Denis refuses to return to their bedroom and insists there is an intruder hiding there. After listening to Denis's description of the intruder, Malcolm laughs, saying: "Why, you twit. That was you!" (16). Gradually, Malcolm persuades Denis that he was merely startled by his own reflection. Although early on Denis retains the capacity for self-recognition, it is clearly on the wane and, as a result, he can no longer orient himself in space and time. The next morning, when Malcolm informs him that his caregiver Yvette is not coming because it is Christmas Day, Denis refuses to believe him and retorts: "I would have remembered that" (17). Both Denis's response and his subsequent aggression signal that his declining ability to identify his reflection is symptomatic of a more widespread degenerative process that transforms individuals into Gothic *doppelgängers* and begets violence.

To soothe Denis's confusion and belligerence, Malcolm slow dances with him to "Heureuse," a French song by Edith Piaf on the record player. The words of the song are reassuring, and initially the couple enjoy moving together in a close embrace: "*Heureuse, comme tout. Hereuse, malgre tout*" ["Happy as anything, / Happy despite anything, / Happy, Happy, Happy … / It must be! I want it! My love, for both of us"] (19).[8] When Denis once again demands to know where Yvette is, however, he quickly becomes enraged. Striking out, his fist meets Malcolm's mouth – "two parts that had never been acquainted even after thirty years" (19). Instinctively Malcolm retaliates, landing a blow on Denis's face that sets the record skipping. Instead of uttering the word "*heureuse*" (happy) the singer mechanically repeats the word "*heure*" (hour) (19–20). As this shift suggests, forgetting transforms the promise of progress and future happiness – "*heureuse comme tout*" into a hellish stasis in which one hour – "*heure*" – is the same as the next.

Until Denis's illness effaces all recognition of self and other, Malcolm continues to empathize with and care for him. Readers learn, for example, that in the years Malcolm had been looking after Denis, "he'd tried very hard to understand how he perceived things, to live the nightmare with him and make it less frightening for them both" (69). Before moving to Canada, Malcolm disassembled their old apartment in Paris, at great cost, and made careful notes "in order to put it back together in Vancouver" (26). Despite Malcolm's efforts to live with Denis in a timeless world, Malcolm discovers that certain forms of decline, namely aging, are an inevitable part of the life course. At one point, when Denis cries out for Malcolm the latter appears and assures him that he is, indeed, there. As proof Malcolm holds his wrist under Denis's nose, so Denis can inhale Malcolm's familiar cologne. Pushing Malcolm's hand away, as if he is being tricked by an imposter, Denis insists that "Malcolm isn't old" (69). For Denis, neither Malcolm's aging body nor his own makes sense; Denis repeatedly flies off the handle when he sees himself in the mirror and throws vases at the glass. As Yvette explains to Malcolm: "He expects to see someone younger" (30). When Denis no longer recognizes his companion of over thirty years, Malcolm realizes he had "forgotten about himself, and now it did seem as if a stranger was standing there on the silver side of the glass" (69). For a time, Malcolm dyes his hair jet black. The deception works and Denis recognizes him again, but, in keeping with the broken mirrors in their apartment, the recognition is fractured and fleeting. Gazing at himself in the cracked mirror, Malcolm acknowledges that he "looked positively Cubist" (32). When he finally makes the difficult decision to place Denis in long-term care, we are told that Malcolm's "centre disappeared. The core of him went and he knew himself to be drifting as if he were made of smoke or vapour or some other intangible substance" (147).

As the passages cited above suggest, *A History of Forgetting* relies on the image of the mirror to evoke the existential crises associated with one's identity fracturing and, ultimately, vanishing not only due to neurological disease but as the result of the breaking of intra- and intersubjective social bonds and of the inexorable passage of time. At one point, Malcolm admits that "it was not the first time he had looked into this very mirror and seen something not quite right" (32). He recalls how, years ago, when they lived in Paris, he noticed that "where the glass met the oval frame there was a liquid-looking discoloration, flat and unreflective as molten lead. In the worst of these patches the paint had chipped away entirely exposing the wood backing and the illusion. Across the whole surface were scattered blemishes like mildew" (33). Rather than buy a new mirror, Malcolm took it to a shop for repair. Seizing the mirror, a craftsman held it aloft, "reflecting side facing Malcolm, Malcolm looking at himself" (33). To Malcolm's horror, before his very eyes, "he disappeared. In one stroke, his face was swept away" (33). Echoing Malcolm's later experience in which he loses his "core," in this scene and others that follow, the mirror signals the unsettling potential for psychological, social, and physical annihilation.

The mirror motif establishes links amidst figurative and literal forms of death early on. For instance, when Malcolm visits the home of his client, Mrs Soloff, who is sitting *shiva* for her husband, he notices that all of the mirrors have been covered. His introduction to this Jewish mourning ritual prompts him to reflect on his own apartment where, owing to Denis's inability to countenance his image, the mirrors are likewise draped with towels. As Malcolm explains, they were also "in mourning, sitting *shiva* on the death of their former life" (45). In this same episode, Malcolm learns from a relative at the *shiva* that the Soloffs first met in a concentration camp. In this way, the narrative subtly connects a range of social and physical deaths to the Holocaust. Although Mrs Soloff never speaks of that time, she still bears a tattooed number on her arm. Later, when Alison fails to recognize its significance and naively enquires about its origins, the amiable and gentle Mrs Soloff, characterized as "dignity personified, with her white hair ... floating in a nimbus around her head" like a halo, uncharacteristically chastises her angrily, telling her in no uncertain terms, "You are a very stupid girl" (124).

As in the first chapter, in which Denis and Malcolm come to blows, Mrs Soloff's hostile response demonstrates how failures of recognition repeatedly lead to breakdowns in communication and usher in violence. This sequence occurs again prior to Christian's death, when Malcolm visits Denis at the care facility to celebrate Christmas. When the elevator doors open, Malcolm witnesses a veritable tower of Babel, as virtually all of the residents suffer from dementia. They forget they are in the present and live in memories of the past. In this regard, they mirror the behaviour of Christian's murderer, who likewise acts out genocidal impulses that came "straight out of the past" (216). Malcolm's confrontation with both the residents and Vorst give the lie to the illusion of social progress and the related illusion of sequential identity or selfhood. These are precious illusions because they imply control, comprehensibility, order, improvement and justice, while defending against an awareness of chaos, confusion, and helplessness. Nevertheless, Malcolm realizes the limitations of the illusion when he must decide which version of Denis is more authentic, his cheerful lover or the raging anti-Semite. As this episode demonstrates, all of the residents have regressed and cease to recognize each other: one patient, Mrs Ross, calls for her mother, who is long dead. Another, Mrs Patterson, imagines that she is a young girl and the Second World War has just started. She encourages Malcolm to join her in waving goodbye to the soldiers. For his part, Denis, who once loved everyone and was beloved by all (23), insists he is in Hell and repeatedly quizzes Malcolm to discern who among his fellow residents are Jews. "Jews are everyone," he warns Malcolm. "For all I know, you could be one, too" (168–9). Although these "lost souls" (166), as Malcolm terms them, are "supposed to sit down together in a spirit of peace and love" (166), their fellowship is irrevocably shattered due to their lack of compassionate recognition. Misrecognition reaches a peak when Denis points his finger at Mrs Ross and shouts, "Jew! Jew!" Mrs Ross begins to scream, spreading panic among the other patients. In the mayhem, Denis wheels on Malcolm, calling him a "*Tapette*!" – "Faggot" – and, biting his cheek, draws blood (170). In the aftermath, some residents pray while others bellow like animals. Nurses scurry from the other floors "to shut down the apocalypse" (170). The biting of Malcolm's cheek, a gesture that fuses animal rage with the consumption of human flesh, recalls Northrop Frye's analysis of the relationship between the Eucharist symbolism and its demonic parody (Frye, *Anatomy* 147–50). According to Frye, in the demonic apocalyptic world we often "find the cannibal feast, the serving up of a child or lover as food" (*The Secular* 118).

This scene is juxtaposed with the account of Christian's murder – yet another example of secular apocalypse – this time seen from the perspective of a nameless witness, who is addressed in the second person as "you." While trawling for sex at night in the park, the unnamed witness encounters three people giving chase to a shrieking boy:

All three barrel across the wet grass, the boy pumping limbs, the other two gaining, one holding out a stick to trip him up. You don't move, either to help him or to retreat. You are frozen where you stand.

From the corner of your eye, a fourth figure. See him moving in the same direction, but in no kind of hurry, stiffly, almost regimental, in the manner of police.

No person permitted in this park.

The boy is still running, then, hooked at the ankle he goes down-face first, almost comically. A hysterical, half-nauseated little laugh slips out of you. And then the joyless robotic kicking, the grunting – their exertion or the boy absorbing blows. *Fucking, fucking, faggot* they chant. When the fourth reaches them, he takes the stick, raises it and, in the air, it glints. Savagely, he brings it down just as two trains smash together. (187)

Owing to its use of the second person, this scene implicates the reader – "You are frozen where you stand" – placing us in the position of someone who is likewise caught in the pattern of repetition and degeneration. The novel reinforces the parallels between the prior episode with Malcolm through the repetition of the word "faggot." I would add that while the trains referred to in the passage recall the trains that delivered people from all across Europe to their deaths, they also serve as a figurative device, akin to the image of the driver's sunglasses, reflexively signaling how the novel as a whole works by forcibly bringing two trains of thought together – the past and the present.

SECTION IV: CHRISTIAN AS A QUEER CHRIST FIGURE

At issue in the novel is, firstly, how to adequately address the complex interrelationship of past (individual and species-wide history) and present, and secondly, how to acknowledge the ways in which we are complicit in failures in recognizing the Other and lapses in seeing our own culpability and violence. Insight into this complexity is precisely Christian's gift and his role in the text entails conveying it to others. When Alison innocently enquires about Mrs Soloff's tattoo, it is Christian who gently offers her a history lesson. Equally important, in contrast to the handsome Denis, who only later in life has a problem with his reflection, Christian, whose face, altered from birth – recalling Malcolm's fleeting experience of "looking positively Cubist" (32)

– *is* the problem in the mirror.[9] Early on readers learn that Christian's eyes are not straight and that his nose is flattened, which causes him to breathe audibly. When Alison goes out with Christian for lunch for the first time, she puzzles over his unusual features:

> Now that he was across from her, she no longer had to avoid looking at him for fear he would think she was trying to figure out the problem on his face. Where to look, though? When he fixed her with the bright tack of his left eye, the right veered off, distractingly. She followed its dead-end gaze, only to abruptly refocus on the left straight-ahead eye again. The moment she did, it veered – a back-and-forth confusion like the old gag where two people jam in a door frame after so many after-yous. Soon she realized she wasn't listening to what he was saying … so she looked elsewhere on his face, to the flattened nose, the nostrils squashed almost to slits. He snuffled when he breathed; he nasalized. The scarred skin above his lip was shiny and pink. (98)

As this passage states, Christian's eye/I is not straight. Figuratively speaking, his eyes signal his status as queer (not straight). Equally important, references to his flattened nose and the snuffling sound of his breath align him with animality. In accordance with the text's attention to detail and its relentless shuttling between the present and the past, in this episode, Christian sits across from a travel poster on the wall, featuring the Eagle's Nest. As Christian explains to Alison, it was "Hitler's infamous hideout" (98–9). Rather than suffer shamefully and silently under Alison's scrutiny and, by extension, the scrutiny of Western culture, which seemingly remains intent on weeding out defective traits, Christian responds by joking: "'You have found me out,' he quips. 'I am a hairdresser with a harelip'" (99). Far from being offended by her probing gaze, Christian assures Alison she will get used to him.

At "Vitae," Christian's clients likewise repeatedly find themselves puzzling over his face. Yet as the narrator explains, they come to the salon "to be offered a pierced, sympathetic ear. For advice, for judgment to be reserved. To confess" (92). This is precisely the service Christian – whose face is "flattened like it was pressed against glass" – offers them (88). For them, Christian is the Other who assures his clients of their difference and perfection. He suffers for their sins. His Gothic role as double is made explicit in his conversation with

Alison when he likens himself to Frankenstein's monster. In keeping with Mary Shelley's story, in which Victor flees from his monstrous "child," Christian's parents likewise abandoned him. "I was quite a shock to them," he tells Alison: "After me, they gave up reproducing" (135). When she asks him where they live, he replies tersely: "Who knows. They do not approve of me and I do not approve of them" (135–6). The betrayal of Christian by his own parents recalls more disturbing events in Germany prior to the Second World War, when parents of children with physical and mental challenges petitioned the government to have their children euthanized (see Wright 105). Visibly different, Christian confesses he is a frequent target of rejection and a host of tactless and cruel remarks. Although Alison cannot imagine anyone purposely trying to hurt Christian, he warns her prophetically, "Sweetie ... We have our enemies" (126).

Although the text aligns Christian with monstrosity, he is simultaneously portrayed as a Christ figure. In this updated version of the biblical story, Christian is betrayed while cruising for sex in a public park. Dressed in his red T-shirt that reads "Worship Me," valentine red Doc Martens, and sporting a dog chain necklace, Christian represents a 1980s incarnation of the Son of God. His identification with Jesus is further evidenced by his motto. As he tells Alison, "Love and life are one. If you separate out love, you're not living. Instead, live every moment for love" (100). True to his credo and his namesake, Christian shows compassion for all of his colleagues. In addition to saving Alison from drinking bleach and endearing himself to her on her first day at "Vitae," Christian befriends Malcolm at the office Christmas party shortly before he is murdered. Playing on the salon décor's allusions, the partygoers reenact the decline and fall of the Roman Empire. At the height of the revelry, Christian dares Malcolm to kiss him under the mistletoe. Without "flinching or showing he was in any way repelled" by his face, Malcolm obliges and kisses Christian firmly on the lips (143). For his part, rather than feel repulsed, Malcolm views this as the first decent thing he has done in a long while. A few days later, Christian shows up unannounced at Malcolm's apartment, bearing croissants and an offer of friendship. In his characteristically camp, self-deprecating fashion, Christian identifies himself over the intercom in the lobby, saying, "It's me, Christian. The *homunculus* you work with" (149). During Christian's brief visit, he flaunts his status as a figure of abjection. Helping himself to a chocolate croissant, at one point, he bites into it and shows

Malcolm the filling, merrily shouting, "Poo!" and laughing his high-pitched laugh (151–2). Seeing that Malcolm is not amused, Christian kindly changes the subject and asks Malcolm to tell him about his life with Denis in Paris. In his account, Malcolm speaks frankly about his difficulties with French anti-Semitism. During their *tête à tête*, how-ever, Malcolm neither reveals that Denis is suffering from dementia nor that he is now living in a care facility. When Christian comments on Denis's good looks, evident in the photographs displayed in the living room, Malcolm insists that he loved Denis not because he was handsome, but because, like Christian, he was "kind" (155). After uttering this statement, Malcolm experiences an epiphany: he real-izes that for all Christian's "pranks and gossip … the little man had the ethos of a saint" (149).

SECTION V: THE LAMB OF GOD AND IMAGES OF THE SACRIFICIAL ANIMAL

In *A History of Forgetting*, homosexuals, Jews, and dogs are identi-fied as figures of abjection that are unjustly marginalized and tar-geted for violence. Not coincidentally, Christian is identified with all three categories. When a new client greets him, for example, saying, "You're Christian, right?'" He responds, "No. I'm Jewish" (92) – an allusion to Christ's originary faith. Readers are also told that "what little remained of Christian's hair he wore duckling-coloured and shaved down close, and now he was pointing to his bald spot, a per-fect yarmulke of flesh" (92).

Perhaps because marginalized individuals in the novel – most obviously Malcolm's elderly female clients – are treated like dogs, or because the word "dog" is a palindrome for God, the narrative repeat-edly associates Christian with canines. More precisely, his flattened nose and tendency to snuffle forge a profound connection between Christian and Denis's beloved dog, Grace. Malcolm brought Grace home at the urging of Denis's caregiver Yvette, who realizes that Malcolm is growing unable to meet Denis' needs. She explains that a dog would help calm Denis. In accordance with Yvette's prediction, Grace brings Denis untold happiness. Due to Denis's memory loss, every time Malcolm returns from the park with Grace, he sees her for the first time and, with every encounter, "he was freshly smitten" (60). Neither judges the other and theirs is a bond forged purely from love. Shortly after Grace joins their lives, Malcolm introduces her to the group of companion animals belonging to his elderly clients who congregate every morning in the park. As Malcolm observes, all of their dogs suffer from various deformities and diseases. Grace, for example, does not have a tail and she is incontinent: the "stump in back of her – the size of a man's thumb severed at the knuckle" wiggles as she pees (58). Mrs Veve's dog, Lady, suffers from a grotesque tumour that hangs from its belly like an enlarged scrotum. Mrs Parker's beloved Chihuahua, Mitzi, is blind, and Mrs Rodick's pug, Hugh, has epilepsy. Far from being ashamed of their pets' defects, however, the women lovingly boast about the creatures' imperfections. For them, their canines' flaws and vulnerabilities enhance their bonds. Although Malcolm longs to tell the group about Grace's incontinence because it truly makes her one of the club, he does not mention it since, for all he knew, "they might be similarly inconvenienced" (57). His insight underscores how aging, a natural form of decline, affects all mortal creatures.

Rather than be repelled by human defects, Malcolm insists that flaws are an inextricable part of beauty. For example, although the owner of "Vitae" makes every effort to enhance her beauty, in Malcolm's eyes her perfection is grotesque. She will never be beautiful because, as Malcolm explains, a "truly beautiful woman acknowledges her flaws, even flaunts them, for they are what make her unique. They grace her character, which is the real seat of beauty" (83). Despite his theoretical understanding of the relationship between human beauty, flaws, and grace, Malcolm nevertheless finds the dogs' bodies and behaviour disgusting. We are told, for instance, that the pug's mouth at the corners "reminded Malcolm of blackened female genitalia" (55). When he looks away, he catches sight of Grace "splayed pornographically as she cleaned herself" (55). Although Mitzi wanders in "a seemingly inoffensive circle," Malcolm has "learned to recognize the signs preliminary to defecation. He had a moment like this every day, when he didn't know *where* to look" (55).

After Denis enters the care facility, Malcolm is similarly ashamed of Denis, who, in keeping with the connections drawn in the novel between mental decline and animality, has taken to defecating in a fellow patient's drawer and stealing someone else's incontinence pants. Even though Yvette tells him that Denis's actions have nothing to do with him, nevertheless Malcolm feels they do: "He felt anything to do with Denis reflected back on him" (158). Unable to "separate himself from Denis' actions and opinions" (158), Malcolm responds by abandoning Denis, rebuffing Grace's pleas for affection, and teasing her cruelly.

As Malcolm's increasingly malicious behaviour toward Grace could be seen to indicate, she serves as a mirror of a personal and societal disavowal of our capacity for degeneration. Sadly, Malcolm's disavowal has the same consequences as that of the young men who killed Christian. On the morning of his departure for Poland, Malcolm has Grace euthanized. As he explains, prior to dropping her off at the vet's, he tied "a new bow on her and wiped her eyes with a cloth. Her pink tongue washed his hands; no end to her forgiveness" (306).[10] Later, however, in Poland, while lying in bed the night before he and Alison drive to Auschwitz, Malcolm cannot sleep. Thinking about Grace, he confesses that she "was haunting him. In every creak, he heard her yelp" (305). Only when it is too late does he realize his error in dismissing Grace as a witless beast and ending her life: "What he'd done was wrong and now, in his regret, he realized he had been wrong about her, too ... He'd considered her brainless and pitied her. All animals he tended to pity – because they cannot read. But can't they? Thinking back on their many hours in the park, he recalled how, let off the lead, she would fly off on a course of delirious sniffing. It reminded him of how he liked to race home to a book. Was it not a form of reading then, this picking up a scent trail, akin, say to Braille? Braille for the nose. Splashed up on the tree trunks, put down in trickles in the grass, there were epics and sonnets, novellas and pornographic tales. Grace had been voracious for it all; she had really been a perfect little companion" (305). After he has Grace put down, Malcolm finds her hair all over his apartment: "A fine layer of hair had settled over it all, as if he had disposed of the dog by plugging in a firecracker and exploding her in the room" (293). This scene presages the roomfuls of hair that he and Alison witness at Auschwitz – hair that belonged to the millions of individuals slaughtered by the Germans. In its treatment of dogs, specifically in the repeated references to canine and human hair, the novel deconstructs the boundary reinforced during the Enlightenment between human and animal, and the claim that both are "beyond language" (Bewell 32). Having no access to language left animals, Jews, and the feeble minded, alike, bereft of the protection, rights, and privileges accorded to human citizens under the law. After she witnesses the warehouse filled with hair at Auschwitz, Alison recalls the first and only time she had been to church as a girl. The Sunday school teacher had told them that "God had counted every hair on their heads" (347).

In blurring the distinction between human and animal, *A History of Forgetting* specifically challenges Western culture's privileging of particular assessments of cognitive ability and valorization of intelligence and IQ scores, the legacy of Enlightenment thinkers such as Locke. In addition to insisting on the intelligence of Christian's killer, at one point, for example, Malcolm acknowledges that Alison is not terribly bright. As he says, she is "no rocket scientist," but he nevertheless maintains that in her "there were qualities equal to intelligence" (267). Alison's dedication to Christian and her grief at his death prompts Malcolm to recall a line from Virginia Woolf's novel *Mrs Dalloway* (1925), "What did the brain matter, compared to the heart." Malcolm "thought it marvelous, marvelous she could care so much" (267–8).

Malcolm's celebration of caring and his insistence that it trumps intelligence, however, raises a question that haunts the novel. What about people such as Denis who, due to illness, lack the ability to recognize and thus care for others – or, for that matter, for themselves? Is society no longer bound to care for them? At bottom, in its treatment of Denis, the text draws our attention to a highly problematic and ultimately unsatisfactory response to this question. In the end Malcolm abandons Denis; his fate is never conclusively narrated. On the one hand, due to its sympathetic treatment of Christian the narrative displaces the fascist ideology that promotes abjection; on the other hand, its treatment of Denis reinstalls Gothic tropes and effaces the humanity of people suffering from dementia. In this way the narrative shows how easy it is to substitute more palatable sacrificial victims – ones who, like Christian and Grace, are blameless and loveable and hence worthy of mourning – for more difficult, "hate-filled" individuals suffering from cognitive decline.

Although the novel draws attention to the implications of this type of substitution, the text never explicitly champions this process, which is everywhere apparent. A passage concerning Denis's affinity for animals perhaps best conveys the facets of this process. Reflecting on Yvette's suggestion that he purchase a dog for Denis, Malcolm realizes that Denis would be thrilled with the idea because he loves all creatures, dead or alive: "He used to cup the summer wasps in his bare hands to release out the window and throw bread crumbs down for the courtyard pigeons. If, on the street, he happened to pass a dog tied to a post, he would always stop to offer it encouragement. As for the rabbits hanging like Mussolini in the market – too late. Denis could only help by elevating them to a higher incarnation in a terrine. In a bowl next to the sink the eel, flayed and segmented, soaked in water, waiting its turn at immortality. The decapitated head floated near the surface, the eyes little sightless beads" (31). What is striking here is the suggestion that animals can be elevated "to a higher incarnation" – a process that neatly sums up the text's treatment of Denis. The last time Malcolm visits Denis at the care facility, he observes that Denis's eyes were "pale and glassy" (284), an image that recalls the eel's "eyes like sightless beads." As Malcolm explains, what he saw now "was vacancy … Here was the ghost at last" (284).

Equally important, by juxtaposing Denis to Christian – a fellow homosexual who serves as a more palatable or "cooked" version of disability, to borrow Lévi-Strauss's term – readers are prompted to consider which characters garner our sympathy. The narrative highlights the difficulty involved in accepting Denis in all his rawness – a man who, due to cognitive decline, defecates in drawers. As the scene in which Malcolm and Christian commune over croissants illustrates, Christian is a mentally agile and intelligent young man who only pretends to eat feces when in fact he is biting into a perfectly respectable and delicious chocolate croissant. In the end, some readers may well find it easier to mourn Christian and Grace rather than Denis, who becomes "unkind" and "unlikeable" (194). In this way, the text encourages readers to ponder the ethical implications of a process of substitution whereby a cognitively disabled elderly homosexual is replaced by a witty, youthful one with a physical disability. This process of substitution recalls the Enlightenment view of idiocy that posits an implicit hierarchy whereby physical differences are located above cognitive challenges that instigate memory loss. As I argue in the next section, this hierarchy is adopted and adapted by the text's repeated suggestion that one of the best ways to prevent degeneration lies in reading and remembering history and, in the process, treating the world as text.

SECTION VI: CONCLUSION:
READING THE WORLD AS SECULAR TEXT

The novel's repeated references to various forms of reading highlight its overriding faith that narratives – ranging from historical works about the Holocaust to Dante's *Inferno* to the Bible to an image of the world itself as text – can relate crucial lessons concerning humanity's capacity for violence and compassion. Owing to the host of intertexts in many languages and to the emphasis on touch, Adderson's narrative underscores that reading is not restricted to the decoding of texts written in English. Put differently, according to the novel, goodness is inextricably connected to the ability to read and reflect on signs and symbols ranging from Mrs Soloff's tattoo to canine scent trails. Without the ability to read history, humanity is doomed to repeat the mistakes of the past. As Alison and Malcolm walk through Auschwitz, they are confronted by a sign that states this explicitly: "The one who does not remember history is bound to live through it again" (341). In keeping with its self-reflexive representations of books and reading, *A History of Forgetting* ultimately constitutes a tribute to the ethical power of the book. After their ghastly tour of Auschwitz, for example, Alison visits a nearby church and sees the priest open the altarpiece. Gradually, it dawns on her that the altarpiece is not a cabinet; instead, "*It was a book*" (346). The beginning is carved on the outside and the ending is the entire central panel. The outside story is one of violence: "a taunting and a flaying, a ghastly drawn-out death, wounds bared then disbelieved – almost the same story she had pored over all winter" (347). The inside story, however, featuring a scene of ecstatic revelation, is one of hope:

> If the beginning was carved on the outside in the near-black wood, and the middle on the two carved and vibrantly painted inside covers, then the ending was the entire huge central panel: a woman falling on her knees. She was the size of a living woman, the crowd around her life-size too. Life-size and seemingly inspirited – Alison saw veins pulsing in legs, throbbing arthritic knuckles, pouching skin. One man was holding the woman as she sank; one, fingers twined together, made a gesture unreadable and strange. Another recoiled, two stared, one staggered. Above, angels winged like birds. The painted middle scenes on the doors were of angelic visitations, the poignant docility of livestock, gifts being given, a radiance in the sky. (346–7)

Although the altarpiece tells the age-old story of violence and revelation in religious terms, *A History of Forgetting* nevertheless insists that the familiar story of violence and healing can be discerned by religious and secular readers alike. After visiting the concentration camp, Alison ponders the nature of faith. As the narrator explains: "How could Alison ever believe in God when not even her mother did, her mother who, of everyone Alison knew, came closest to being

a saint? How to believe in anything after the Auschwitz Muzeum?"
(347). After she returns from church as a child and asks her mother
if God really counts every hair on their heads, her mother replies:
"Gosh ... You'd think he'd have better things to do" (347). In answer
to her daughter's second question as to whether she believes in God,
Alison's mother replies: "I just add that extra letter. I believe in Good"
(347). In keeping with this response, *A History of Forgetting*'s message is legible to anyone prepared to transform ghosts into ancestors;
this entails looking beyond the trappings of the Gothic, learning the
lessons of history, and practicing goodness.

   After she returns from church Alison finds Malcolm, who has just
committed a failed suicide attempt. Around him is a dark wet stain
"flecked with white powder and broken bits of half-dissolved pills"
(348). Instinctively, Alison takes Malcolm to the sink where she proceeds to wash his hair – a secular baptism of sorts. As the noxious
black dye washes away, Malcolm feels as if he were "being lifted
up ... The terrible weight of all that had happened was being taken
from him, if only for this moment ... In the mirror, she saw herself
rocking him" (350). Although this image recalls pictures and sculp-
tures of the Virgin Mary holding the dead body of Jesus Christ in her
arms, this pietà nevertheless remains within the novel's overarching
secular framework – expressed as a shift from God to goodness. It
is also a shift from filiation to affiliation, providing an alternative to
the Freudian model that dooms the younger generation to revolting
against the previous generation (see Woodward, "Inventing" 163).

   At bottom, in its portrayal of Alison's getting of wisdom, the novel
highlights its debt to Locke's Enlightenment view of humanity, which
argues that people learn not through Divine inspiration, but instead
through sensation and reflection. Equally important, despite Sontag's
injunction to interpret illness without the aid of metaphor, *A History
of Forgetting* repeatedly illustrates that in the ongoing war against
dementia, physicians and authors alike continue to rely on Gothic
and apocalyptic narrative structures. Adopting a critical stance does
not entail abandoning metaphor but rather using the Gothic as an
opportunity to reflect on history – in this case, the history of earlier wars against dementia. As *A History of Forgetting* hauntingly
reminds us, however, in keeping with the symbol of the ouroboros
each seemingly new attempt to tell the story of dementia is, in part, a
retelling of a history we have forgotten.

9

Unburying the Living in Jane Rule's *Memory Board* and Selected Stories by Alice Munro

As seen in previous chapters, the Gothic horror associated with the threat of dementia has prompted some contemporary Canadian writers to reflect on prior historical moments when considerations of mental and physical imperfections were likewise a paramount social concern. *A History of Forgetting*, for example, returns readers to the crematoriums of Auschwitz to analyze Western society's apocalyptic response to intellectual and physical disabilities. This chapter continues to analyze texts by Canadian writers that offer alternatives to Gothic and apocalyptic portrayals of dementia and the concomitant desire to expel the Other – alternatives that have the added advantage of transcending Freud's binary and familial Oedipal intergenerational model. This model is limited because it offers only the extreme passions of love and hate as affective options and, worse, it posits death as the sole outcome of the supposedly inevitable battle between youth and age. Drawing on works ranging from Jane Rule's novel *Memory Board* (1987) to a selection of stories from the works of Alice Munro, including "The Dance of the Happy Shades" (1968), "The Bear Came over the Mountain" (1999), and "In Sight of the Lake" (2012), I explore how Rule's and Munro's texts likewise demonstrate their engagement with the historical contexts in which they were written as they attempt to subvert the often unspoken links between cognitive decline and Gothic horror. Whereas Rule's fiction conveys a utopian version of history, Munro's short stories offer realist, historical accounts of dementia that contain glimpses of prior modes of resistance to Gothic portrayals of dementia – modes that have been eclipsed by the contemporary biomedical model. These moments of resistance include perceiving individuals suffering from dementia not as disabled but as enigmatic and gifted figures. Munro's fictions also echo the formal and philosophical insights of the Surrealists in the early twentieth century, who insisted that madness highlights the centrality of the imagination.

Written during the AIDS crisis in the 1980s, Rule's utopian novel portrays a Canadian family embracing homosexuals who were previously stigmatized and rejected. Whereas Rule's novel maintains an overtly progressive agenda, Munro's stories do not explicitly represent this type of utopian societal transformation or a righting of past wrongs. Instead, Munro's fictions rely on irony and ironic reversals to afford alternative perspectives on disability and dementia. For example "Dance of the Happy Shades," published in her first collection of the same title, highlights the similarities and differences between children with Down syndrome and other intellectual disabilities and the frail elderly coping with dementia. At the time, views of cognitive disability were shifting due to the effect of the deinstitutionalization movement in the late 1960s, and children with cognitive challenges were no longer viewed as figures of abjection who should be hidden away in asylums. In contrast to "Dance of the Happy Shades," which charts the widening gap between society's treatment of cognitively disabled children and elders, "The Bear Came over the Mountain," from Munro's collection *Hateship, Friendship, Courtship, Loveship, Marriage* (2001), focuses exclusively on the ontological and epistemological ironies associated with later-life dementia. Whereas Gothic portrayals of dementia typically chart the obliteration of selfhood and the transformation of the sufferer into a monster, Munro's stories about late-onset dementia retain the ironic possibility that the markers of personhood and agency persist despite the losses and corrosive stigma associated with dementia. Munro's fictions keep this possibility alive. They also emphasize the fragility and "ontological vulnerability" that underlies all human existence – the awareness that we begin life as infants lacking in control and that throughout the life course, we have an organic propensity to disease and sickness; and, as a result, death and dying are inescapable. Simply put, all bodies "are subject to impairment and disability" (Turner 29). This chapter concludes with a close reading of Munro's recent story "In Sight of the Lake" (2012) because of all her stories to date, it provides the most powerful counter-argument to portrayals of later life as a Gothic state of abject "unbecoming," what sociologists Paul Higgs and Chris Gilleard have recently termed "a black hole" ("Aging without Agency" 121).

Before turning to Rule's and Munro's texts, I want to consider the concepts of the third and fourth age in reference to the human life-span, which I briefly discussed in the introduction, as well as Higgs and Gilleard's suggestion that the metaphor of the black hole best captures the horrors associated with the fourth age. In their writings, Higgs and Gilleard distinguish between what they term the third and fourth age, and they invoke the related metaphors of the "event horizon" and the "black hole" to describe society's affectively charged response to the transformations that occur when elderly people succumb to profound mental or physical frailty. As they confess, the metaphor of the black hole "might seem too strong but our object in using it is to convey the inherent unknowability of the fourth age" (*Rethinking* 16). Glossing the term, Higgs and Gilleard note that in astronomy, "a black hole creates a massive gravitational pull that sucks in every phenomenon of the 'event horizon' which is a point where light disappears completely. Any light emitted from beyond this horizon can never reach the observer" (16). In essence these cosmic metaphors align the fourth age with something sublime, mysterious, and dark, but also lifeless and all-consuming – an enormous sphere of nothing, a void that sucks everything around it into itself. Their metaphors surpass mere declinist ideology and instead index what Elinor Fuchs refers to as "the power and persistence of the Sublime of Age, a visceral horror of physical decrepitude" ("Estragement" 70).

According to Higgs and Gilleard, the third age constitutes a cultural field associated with "the development of generational lifestyles whose origins can be traced to 1960s youth culture with its emphasis on choice, autonomy and self-expression" ("Aging without Agency" 122). They argue further that due to a set of developments that include "the narrowing of mortality within the life space, the expanding possibilities of not appearing or not performing as 'old,'" ("Aging, Abjection" 138), and the efforts to promote a more positive image of "normal" aging, the fourth age has been increasingly Gothicized and construed as a locus devoid of self-consciousness and choice: "It is when people are no longer 'getting by,' when they are seen as not managing the daily round, when they become third persons in others' age-based discourse, within others' rules, that they become subjects of a fourth age. At this point an 'event horizon' is passed, beyond which the everyday round cannot situate a frame of reference from which individual agency is interpreted. It is the combination of a public failure of self-management and the securing of this failure by institutional forms of care that a key boundary is passed" ("Aging without Agency" 122).

In their writings on the fourth age, Higgs and Gilleard underscore the deleterious effects of institutionalization and the role it plays in creating a Gothic social imaginary: "The irreversibility of nursing home placement, the disappearance of any personal exchange in the processes of admission, and the 'deprivatization of experience' that results from admission (Gubrium and Holstein, 1999) create an immense negative force upon both the third age that surrounds but remains imperceptive of it and the general attitude to old age. In short, the fourth age acts as a metaphorical black hole of aging" (125). They invoke the metaphor of the black hole not because it represents the Truth, but because it captures society's affective response and fantasies – what they term the "social imaginary" – associated with later-life. I would argue further that this particular expression of the social imaginary is drawn from high Gothic, which, as noted in the introduction, emphasizes horrifying evil and monstrous transformations.

As Higgs and Gilleard explain, however, the fourth age "is neither an inevitable nor an inescapable stage of life"; instead it can be understood "as a form of social imaginary, coordinated by our collective understandings of frailty and abjection and realized through the social institutions that develop in response to those understandings" ("Aging, Abjection" 140). Rather than view the third and fourth age in the traditional sense as "stages of life," they suggest they are more properly understood as "contested cultural spaces," with the latter's social meaning derived from at least two basic societal changes: "the 'densification' of old age (through general improvements in mortality, institutional policies and practices) and the objectification of frailty and abjection that arises from viewing and/or listening to the narratives of older people in care" (ibid.).

Fiction and the psychological products of fantasy play a central role in the construction of the social imaginary of the fourth age since, as Higgs and Gilleard maintain, it is generated solely on the basis of external perspectives and third-party narratives. In this regard it mirrors the third-person stance of biomedical models: "To many people in or approaching 'later' life, the position of those in the fourth age can be likened to that of an object that has strayed too close to the event horizon and has now gone over it, beyond any chance of return. Equally, no light shines back once the event horizon is traversed. In the absence of any reflexive return it becomes impossible to separate what is projected into it and what occurs within it" ("Aging without Agency" 125). As this passage indicates, straying "too close to the event horizon" describes a shift in narrative perspective such that one becomes the object of third-person narratives and third-party actions, rather than the author of a first-person account that articulates one's own thoughts and desires. One is no longer the hero of one's own story. This shift results in one becoming "'lost' from citizenship and the 'civilised'" ("Frailty" 15). I cite Higgs and Gilleard's insights at length because, on the one hand, they recall the Enlightenment view of the "idiot" as located "outside language" (see Bewell 57). On the other hand, Higgs and Gilleard also stress the importance of narrative perspective and metaphor – the very terrain on which Rule's and Munro's fiction contests the prevailing social imaginary of the fourth age as a black hole.

SECTION I: *MEMORY BOARD* – UNBURYING THE GOTHIC MONSTER

Jane Rule's *Memory Board* has many similarities to Caroline Adderson's novel *A History of Forgetting*. For one, Rule's and Adderson's narratives are set in Vancouver during the 1980s and explore homosexual relationships in which one partner suffers from Alzheimer's. Whereas *A History of Forgetting* highlights the shift from the third to the fourth age by ultimately positioning Malcolm's lover Denis as the monstrous Other and excising him from the narrative, *Memory Board* offers an alternative response to the challenges posed by (queer) aging. Structurally and thematically, *Memory Board* portrays the acceptance of physical and mental vulnerability and promotes the adoption of nurturing roles by people in the third age. Equally important, the novel suggests that when men assume these roles it serves as a much-needed corrective to Western society's privileging of the fantasy of the immortal, autonomous, physically, and cognitively flawless male/hero/human. In keeping with Adderson's *A History of Forgetting*, *Memory Board* emphasizes alternatives to Freud's binary Oedipal model of intergenerational relationships – a model that was graphically portrayed in *Scar Tissue*.

   Memory Board portrays the relationship between two twins, David and Diana, born in Vancouver in 1921. As children, David and Diana are inseparable. Gradually, however, they grow apart. Early on, their estrangement is instigated by their entry into primary school.

Succumbing to peer pressure, David adopts a masculine gender role, which entails showing contempt for girls including Diana. Later, the twins experience a geographic separation when Diana volunteers oversees to aid in the war effort. While stationed in London, she meets her long-time companion, Constance. After falling in love with each other in their early twenties, Diana and Constance never part. By contrast, Diana and David's relationship is almost irrevocably severed when David marries Patricia, a virulently homophobic woman, who forces David to choose between her or his sister.

The novel opens the year following Patricia's death in 1986 when, after four decades of virtual silence, David reaches out to Diana. While Patricia was alive, David made furtive, yearly birthday visits to exchange gifts with Diana. Afterward, "he went back to a life from which she and Constance were entirely excluded" (27). Readers learn that Diana "had never laid eyes on his two daughters. She did not even know their married names or how many grandchildren he had" (27). In its portrayal of cognitive impairment, *Memory Board* juxtaposes Constance's late-onset dementia to David's forty-year estrangement from his sister and her partner, instigated by the shame and prejudice imposed by David's wife. As David explains, he, his adult children, and his grandchildren, who have never met Diana or Constance, must unlearn the "cruel pieties" they were taught by Patricia. The narrative forcibly conveys the malignant aspects of Patricia's homophobia when Diana confesses that even though Patricia has been dead a full year, she is "lodged in Diana's memory like a tumor" (25).

Rather than portray the ostracism of those deemed Other, *Memory Board* depicts characters who make the effort to recognize the living who have been subjected to an unjust social death. In keeping with the Gothic trope of live burial,[1] which in Rule's and Adderson's novels is instigated by the stigma associated with both homosexuality and dementia, *Memory Board* emphasizes recognizing the Other. In the narrative's subversion of the Gothic, recognizing the Other is represented as excavating the living, a motif that recalls Orpheus's rescue of Eurydice. The text highlights the act of unburying early on when Diana recalls how she and Constance first met during the Blitz. As Diana explains, she was there when the bomb fell that killed Constance's mother and sister and buried Constance for forty-eight hours. Part of the rescue team that unearthed the traumatized girl, Diana literally excavates Constance – an experience that later in life, Diana associates with both a release from prison and a birth:

"The arthritic ache in her [Diana's] hands could make her think it was only yesterday that she had dug painfully with them through the rubble to deliver this beloved woman who had delivered Diana from the prison of her desire. 'Constance, Constance, Constance,' she kept calling. 'I will get you out.' But first there had been the mother, then the sister, stillbirths both, and only hours later, Constance, alive" (44–5). This traumatic event plays a profound role in Diana's subsequent decision to study medicine and, equally significant, to specialize in obstetrics. By emphasizing Diana's work as a gynecologist, *Memory Board* self-consciously raises the issue of individual, and by extension social, forms of reproduction and the challenges posed to reproduction by queer forms of subjectivity associated with both homosexuality and dementia. Put differently, like *A History of Forgetting*, *Memory Board* also invites readers to consider the prejudices that govern society's views concerning who should and should not be allowed to reproduce and, by extension, who should and should not be allowed to live.[2]

As disability scholars observe, for the first half of the twentieth century these discussions invariably concerned reproduction and drew on the science of eugenics. In this era, eugenics – "the science of improving the stock" – was brought to bear on the future of the nation (in Kühl 4). Some eugenicists, however, championed the need to prevent the reproduction of the "unfit" to "free future generations from avoidable genetically transmitted handicaps" (ibid. 4, 5).

Both books likewise link the fate of homosexuals to that of cognitively challenged individuals, based on the fact that historically both groups were denied the status of persons or citizens; both were deemed "'lost' from citizenship and the 'civilised'" (Higgs and Gilleard, "Frailty" 15). *Memory Board*'s concern with who does or does not count as a "real" person is forcibly underscored early on, during David's reunion with Diana a year after Patricia's death. At one point during their conversation, David asks Diana, "Am I real to you?" (32). After they part, Diana admits that she was unable to provide him with an answer "that was of any help to him" (32). She also realizes that she longed to ask him the same question. *Memory Board* traces David's and Diana's efforts to recognize each other and, equally important, Constance's humanity. At the end of the novel, David decides to move in with Diana to help her look after Constance. For her part Diana is grateful, but she is also quite surprised that David would choose to move out of his daughter's house "enlivened by a growing family" into what Diana terms "this mortal climate" (315). Rather than maintaining an alliance with youth and socially sanctioned modes of reproduction, David chooses instead to live with his aged, childless, lesbian sister and her lover in order to bring comfort to both women. In keeping with other plot points, this episode highlights the novel's explicitly utopian vision, in which resources and respect are lovingly directed toward those whom society deems abject.

Equally significant and, some might argue, equally utopian, David's capacity to recognize Constance's humanity is not predicated on her ability to recognize him. For instance, when Constance's illness progresses to the point that she no longer knows who David is, rather than feel effaced, he states that he "had always known his love for Constance had to be entirely independent of any recognition from her" (287). His predicament recalls very similar challenging moments in *Scar Tissue* and *A History of Forgetting* when the characters suffering from dementia lose the ability to recognize their caregivers. In the case of *A History of Forgetting*, I argued that the narrative raises a crucial, ethically charged question about society's responsibility to care for people who, due to illness can no longer recognize or care for others – or, for that matter, for themselves. Whereas both Ignatieff's narrator and Adderson's protagonists feel utterly effaced when they are no longer recognized – a feeling that profoundly undermines their ability to continue to look after their loved ones – Rule's idealistic novel highlights David's ability to care for Constance independent of her recognition.

On a related and equally hopeful note, rather than maintain a singular and unchanging identity in relation to the individual coping with dementia, *Memory Board* portrays Constance's caregivers gracefully acquiescing to the transformations of their identities instigated by her illness. David, for instance, allows his identity and the roles he plays to shift according to Constance's needs. When the latter mistakes David for "the plumber or the garbage man or the gardener, he quietly took on those roles, not with any archness or flamboyance but with an understated gentleness which was meant to be reassuring to her and was" (310). As a result, rather than treat Constance as a Gothic victim under house arrest with David and Diana acting as her prison guards, David's "ever-present changing made him appear to Constance as a temporary fact of life rather than an established custodian" (310).

David's ability to adopt different roles and to act as a gentle and reassuring presence supports Diana's hypothesis concerning the potential transformation of the heroic masculine role that predominated during the war years. At one point, David's grandsons visit Diana's house to help install new locks on the doors. Watching them at work, Diana marvels at their astonishing gentleness, which she attributes to the fact that they were born after the Second World War and are part of a new generation that must contend with the threat of a nuclear war: "These two had been allowed to grow up without the fact of war, instead with the threat of such a war that there would be no place for death-defying heroic fantasies, and they seemed to her gentler, more domestic creatures than her own generation had been, not soft, no, but their strength given to mending, moving, making things. They were great docile beings who conferred authority on their elders as if it were a gift from them rather than a yoke the young were forced to bear" (306). The images afforded in this passage of the pervasive shattering of "death-defying heroic fantasies" – and, one presumes, the concomitant acceptance of human beings' ontological vulnerability – and of young men "mending, moving, and making things" offer additional contrasts to *A History of Forgetting*. As we saw in the previous chapter, although Adderson's narrative focuses on decline and degeneration, it locates hope for regeneration primarily in the form of the young female character Alison who, by the end of the novel, has assumed the role of an enlightened, caring citizen. However, as evidenced by her gesture of cradling Malcolm's body and washing his hair, which strongly recalls the pietà, Alison assumes a very traditional feminine role. By contrast, *Memory Board* addresses the need to deconstruct the role of the patriarchal hero-human and, by extension, the Oedipal model of intergenerational conflict.

In keeping with its emphasis on unburying and the transformation of social roles and conservative attitudes, in its account of the long-term relationship between Diana and Constance, *Memory Board* insists on the endurance of the latter's personhood despite her illness. In the novel's final scene, for example, sixty-five-year-old Diana ponders the aptness of Constance's name. Diana muses that Constance was and remains "constant in will to herself even now against the blanks, the confusions, the terrors" (322). In contrast to the uncanny [*unheimlich*] horrors portrayed in both *Scar Tissue* and *A History of Forgetting*, *Memory Board* concludes with a *heimlich* scene in which Diana and Constance enjoy an intimate moment in their home.

Whereas, as Eve Kosofsky Sedgwick astutely observes, Gothic texts
rely on the trope of live burial, *Memory Board* eschews the Gothic
in favour of a realism infused with utopian political dimensions
to formally and thematically resist burying stigmatized characters
suffering from dementia.[3]

SECTION II: "DANCE OF THE HAPPY SHADES" – DECONSTRUCTING THE GOTHIC THROUGH IRONY

Viewed in light of the pervasive anti-Gothic motif of rescuing people
suffering from dementia from the land of the dead, it is significant
that the title story of Munro's first short story collection, *Dance of
the Happy Shades*, is drawn from the myth of Orpheus and Eurydice,
which relates the hero's failed quest to rescue his beloved, who is condemned to live in the underworld.[4] The title of Munro's story refers
to a far more prosaic allusion to the myth: a piano piece played at a
children's music recital by a girl with a cognitive impairment. Like *A
History of Forgetting*, Munro's narrative draws connections between
society's treatment of children living with cognitive impairment and
elderly individuals with dementia; both groups are silenced and typically hidden from view – a form of live burial.

Munro's story is set in the first half of the twentieth century when
the parents of children with Down syndrome were advised to institutionalize their child at birth, and when physicians routinely informed
parents that their child might never talk and could not be taught. As
Mark Jackson observes, "permanent segregation of the feeble minded
in purpose-built colonies, and the separation of the sexes within those
colonies, not only served as a means of effectively limiting the propagation of degenerates, but also crucially established a convenient
physical and ideological distance between the healthy middle classes,
on the one hand, and the polluted and contaminated 'residuum,'
on the other" (149). The radical challenge posed by "Dance of the
Happy Shades" is perhaps best understood when one considers that
Munro first published the story in the *New Yorker* in 1961, when
there were few literary models for representing cognitively disabled
children. The only serious, literary work in which Down syndrome
figured was William Faulkner's portrayal of Benjy Compson in *The
Sound and the Fury* (1929).[5]

Beyond the realm of literature, as Aldred Neufeldt observes, in
Canada prior to the 1960s "mental retardation, as it was then known,

was characterized by a sense of shame and social stigma felt by families and a lack of concerted interest on the part of both professionals of all kinds and policy makers ... The fact that parents of children with intellectual impairments neither knew of each other, nor were emboldened to take collective action until after WWII speaks volumes about the shame and neglect attached to the condition" (20). Children with cognitive impairments were sent away to live in small residential schools (the first was built in Orillia, ON in 1888); and while the "original intent was laudable, the residential 'schools' rapidly deteriorated into what became 'human warehouses' that were the subject of much attention by advocates in succeeding decades" (17). These overarching historical dimensions provide the background for my reading of "Dance of the Happy Shades," a domestic narrative that portrays a series of surprising events which transpire at Miss Marsalles's annual piano recital.

The story is related from the perspective of the adolescent, middle-class narrator, who is Miss Marsalles's pupil (as was her mother before her). Early on, readers learn that neither the young performers nor their well-heeled, young mothers are looking forward to the prospect of attending yet another recital at Miss Marsalles's home. Over the years, Miss Marsalles has moved from her tiny Rosedale home to ever more cramped accommodations. In this way, the narrative draws a parallel between her economic decline and her aging body. The narrator's mother insists that Miss Marsalles is simply getting *"too old"* (211). She also complains that the last three parties were "rather squashed" (211) and that this year, Miss Marsalles has moved to an even tinier home in a seedy part of town. Equally distressing and potentially one of the causes of the economic decline, Miss Marsalles's older sister, once a fixture at her annual recital, is now bedridden following a stroke that has left her cognitively impaired and unable to speak. In keeping with Locke's definition of the "idiot," she is located "outside of language" (Bewell 57). Never appearing in the story, the sister remains a haunting, Gothic figure of mental and physical age-related degeneration.

The themes of decay and degeneration pervade the story, which highlights society's tendency to stigmatize and expel those experiencing economic, physical, and cognitive decline. The story's blurring of these categories reflects shifts that occurred during the first half of the twentieth century when rather than view social pathology as inhering solely in socio-economic conditions – as a problem associated

with "the poor" – the rhetoric was adapted to convey a new conception of a social pathology "clearly located in the *biological* nature of
a distinct 'class' of the population" – the newly designated category
of the "feeble minded" (Jackson 2; my emphasis).

Overarching anxieties about physical aging and decay are introduced in Munro's story early on, with the partygoers' concern that
the food, which has been set out early in the day, will spoil in the heat.
The related threat of cognitive degeneration is likewise introduced
at the start when the narrator and her mother meet Miss Marsalles's
neighbour, Mrs Clegg, and the latter whispers that Miss Marsalles's
sister will not be joining them. "Yes, it's a shame," Mrs Clegg confides,
"She lost her powers of speech, you know. Her powers of control
generally, she lost" (218). In this instance, as in Munro's later story
entitled "Powers," "Dance of the Happy Shades" draws attention to
those who are rendered mute and whose cognitive fitness has waned
– variables that potentially doom individuals to a social death. The
silencing of people who are ill coupled with the surprising events that
unfold in Munro's story recall Lambek's insight, noted earlier, that
irony entails "the recognition that some of the potentially participatory voices or meanings are silent, missing, unheard, or not fully
articulate, and that voices or utterances appearing to speak for totality or truth offer only single perspectives" (*Irony* 6). Munro's narrative highlights the divisive and corrosive power of this type of limited
representation which, mirroring apocalypse's Manichean division
and the supposed gap between the third and fourth ages, induces a
select group to pity another, thereby ostracizing and demeaning those
who are stigmatized by placing them beyond the proverbial pale.

Despite her guests' barely veiled desire to be over and done with
the dreadful ritual, for reasons that are not immediately apparent,
Miss Marsalles insists on making everyone wait. When she enters the
house, the narrator senses that Miss Marsalles "was looking beyond
us as she kissed us; she was looking up the street for someone who
had not yet arrived" (217). Only when the narrator is playing her
piece does the explanation arrive for Miss Marsalles's delay. Looking
out of the corner of her eye, the narrator sees "a whole procession of
children, eight or ten in all, with a red-haired woman in something
like a uniform, mounting the front step" (220). The arrival of the
latecomers, which serves as a sign of their stereotypical slowness – as
latecomers, they are literally retarded – ushers in "a peculiarly concentrated silence" (221). The narrator remarks further on her sense

that something "has happened, something unforeseen, perhaps something disastrous" (221). Only when she returns to her seat is she able to scrutinize the unusual features of the children. Her attention is caught by the singular profile of a boy about nine or ten, who is walking toward the piano. As he looks up at Miss Marsalles, the narrator observes his "heavy, unfinished features, the abnormally small and slanting eyes" (221). Gazing at the rest of the children, she sees the same profile repeated two or three times – a repetition that enhances the story's emphasis on ironic doubleness and mimicry. Munro's story does not rely on these visual and corporeal stock images to identify the less than human. Instead the narrative combines these markers of difference with evidence of the children's musical ability. This pairing challenges the reductive visual logic that supported society's decision to banish these children to institutions.

In answer to the narrator's mother's shrill question, "Who are they?" (221), Mrs Clegg explains that they are from the class that Miss Marsalles has out at the Green Hill School. "They're nice little things," Miss Clegg says, "and some of them quite musical but of course they're not all there" (221). Throughout the story, the connection between Miss Marsalles's sister and the children remains implicit. Yet both the elderly woman suffering from cognitive decline and these youngsters are aligned with degeneration (the antithesis of evolution) and are deemed non-persons: "unfinished" "things" who are supposedly "not all there." Both groups are also expected to remain hidden, secluded in private bedrooms or asylums and thereby complying with their social death. In keeping with the theme of degeneration, Miss Marsalles's sister who has lost her powers of speech is etymologically likened to an "infant," a word derived from the Greek term meaning "not-speaking." By stressing the silence of Miss Marsalles and the children in contrast to the vocal and shaming commentary of Mrs Clegg and the outraged mothers in the audience, the story underscores who has the power to control the social and affective meanings of dementia. As Lambek insists, however, these utterances "offer only single perspectives." By relating events from the more open-minded perspective of the youthful narrator, "Dance of the Happy Shades" casts doubt on the adults' deeply entrenched, negative perceptions of both elders and children with cognitive impairment.[6]

The mothers' response to the children from Green Hill – a combination of pity and disgust – recalls Jackson's insight that those "inhabiting the borderlands of imbecility were both pitied and considered a danger to the State" (1). When the children from Green Hill first make their appearance, the narrator states that the adults are almost audible in saying to themselves: "*No, I know it is not right to be repelled by such children and I am not repelled, but nobody told me I was going to come here to listen to a procession of little – little idiots for that's what they are*" (222). By parading rather than effacing the children from Green Hill, "Dance of the Happy Shades" recalls Helen's experience in "The Peace of Utrecht." As noted in chapter three, Helen and Maddy feel as if they are "accompanying a particularly tasteless sideshow" when they appear in public with their mother, whose battle with Parkinson's results in her daughters' paralyzing shame. The parade of children with Down syndrome also echoes *A History of Forgetting*'s emphasis on Christian's facial deformity. These narratives' displays of difference are significant because, as historians note, the cause of eugenics was propelled to a great extent "by the visual aversion to 'the unfit,' giving rise to legal support for segregating them from society, as well as preventing their future propagation" (Brave and Slyva 35).

The mothers' disgust also recalls Leo Nascher's opinion, cited in chapter three, that the appearance of cognitively challenged individuals is "repellent both to the esthetic sense and to the sense of independence, that sense or mental attitude that the human race holds toward the self-reliant and self-dependent" (v–vi). Those who adopt this view might argue that the mothers' outrage and disgust constitute involuntary, universal human affects – instinctual responses to the abject. Yet this essentialist view was contested in the eighteenth century when Locke initially forged the category of the idiot and made it central to his definition of man. Wordsworth, for example, contends that "the loathing and disgust which many peo[ple] have at the sight of an Idiot, is a feeling which, though having som[e] foundation in human nature is not necessarily attached to it in any vi[tal] degree, but is owing, in a great measure to a false delicacy, and if I [may] say it without rudeness, a certain want of comprehensiveness of think[ing] and feeling" (in Bewell 54). Far from imposing a utopian resolution to this moral conflict, the narrative illustrates instead that non-judgmental and non-violent approaches to dementia have always shadowed the dominant response of fear and revulsion. Both the dissenting views of the narrator and the presence of the accepting and compassionate Miss Marsalles introduce an alternative, ironic approach to cognitive disability within the narrative. Despite the mothers' attempt to stigmatize the children from Green Hill, and thereby create a division between their children and the latecomers, the narrator insists that the latter do not play any worse than the regular students. Nevertheless, she goes on to admit that there is "an atmosphere in the room of some freakish inescapable dream" (222). Her use of the words "freakish" and "dream" indicate, however, that from the perspective of the narrator and the mothers, neither Miss Marsalles's sister nor these children occupy the real world (in which "neurotypical" individuals are respected and those deemed "non-neurotypical" remain hidden in asylums) and the unreal world (in which people with dementia mingle freely with "neurotypicals" and are accorded the same respect).

Recalling my discussion in chapter five of the surreal aspects of "Powers," I would suggest that in Munro's fiction references to dreams and the eruption of surreal elements effectively highlight the limits of representation and society's efforts to master the Other. As philosopher and gender critic Judith Butler explains: "For representation to convey the human, representation must not only fail, but it must show its failure. There is something unrepresentable that we nevertheless seek to represent, and that paradox must be retained in the representation we give" (144). Munro's narrative exposes this failure most forcibly when it relates how, as they listen to Dolores Boyle perform "The Dance of the Happy Shades," the mothers sit speechless, "caught with a look of protest on their faces, a more profound anxiety than before, as if reminded of something that they had forgotten they had forgotten" (233). Prior systems of representation explicitly fail because in this uncanny moment, they forget to forget (i.e. they no longer repress their awareness and thus fleetingly remember) that the division between "feeble-minded" and neurotypical individuals was, in fact, "sheer invention" (Goodey 215) – a historical artifact of the eighteenth century that designated specific groups as non-citizens who existed outside of the law. Equally relevant, the story's description of the mothers' plight also resonates with common descriptions of advanced dementia, which likewise causes people to "forget that they have forgotten." Viewed in this light, the mother's cognitive lapse momentarily aligns them with individuals with dementia, further eliding the division between neurotypical and non-neurotypical behaviour. Rather than condemn the mothers for their response and invite the reader to stand apart from them in harsh and superior judgment, Munro's narrative simply alludes to an alternative response akin to Wordsworth's view.

In Munro's texts, dreams, dream-like states, and other countries frequently serve as catalysts for irony by highlighting the world of fantasy versus reality and by blurring the boundary between the two. In addition to highlighting the potential ironic inversion of real versus imagined worlds, dreams also prompt Munro's characters to reflect on the supplemental, existential ironies that attend the natural passage of time that renders certain views and ways of life obsolete.[7] In Munro's fiction, life's social rhythms and conventions can change for the better. Ironically it is Dolores, whose name is from the Latin word for "sorrows," who conveys the possibility of the freedom of a great unemotional happiness. Although the mystery of her music is never resolved, it offers insight into a non-egocentric form of happiness that is not restricted by the notion of a rational self. In portraying Dolores as an enigma, Munro recalls Wordsworth's representation of the idiot as a "figure of mystery, and thus of our own limits of understanding, recalling Renaissance notions of divine folly" (Andrews 74).[8]

When faced with the mothers' palpable disgust and dismay, however, Miss Marsalles refuses to abide by the implicit rules of the real world; she is neither shamed by nor projects an iota of shame onto the children. We are told, for example, that she takes the first boy's hand and smiles at him "and there is no twitch of his hand, no embarrassed movement of her head to disown this smile" (222). Rather than acquiesce to the social death of people with dementia, Miss Marsalles says each child's name as if it were "a cause for celebration" (222). Moreover, for her, the bravura performance of Dolores Boyle, in particular, is "something she always expected, and she finds it natural and satisfying" (223). In essence, her decision to include the children from Green Hill in the recital represents what Canadian writer and literary critic Robert Kroetsch termed "unhiding the hidden."[9] Her inclusive gesture also reflects the changing zeitgeist, specifically, the transformation of the social imaginary that, prior to the 1960s, deemed children with cognitive impairments "'lost' from citizenship and the 'civilised'" (Higgs and Gilleard, "Frailty" 15).

In considering Munro's ironic aesthetics, it is significant that the story's emphasis on performance, specifically the parade – figured in "Dance of the Happy Shades" as a Bakhtinian, carnivalesque "procession of little idiots" – constitutes one of Munro's signature motifs

(Redekop xiii). In Munro's fiction, the parade allows for an often ironic comparison between two world views because it produces a "tableau effect," in which "old conventions are briefly held still for us so that we may examine their workings" (xiii). Whereas Magdalene Redekop has focused on how Munro's stories invoke the parade and play with both the masquerade and mimicry to deconstruct the idealized maternal figure, I argue that her stories rely on these elements to challenge socially constructed notions of disability.

According to French feminist philosopher Luce Irigaray, the goal of the mimic is to "'make visible' by an effect of playful repetition, what was supposed to remain invisible" (76). With the introduction of Dolores, a preternaturally gifted musician, "Dance of the Happy Shades" "makes visible" and "audible" both the outdated views of the mothers and the newly emergent subject position of the Other, a child with an intellectual disability. In figuratively and literally staging the appearance of Dolores and by demonstrating her ability, in the mother's eyes, to mimic and indeed exceed the musical ability of neurotypical children, "Dance of the Happy Shades" offers its most emphatic challenge to Gothic representations – the live burial – of people coping with cognitive disability.

By flaunting the demand for the segregation of the "unfit," and by portraying a child with an intellectual disability as a brilliant musician whose abilities far surpass that of neurotypical children, Munro's text signals its debt to the larger disability movements that articulated the rights of people with cognitive disabilities. As scholars observe, the disability movement was founded "on the transformative and liberation politics of the 1960s new left movements" (Chivers "Barrier" 307; see also Neufeldt). These changes affected not only people with disabilities but also the meanings and linkages between youth and elderly people coping with disability. As Higgs and Gilleard observe, in the case of disability organizations, the historical alliance with the youth movements of the 1960s rendered suspect any close alliance with the old" ("Frailty, Disability" 482). Leni Marshall observes, for example, that whereas "a sizable number of people identify with disability-focused alliances," there is "not a broadly accepted Elder culture with which people connect" (25). As a result, in specific contexts, "people with disabilities have a higher level of social visibility than do people of advanced age" (25). Marshall refers to the "hypervisibility of bodies with disabilities" (26; see also 27). Moreover, as both disability and chronic illness movements increasingly relied on first-person narratives to contest the dominance of biomedical worldviews, the newly emergent, citizen/subject positions associated with not only disability, but also with older age and chronic illness were gradually disaggregated from the social imaginary of age-related dementia and Alzheimer's disease. People who identified as disabled, as aged but otherwise healthy "zoomers,"[10] or as coping with a chronic illness all successfully transformed their objectification through narrative and used their status as oppressed subjects as a platform to claim rights, recognition, and respect. In keeping with these socio-historical shifts, Munro's narrative figuratively rescues the children from the land of the dead, whereas Miss Marsalles's sister and, by extension, citizens coping with age-related dementia remain absent and threatening figures, images of "future dependency, decrepitude and death" ("Frailty, Disability," 484).

As noted earlier, the title "Dance of the Happy Shades" alludes to the myth of Orpheus and Eurydice, emphasizing once again the utopian impulse in both Rule's and Munro's fiction to deconstruct the Gothic and unearth the living. The Gothic allusions to ghosts or shades, the title's reference to the French word "*heureuse*," and the story's reference to music also recall the analysis in the previous chapter of the emphasis in *A History of Forgetting* on the play on "*heureuse*" and "*heure*" in the couple's favourite song. As I noted, in the opening pages of Adderson's novel Denis lashes out at Malcolm, causing the record player in Malcolm and Denis's apartment to begin to skip. Instead of singing the word "*heureuse*" (happy), the singer on the record mechanically repeats the word "*heure*" (19–20). As I argued, this scene suggests that dementia transforms the promise of progress and future happiness – "*heureuse comme tout*" – into a hellish stasis in which one hour – "*heure*" – is the same as the next. In Munro's short story, however, the opposite proves true. Instead, a child with dementia *and* a profound musical gift transforms an unvarying set of hours spent in Miss Marsalles's living room, listening to an endless stream of unmusical children bang out the same ditties, into an epiphanic experience.

Ironically, in a narrative that features silent, cognitively challenged children and elderly individuals, at the end of the story it is the mothers who are rendered speechless. Paralyzed and silent, they find themselves in the same position as Miss Marsalles's sister who due to a stroke also lost her powers of speech. More precisely, the women find themselves unable to utter the words "*Poor Miss Marsalles*" (224).

They have lost their "powers of control generally" and, as a result, they can neither shame Miss Marsalles nor dismiss the revelation afforded by the children from Green Hill School. The story's final sentence highlights the power of art to effect this revelation. As the narrator says: "It is the Dance of the Happy Shades that prevents us, it is that one communiqué from the other country where she lives" (224). Having witnessed Dolores Boyles's capacity for artistic genius the mothers can no longer fully control the meaning of cognitive impairment, nor reduce it to a pathology that eclipses an individual's humanity or her capacity for creative expression.

Despite this ironic reversal, the story nevertheless demonstrates that the meanings attributed to dementia are not the same for the young and old. The narrator's reference, for example, to "the other country" where the elderly Miss Marsalles lives recalls William Butler Yeats's poem "Sailing to Byzantium" (1928), whose opening lines proclaim: "This is no country for old men." Viewed in this light, "Dance of the Happy Shades" offers a partial counter-argument to Yeats's resigned acquiescence to enforced exile. On one level, Munro's narrative suggests that people who mistakenly equate genius with wholeness, wealth, and physical and mental perfection may find themselves silenced and exiled from a vital source of human creativity.

Although this insight potentially includes both younger and older individuals coping with cognitive decline, as noted above, later-life dementia became increasingly disaggregated from the positive recasting of disability, chronic illness, and the third age. In her later writings, Munro "plays" with the prevailing social imaginary, which conceives of dementia as a black hole from which no light escapes. Rather than offer the Truth concerning the experience of later-life dementia, her stories concede to the fact that we are always fabricating stories. In "The Bear Came over the Mountain" and, even more forcibly, in her recent story "In Sight of the Lake," Munro relies on irony and the formal and thematic motif of the joke to highlight the limitations of our current Gothic view of dementia and to offer more playful and palatable alternatives to the metaphor of the black hole.

SECTION III: IRONY AND AMBIGUITY – "THE BEAR CAME OVER THE MOUNTAIN"

"The Bear Came over the Mountain" is a story that offers a fascinating account of a marriage of almost fifty years troubled by what might best be described as an ongoing crisis of pathological forgetting. The story traces the experiences of Grant, a former university professor and self-confessed philanderer, who witnesses his wife Fiona's rapid cognitive decline due to Alzheimer's disease. Knowing that her condition will only worsen, seventy-year-old Fiona voluntarily commits herself to Meadowlake, a residential care facility. The institution's policy stipulates that new residents are not allowed visitors for one month. When Grant visits his wife after the prescribed separation, he is shocked to discover that Fiona has formed a passionate attachment to a temporary resident named Aubrey. Equally disconcerting to Grant, Fiona treats him as if he is a new resident, offering him a cup of tea – a beverage he never drinks – and she spends the rest of her time fawning over Aubrey at his bridge game. The transference of her affection suggests that she has seemingly completely forgotten her attachment to Grant and their life together. Rather than accept that he has been erased from Fiona's memory, Grant wonders whether his wife, known for her humour and ironic approach to life, is willfully playing an elaborate trick on him.

In effect Grant cannot decide if Fiona's feelings for Aubrey spring from her illness or if they are a purposefully ironic and wounding commentary on his own multiple past infidelities. Equally ironic, as Sally Chivers argues, Grant "cares too much now that Fiona no longer desires his attention and now that he has, in a sense, left her" (*Silvering* 91). Readers grapple with similar questions: does Fiona's behaviour relate to the past, namely her knowledge of Grant's infidelities and their previous relationship, or does it represent an eruption of desire in the present that signals a complete break with the past and past selves? In Munro's story, it is never clear if, due to illness, Fiona ceases to act rationally and to exert her will. We are left equally uncertain as to whether her husband, Grant, her putative rational caregiver, acts in accordance with reason or passion throughout their relationship. As Chivers observes, "as Fiona changes more and becomes less reliable, Grant settles into his own unchanging ways, which ironically involve unreliability as a monogamous spouse in order to express his undying devotion" (*Silvering* 92). Put differently, Munro's story, which charts Fiona's experience of cognitive decline, uses irony and ambiguity to subvert Gothic and apocalyptic portrayals of dementia by attributing potential agency to Fiona and by calling into question the integrity of the supposedly rational, healthy, and normal care providers. In keeping with "A Dance of the Happy Shades," "The

Bear Came over the Mountain" offers ambiguous and ironic communiqués from Munro country where agency, creative expression, and human imperfection – most notably dementia – co-exist.

As I have shown in previous chapters, a shadowy uncertainty seems to characterize Alzheimer's from both a scientific and a philosophical perspective. This uncertainty seems to produce appropriately complex narratives that break down the division between certain broad concepts that are normally categorized separately. In *A History of Forgetting*, for example, the rather dubious separation of past and present is replaced by a kind of surreal, blurring effect in which time intrudes, disappears, or falls out of sequence. "The Bear Came over the Mountain" emphasizes that personal identity is constructed and deconstructed within a temporal framework that, at times, seems fractured. For elderly individuals, in particular, the temporal framework is inherently fragile and fissured. In "The Bear Came over the Mountain" Alzheimer's merely exacerbates the fracturing of time and personhood. Fiona's erratic behaviour prompts Grant to wonder if the Fiona who now loves Aubrey is really his wife of almost fifty years.

In his essay on his father's struggle with Alzheimer's, Jonathan Franzen bemoans the fact that the media typically portrays the illness as a terrifying scourge that "refracts death into a spectrum of its otherwise tightly conjoined parts – death of autonomy, death of memory, death of self-consciousness, death of personality, death of body" (89). Franzen observes further that both the media and biomedical reports subscribe to the "most common trope of Alzheimer's: that its particular sadness and horror stem from the sufferer's loss of his or her 'self' long before the body dies" (89). In response to this tidy mechanistic model – a response that is based on his experience with his father who suffered from Alzheimer's – Franzen insists that his father's brain was not "simply a computation device running gradually and inexorably amok" (89). Equally important, he wonders whether the various deaths cited earlier – of autonomy, of memory, of self-consciousness, of personality, of body – "can ever really be so separated, and whether memory and consciousness have such secure title, after all, to the seat of selfhood" (89). The ambiguity concerning the nature and locus of the father's selfhood provides the foundation for irony in Franzen's writing. "The Bear Came over the Mountain" similarly highlights the ironies associated with illness and, in the process, diminishes dementia's corrosive impact as a Gothic, "identity-spoiling" disease that effaces the possibility of choice.

Indeed as I have shown, Alzheimer's constitutes an illness of which ambiguity seems almost a defining factor. As Sarah Powell observes:

> With many medical challenges, it is possible to point precisely to what a healthy body looks like in comparison to the unhealthy body that requires medical attention. This is how a diagnosis is reached. However, unlike in the case of most other medical problems, there is no base test for what the healthy or normal person without Alzheimer's should look like. A non-cancerous body vs. a cancerous body or an intact leg vs. one that is broken is a visible distinction not available in cases of Alzheimer's, of which definitive biological proof can normally only be given after post-mortem exams. Alzheimer's is instead diagnosed by what amounts to a very complex and methodical form of conjecture; its presence is detected through the observation of cognitive and behavioural abnormality. The problem with a method of diagnosis that relies on symptomatology in the case of this particular illness is that the way in which Alzheimer's presents in different individuals is highly variable and unpredictable, but so, too, is healthy behaviour. This confusion around the distinction between normal and abnormal behaviour results in the diagnosis of Alzheimer's being largely determined through a series of cognitive behavioural tipping points, between forgetfulness and memory loss, confusion and disorientation, and illness and selfhood. As Grant wonders of Fiona in *Away From Her*, Sarah Polley's adaptation of Munro's story: "What if this is just her? Just being herself?"[11]

At bottom, Munro's story explores the instability and limits of diagnosis and the near impossibility at times of distinguishing between illness and selfhood by situating her story so that it balances on the liminal tipping point.

As noted in the introduction, Linda Hutcheon argues that irony oscillates in semantic terms between the simultaneous "perception of the said and the unsaid" (*Irony's* 39) – between literal and inferred meanings. In Munro's story Alzheimer's serves as a catalyst for the creation of irony in a narrative that raises questions about remembering and forgetting, fidelity and infidelity, the instability of meaning, the workings of ironic discourse, and the transference of desire. Grant's view of Fiona accommodates irony, renders her behaviour meaningful and, equally important, implicates Grant – an adulterer – as a person prone to passionate breaks in his consciousness, and hence his rational self. His passionate episodes, which eclipse his ability to reason, make it difficult if not impossible to distinguish between normative and pathological episodes of forgetting.

"The Bear Came over the Mountain" is focalized by an apparently shameless husband who is, nevertheless, plagued by guilty dreams of his adulterous behaviour. At one point, readers are told that Grant hauls himself out of a dream and sets about "separating what was real from what was not." As he recalls: "There had been a letter, and the word 'rat' had appeared in black paint on his office door, and Fiona, on being told that a girl had suffered from a bad crush on him, had said pretty much what she said in the dream [...] and nobody had committed suicide. Grant hadn't been disgraced. In fact, he had got off easy when you thought of what might have happened just a couple of years later. But word got around. Cold shoulders became conspicuous" (284). This passage, with its emphasis on graffiti, underscores the narrative's overarching insistence on the power of language to stigmatize an individual. In his role as focalizer, Grant repeatedly presents himself and his predicament in the most favourable light. As the passage cited above and others also illustrate, however, his ongoing habit of objectifying women undercuts his self-presentation as a man of integrity. Grant admits that when he and his colleagues were busy having affairs during the 1960s, Fiona was the one who showed no interest in partaking in the social games of the times. In fact Fiona, who is by turns serious and ironic, is the one woman whom Grant cannot entirely fathom or control.

Munro's story opens with Grant's recollection of Fiona's childhood home and how they met in the town where they both went to university. As a young man, Grant was struck by Fiona's wealth, her irreverence for the things that other people took seriously, her fondness for jokes and generally ironic approach to life: "Sororities were a joke to her, and so was politics" (274). She made fun of the men who were courting her, including Grant, "drolly repeat[ing] some of his small-town phrases" (274). In light of Fiona's "superior" class and sophistication, Grant was surprised that she was interested in him and he thought "maybe she was joking when she proposed to him" (276) on a beach, shouting over the waves: "Do you think it would be fun … Do you think it would be fun if we got married?" Gazing at Fiona, now seventy years old, Grant muses that she looked just like herself – "direct and vague as in fact she was, sweet and ironic" (276).

Grant's musings on the gradual and insidious appearance of Fiona's symptoms likewise support his view that Fiona may be playing a trick on him. He recalls how once she went for a walk across the fields and came home by the fence line. On her return, she drolly remarked that "she'd counted on fences always taking you somewhere" (276). Reflecting on her comment, Grant admits that it "was hard to figure out. She'd said that about fences as if it were a joke" (277). He is equally at a loss when she dismisses her symptoms: "I don't think it's anything to worry about … I expect I'm just losing my mind" (277). Recalling their first visit to the doctor, Grant describes how he tried "without success to explain how Fiona's surprise and apologies now seemed somehow like routine courtesy, not quite concealing a private amusement. As if she'd stumbled on some unexpected adventure. Or begun playing a game that she hoped he would catch on to" (277). In keeping with Franzen's refusal to view his father's brain as a clock winding inexorably down, Grant similarly assumes that Fiona is playing a strange and potentially wounding game. When he drives her to Meadowlake, she reminds him of the time they had gone skiing at night. "If she could remember that, so vividly and correctly," Grant muses, "could there really be so much the matter with her?" (279).

For Grant, the game of communication continues, although under a different guise. Viewed in this light, the text's repeated references to bridge games emphasize the intersubjective aspects of the production of meaning and identity. As noted earlier, when Grant first visits Fiona he finds her hovering over Aubrey at the bridge table. To his dismay, Grant finds himself the unwelcome intruder and the other players look at him with displeasure. Only Fiona greets him warmly: "'Bridge,' she whispered. 'Deadly serious. They're quite rabid about it'" (288). After offering him a cup of tea – which, as noted, he never drinks – Fiona gazes in Aubrey's direction: "I better go back," she says, "He thinks he can't play without me sitting there. It's silly, I hardly know the game anymore" (288). As well as raising questions about her competence, her comments remind us that no one can play the game of generating meaning without the other's presence. Aubrey seemingly depends on Fiona's role as witness to enable him to inhabit his role as a player, an ironic echo of her relationship to Grant. In both instances, the men cannot maintain their identity without Fiona acting as a witness to their games. In effect, her agency and her actions highlight the intersubjective foundation of identity. As represented in the story, this factor, together with the affective and embodied nature of memory and the instabilities associated with Alzheimer's, undermines the Enlightenment notion of the autonomous, rational self.

Munro's text continues to underscore the intersubjective facet of selfhood when Fiona, before returning to the game, tries to console Grant: "It must all seem strange to you but you'll be surprised how soon you get used to it. You'll get to know who everybody is. Except that some of them are pretty well off in the clouds, you know – you can't expect them all to get to know who you are" (288). Again, like the wise fool in a Shakespearian play, Fiona's words are instructive. If, as Jesse Ballenger insists, Alzheimer's "affects us all" (*Self* 153), then her cognitive impairment and institutionalization are, indeed, equally his experience; Grant is thus akin to a new resident who must work at understanding the Other (his transformed wife and, due to the reciprocal nature of their roles, himself).[12]

For his part, Grant reflects on Fiona's words of wisdom during their first brief exchange to determine whether he accurately detected the ironic marker: "She had given herself away by that little pretense at the end, talking to him as if she thought perhaps he was a new resident. If it was a pretense" (291). The sly strangeness of Fiona's statements and behaviour eventually prompt Grant to quiz Fiona's nurse, Kristy: "Does she even know who I am?" he wonders, admitting to himself that for his part, he cannot decide: "She could have been playing a joke. It would not be unlike her" (290–1).

Further surprising complications arise when Aubrey's wife, Marian, decides to take him back home. Aubrey's departure plunges Fiona into a life-threatening depression. In an effort to help her, Grant pays Aubrey's wife a visit. Marian mistakenly assumes that Grant has arrived to castigate her for allowing Aubrey to "molest" his wife. Quite the opposite, Grant hopes to persuade Marian to return Aubrey to Meadowlake and to Fiona. During their meeting, comic reversals abound: Grant praises Marian for being "noble and good" (16) and caring for her husband at home, but she promptly informs him that she simply cannot afford to keep him in an institution. Grant assumes that Marian will dismiss him as a "silly person ... who didn't have to worry about holding on to his house and could go around dreaming up the fine generous schemes that he believed would make another person happy" (16). Instead, Grant awakens Marian's sexual interest, and when he returns home he finds a message from her on his answering machine inviting him to a dance for "singles" at the Legion.

Munro's story never reveals what transpires between Grant and Marian. The story concludes with Grant delivering Aubrey to Meadowlake. "Fiona," Grant says, "I've brought a surprise for you. Do you remember Aubrey?" (18). Rather than elicit joy, however, Grant's surprise gift devastates Fiona and, for the first time since she became a resident at Meadowlake Fiona seems to remember Grant. "You've been gone a long time," she remarks. "You could have just driven away ... Just driven away without a care in the world and forsook me. Forsooken me. Forsaken" (18). It is unclear if she is referring to Grant's reaction to her recent infidelity, to her illness, or to *his* past infidelities. The story concludes ambiguously with Grant's response. He presses his cheek against Fiona's withered visage and murmurs: "Not a chance" (322). Like Fiona's remark, Grant's comment remains opaque; although he seems to be professing his love for her, it is also quite possible that he has just been unfaithful to her again and he is satisfied to have Fiona out of the way so that he can pursue his affair with Marian.[13]

The structure of Munro's narrative repeatedly draws an ironic parallel between Fiona's memory loss and surprising attachment to Aubrey and Grant's prior infidelities, which he chose to "forget" and which Fiona had also learned long ago to "forget." Put differently, the narrative effects a chiasmatic reversal. Initially, Grant occupies an elevated position due to his status as the supposedly cognitively healthy caregiver whose selfhood remains intact, whereas Fiona is vulnerable to stigma due to her dementia. By the end of the story, however, the revelation of Grant's adulterous behaviour renders him vulnerable to stigma. Although his habit of trawling among his students for sex was acceptable in the 1960s, the times have changed. The times have also changed with respect to the society's response to dementing illness.

While acknowledging the complexity of the dénouement of Munro's story, some critics have nevertheless ultimately viewed Grant as absolutely selfless in returning Fiona's lover, Aubrey, to Meadowlake. Héliane Ventura, for example, describes the story as "a reconfiguration of love at twilight" (n.p.). Yet such readings, which split Grant's character simply into the formerly unfaithful spouse and the newly redeemed husband are not supported by the text; nor do they do justice to the ongoing ironic oscillations in Grant's character that persist to the end. In the final version of the story, Munro added sections in which Grant reflects on what he stands to gain from using his sexual allure to convince Marian to return Aubrey to the nursing home.[14] Figuring Marian out, he suggests, would be like "biting into a litchi nut" with an "oddly artificial allure" (317). The fact that his sexual satisfaction remains at stake is further clarified when, elaborating on this sexist conceit, Grant insists that his plan "would not work – unless he could get more satisfaction than he foresaw, finding the stone of blameless self-interest inside her robust pulp" (319). The narrative also juxtaposes the final scene in which Grant seemingly selflessly appears with Aubrey in tow to Grant's prior lustful contemplation of "the practical sensuality of [Marian's] ... cat's tongue. Her gemstone eyes" (321). These are not the rational, objective thoughts of a self-sacrificing husband.

As both "The Peace of Utrecht," Munro's earlier story concerning her mother's dementing illness, and "The Bear Came over the Mountain" indicate, within Canadian literary works people struggling with dementia are neither depicted nor perceived solely as nonpersons lacking in agency, ontological "black holes." In "The Bear Came over the Mountain" the narrative's ambiguous treatment of Fiona's dementia, specifically her capacity to remember fragments of her past, including Grant's affairs, makes it impossible for readers to perceive her as a powerless victim lacking in selfhood – or to borrow Franzen's metaphor, a clock winding down. Like Franzen's essay, Munro's narrative's extended ambiguity and ironic doubling also call into question medical myths about loss of self and subjectivity through aging and age-related dementia.[15]

To summarize thus far, whereas Rule's fiction relies on a utopian vision to deconstruct Gothic portrayals of both queer aging and dementia, in "The Dance of the Happy Shades" and "The Bear Came over the Mountain" Munro uses her distinct, trickster-inspired, ironic style to interrogate the stigmatizing of people coping with dementia. In the final section of this chapter, I turn to Munro's recent story "In Sight of the Lake" because it adds important philosophical and aesthetic dimensions to my analysis. In contrast to Munro's previous stories, "In Sight of the Lake" offers insight (pun intended) into the mind of an elderly woman coping with symptoms of dementia and hysteria. Equally important, the story incorporates surreal elements to bring the reader into the mind of the protagonist. Although entirely Munro's fantasy of what goes on in her character's mind, this vision offers an alternative to the paranoid Gothic representation of the fourth age. Taken together, the narrative's focalization and its reliance on surrealism to re-create the experiences of dementia and hysteria constitute Munro's most profound challenge to date of the Gothic metaphor of dementia as a black hole.

SECTION IV – "IN SIGHT OF THE LAKE": THE JOKE IS ON US

The opening sentence in "In Sight of the Lake" – "A woman goes to her doctor to have a prescription renewed" – relies on the diction and cadence of a joke, including the deferred expectation of a punchline.[16] From the start, readers are alerted to the story's central organizing principle and its overarching thematic concern with the nature of jokes and tricks. The story offers an account of a woman named Nancy, who has been referred to a specialist due to her memory problems. Rather than make her way to the specialist's office early in the morning, Nancy decides to travel to the nearby village a few days beforehand to avoid running around and getting lost when she is in a hurry to get there in the morning. Due to a series of errors, however, Nancy cannot find the specialist's office. When looking for the doctor's name and address, for example, she discovers that she has misplaced the information. Examining the scrap of paper she finds in her pocket, she realizes to her dismay that the only thing written on it is the shoe size of her husband's sister, who is dead. Following this mishap, increasingly strange and surreal phenomena characterize her trip, ranging from the sight of clocks that no longer tell the time, to a boy riding his bicycle backwards, to a strange, lush, private garden filled with flowers that burst from between the paths and from the grass.[17] Toward the conclusion Nancy, like Alice in Wonderland, has tumbled down the proverbial rabbit hole and is hopelessly lost. In an attempt to find her way to the doctor, she strikes up a conversation with a man who tends the exotic flower garden. When she asks him for directions to the specialist's office, he wisely suggests that she look for the specialist at the Lakeview Rest Home. To her chagrin, however, Nancy realizes that rather than respond to him properly, she merely echoes his words. The story concludes with Nancy, who has made her way to the Rest Home, alone at night in an empty corridor of the institution, hysterically calling for help. In the end, help of a sort arrives. An orderly named Sandy chides Nancy for creating a scene. At this point readers are shocked to discover that Nancy is, in fact, a resident of the Home, and that the preceding events were merely her subjective fantasy. "What are we going to do with you?" says Sandy. "All we want is to get you into your nightie. And you go and carry on like a chicken that's scared of being et for dinner" (232).

As this brief plot summary indicates, the story relies on the clichéd formal ending of "it was all a dream" to prompt readers to relate to Nancy as a subject rather than the object of the gaze. Indeed, as she embarks on her quest and we follow her on her journey until the final, shocking revelation of her status as a patient in the nursing home, we literally see through her eyes, as she surveys the town and its inhabitants. As Magdalene Redekop astutely observes, Munro's principal tactic for subverting the tendency to turn female bodies into objects is to portray them in the act of looking. Redekop argues further that for the woman who subjects others to her gaze, "nothing less than the survival of her self is at stake" (5). Like any confident tourist visiting a small town, Nancy displays all of the markers of robust subjectivity: she makes choices, she generates several hypotheses concerning the most likely location of the specialist and she tests them, she is emotionally attuned to her surroundings, and she expresses her judgments freely.

She is also demonstrably playful, but understandably would prefer to be the one making the jokes rather than serving as the butt of other people's jokes. When she first catches sight of the nursing home, for example, she notices that the floor "is all silvery tiles, the sort that children love to slide on" (229). For a moment, "she thinks of the patients sliding and slipping for pleasure and the idea makes her light-hearted" (229). As the narrator explains, she holds an internal colloquy on the topic of whether or not she should give it a try, but, ultimately, decides against it: "'I didn't dare try it myself,' she says in a charming voice to somebody in her head, perhaps her husband. 'It wouldn't have done, would it? I could have found myself in front of the doctor, the very one who was getting ready to test my mental stability. And then what would he have to say?'" (229). From the start, however, readers recognize that life has already played a trick on Nancy and shamed her because when she goes to see her doctor, the latter is not there. We are told that "It's her day off. In fact the woman

has got the day wrong, she has mixed up Monday with Tuesday"
(217). Nancy's error pertains to the very issue that she had wanted to
raise with her doctor: "She has wondered if her mind is slipping a bit"
(212). Anxious about her memory slips, Nancy secretly hopes that
her doctor will laugh off her concerns. Instead, the doctor's assistant phones to tell Nancy that an appointment has been made with
a specialist. During their conversation, Nancy continues to yearn
for reassurance, for someone to understand, and simultaneously to
reduce her anxiety by making light of her problem. When the assistant explains that the specialist "deals with elderly patients," Nancy
replies, "Indeed. Elderly patients who are off their nut" (212). For
Nancy, it is a tremendous relief when she manages to get someone
to laugh with her rather than at her (218).

In addition to highlighting Nancy's desire to remain in control and
maintain her independence, the story – which is narrated in the third
person but focalized from Nancy's perspective – affords tremendous
insight into Nancy's emotional sensitivity and her desire to avoid
being shamed, which creates an empathetic bond between reader
and character. Throughout the story Nancy's emotions, particularly
her anxiety, remain palpable. For example, Nancy decides to visit the
town prior to her appointment precisely because she wants to ensure
that there will be "no danger of her arriving all flustered or even a
little late, creating a bad impression right off the bat" (218).[18] Later,
when she takes leave of the man who tends the lovely garden and
heads off to the Lakeview Rest Home, she worries that she will not
be able to find her keys: "She can feel the approach of familiar, tire-
some panic. But then she finds them, in her pocket" (228). Finally,
as she drives away, she catches sight of the gardener talking to some
of the townspeople and wonders if their conversation concerns her:
"Maybe a remark to be made, some joke about her vagueness or sil-
liness. Or just her age. A mark against her" (228). As these passages
suggest, Nancy desires more than anything to be in control, to be the
one "making a silly joke" (227). By conveying Nancy's thoughts as
she grows ever more desperate to orient herself and to avoid being
mocked, readers appreciate what it must be like not merely to be
lost (disoriented), but also to have lost face and, as a corollary, in the
words of Auguste D., to have "lost" oneself.[19] When the punch line
of the story hits home, readers recognize that despite her persistent
worries about being caught "slipping," all along Nancy has been in
the same position as Auguste D. and Miss Marsalles' sister, women

who in the eyes of others have demonstrably lost their "powers of control" (218). In the words of Gilleard and Higgs, they are "'lost' from citizenship and the 'civilized'" ("Frailty" 15).

On the one hand, the conclusion demonstrates irrefutably that Nancy's powers are severely restricted since she seemingly cannot put on her own nightie. Equally relevant, throughout the text are clues – most obviously the references to the broken clocks and chipped crockery – that serve as objective correlatives for Nancy's status as a broken object. On the other hand, in keeping with the doubled structure of irony, these clues remain in the background while in the foreground Nancy focalizes her journey through her surreal dream world. In the end, when the perspective shifts, the Gothic returns with a vengeance, but its status as a social imaginary and its external origins are highlighted by the fact that it is supplied by the reader. Simply put, readers have more insight into Nancy's abject position within the nursing home than Nancy herself; hence, readers impose a Gothic point of view. In her thoughts, Nancy remains a subject who chooses to leave the Lakeview Rest Home. In keeping with the story's reliance on dramatic irony and its emphasis on the external origins of the Gothic social imaginary, readers must ignore the awareness of Nancy's sense of personhood and agency to view her as an object.

In light of the story's engagement with the Female Gothic,[20] it is no coincidence that the image of the helpless woman, often garbed only in a nightie, serves as a recurring motif in this story and, indeed, in virtually all of the works we have considered, including the nonfictional case study of Auguste D. The pervasiveness of this image of female helplessness and confinement suggests that it is integral to Western society's Gothic social imaginary of the fourth age. I would argue further that both the figure of the helpless woman and the allusions to hysteria in the closing paragraph of "In Sight of the Lake" remind us further that, as I noted in chapter one, the Gothic social imaginary of the fourth age draws on some of the same fears and desires inherent in the late-nineteenth and early twentieth century hysteria diagnosis.[21]

By juxtaposing hysteria and age-related dementia and linking them to the locus of the asylum, "In Sight of the Lake" highlights the origins and structure of the social imaginary of the fourth age, which derives its affective power from the ongoing stigma and pathologization of women's supposedly inherently diseased minds and bodies. Rather than reinstall this stigma, "In Sight of the Lake" uses Munrovian irony to drive home the awareness that in discussions of later-life dementia, and even in seemingly factual medical accounts, fantasy and storytelling play a crucial role. Equally important, Munro's narrative demonstrates that the voices and insights of the people most affected by our fantasies are missing. "In Sight of the Lake" effects a vertiginous shift in perspective that plunges the reader into the world of dreams. In the end, the reader returns to "the real world" only to realize that she is still within a dream; the ending of the story, which locates the reader in the nursing home, is still part of Munro's fiction.

Rather than serve as a joke solely on Nancy – a mark against her alone – the narrative plays an elaborate trick on the reader by destabilizing her sense of what is real and what is imagined and by showing how both are mutually constitutive. Readers are left to consider whether the world we currently live in is, in part, a dream in which we all slip and slide, and where failure and mortality are not accidents but rather part of the life course and meaningful components of both personal and social narratives. It is sobering, in this regard, to recognize that one out of three people over eighty-five has dementia, which raises the perennial question of whether the illness springs from disease or from the natural course of aging. Viewed in light of Munro's oeuvre as a whole, Nancy's failed quest to meet the elderly specialist – who will supposedly grant an objective diagnosis of her illness – recalls the conclusion of "Powers." Both stories feature protagonists named Nancy who indulge in imaginative fantasies of agency and repair. As in "Powers," "In Sight of the Lake" emphasizes the fact that characters and readers alike remain helpless to alter the course of certain events.

Far from inviting the reader to dismiss these characters as failed or deluded questers, Munro's stories admit the reader into a larger community of vulnerability, risk, and failure. As Redekop maintains, the "backdrop of Munro's comic performances is black" (237). False comforts "are seen through, but there is no true comfort simply in debunking the false ones. The comfort, rather, comes from our sense of participating in a community that has mutual fears and desires" (237). Equally crucial, instead of castigating readers for ignoring the real world like some prim school marm "In Sight of the Lake" relies on a third-person narrator to highlight the complexity and insights afforded by dreams and, more generally, the imagination. "You must have had a dream," Sandy says to Nancy, "What did you dream about now?" (232). Although these words are addressed to Nancy, they also implicate the reader who has shared Nancy's dream.

In the final section of this chapter, I want to analyze some of the implications of Munro's reliance on dreams and, more precisely, on the elements of surrealism within the tests that figure Nancy's later-life dementia. In brief, the Surrealist movement, which began in the 1920s and whose members were initially concentrated in Paris, developed out of the earlier Dada activities, a movement whose beginnings coincided with the onset of the First World War. The Dadaists believed that the reason and logic of bourgeois capitalist society had led people into war. They represented their rejection of that ideology in artistic expressions that appeared to eschew logic and embrace chaos and irrationality. The Surrealists likewise rejected conventional notions of madness and frequently relied on the practices of free association, automatic writing, and dream analysis in their attempts to alter civilization and liberate the imagination. Although both Dadaists and Surrealists maintained in common the rejection of logic and reason, the followers of both groups eventually separated. Equally important, unlike the Dadaists, the Surrealists were profoundly influenced by the writings of Sigmund Freud, specifically his notion of the unconscious.

On the one hand, the repeated mention of the broken clocks in "In Sight of the Lake" may remind some readers of the clock-drawing test used to screen for cognitive impairment and dementia. Such tests transform subjects into numerical scores that determine their "citizenship," in Sontag's terms, as either impaired or neurotypical, ill or well. On the other hand, for readers with only a passing familiarity with the Surrealist movement, Munro's allusion to broken clocks may also bring to mind Salvador Dalí's famous painting of melting clocks, "The Persistence of Memory" (1931), which features three large clock faces draped over various objects – a tree branch, a table, and what appears to be a white cloth laying on the ground. Similarly, the image of the boy riding backward together with Nancy's internal colloquy recall Dalí's equally evocative painting, "Sentimental Colloquy" (1944). At the centre of this painting is a blue grand piano sitting on what appears to be an immense cream-coloured plank floor that runs from the foreground to the vanishing point. The piano's cracked top board thrusts upward toward the upper edge of the frame. Water pours through the immense crack, transforming the broken instrument into a fountain. In the foreground and the background, skeletal figures ride bicycles across the plank floor in neat rows, forming a grid, with their white veil-like capes trailing behind them.

In drawing these associations, I am not suggesting that there is a one-to-one correspondence between the verbal images Munro generates in her narrative and those found in Dalí's art. Instead I am arguing that the narrative's depiction of surrealist images highlights a debt to a movement that prized the individual imagination and famously did not pathologize altered states of consciousness. Far from positing that Munro was conscious of these connections, I am comparing the rejection of logic and reason, in an effort to liberate the imagination, in surrealism and "In Sight of the Lake" in order to highlight an important alternative to Gothic constructions of the fourth age as a black hole.

It is significant in this regard that André Breton (1896–1966), one of the founding fathers of the Surrealist movement, was a physician who trained in psychiatry. During the war, Breton worked in an asylum where he treated soldiers for shellshock, which according to Charcot and Freud was a form of hysteria. In treating his patients, Breton notably listened carefully to their fantasies and prized their imagination. In his first *Surrealist Manifesto* (1924), Breton championed the power of the imagination to liberate individuals from the corrosive effect of shame and from society's deathly rules and conventions. As he states: "Amidst all the shame we are heir to, it is well to recognize that the widest freedom of spirit remains to us. It is up to us not to abuse it in any serious manner. To make a slave of the imagination, even though what is vulgarly called happiness is at stake, is to fail profoundly to do justice to one's deepest self. Only imagination realises the possible in me, and it is enough to lift for a moment the dreadful proscription."[22] Breton also argued that those deemed mad should not be confined within asylums or denied their liberty simply because they had retreated into their imaginations. He argued, instead, that this faculty represents the most vital core of our humanity. Moreover, for people unjustly confined, the imagination provides great solace:

> Everyone knows, in fact, that the mad owe their incarceration to a number of legally reprehensible actions, and that were it not for those actions, their liberty (or what we see as their liberty) would not be at risk. They may be, in some measure, victims of their imagination, I am prepared to concede that, in the way that it induces them not to observe certain rules, without which the species feels threatened, which it pays us all to be aware of. But

the profound indifference they show for the judgment we pass on them, and even the various punishments inflicted on them, allows us to suppose that they derive great solace from imagination, that they enjoy their delirium enough to endure the fact that it is only of value to themselves. And, indeed, hallucinations, illusions etc. are no slight source of pleasure. (in Kline n.p.)

Breton made the equally bold claim that rather than view error as a sign of degeneration, pathology, or a loss of control, it is perhaps more appropriate to see error – which, as noted, Munro's story aligns with losing one's way and slipping and sliding – as fundamental to human creativity and play. "Is not the possibility of error, for the spirit," Breton asks, "rather a circumstance conducive to its well-being?" (ibid.).

Reading "In Sight of the Lake" in light of its surrealism offers insight into prior moments of resistance to earlier Gothic social imaginaries concerning mental illness. It would seem that from the late nineteenth century to the present, Western society oscillates between two fantasies – a utopian image of enduring personhood or a dystopian image of a black hole. This tendency toward splitting recalls Sontag's famous opening to *Illness as Metaphor*: "Illness is the night-side of life, a more onerous citizenship. Everyone who is born holds dual citizenship, in the kingdom of the well and in the kingdom of the sick. Although we all prefer to use only the good passport, sooner or later each of us is obliged, at least for a spell, to identify ourselves as citizens of that other place" (1). As Rule's and Munro's texts illustrate, however, both forms of citizenship are determined by societal fears and desires rather than solely on the basis of biomedical fact. As Jay Ingram insists, there is "no chasm between normal mental functioning and Alzheimer's disease" (122). Instead, "there is, at best, a blurred line between normal cognition, mild impairment and full-on dementia" (123).

In *Memory Board,* a compassionate bid is made to allow those with a "bad" passport to enjoy the rights and privileges accorded to those blessed with a "good" passport. By contrast, in "Dance of the Happy Shades" and "The Bear Came over the Mountain," Munro relies on the tropes of mimicry and irony to undermine the authenticity of both good and bad passports and the efficacy of policing the border between the countries of the well and the sick. In the story "In Sight of the Lake," the narrative imaginatively reconfigures, and for a time replaces, the prevailing Gothic map of the kingdom of the sick, with an alternative yet equally imaginative map.[23] Thanks to this playful act of substitution, readers can revise their understanding of the fourth age as a black hole populated by "orphaned" bodies (Gilleard and Higgs, "Frailty, Disability" 485).

Munro's evocation of a surreal landscape recalls Fuchs's fascinating observation concerning dramatic presentations of old age that resist declinist ideology by invoking an alien landscape. As Fuchs explains, "These places suggest to me ... an immensity of the conscious experience of age barely glimpsed in the discourse of normative life, where the failing body-as-decline numbly presides" ("Estragement" 77). Fuchs argues further that "these places and their developmental import ... have frequently been missed by actors, directors, spectators and critics alike" (77). Munro's fiction – which epitomizes the growing resistance to Gothic and apocalyptic biomedical narratives of dementia in Canada since 2010 – prompts readers to enter these strange, hidden landscapes, and, equally important, to take what Thomas Kitwood called "a person-centered approach"[24] to their inhabitants. In Munro's stories readers encounter elderly women, many of whom are isolated and anxious, dreaming of more inclusive social imaginaries, towns with gardens where everyone is "welcome to rest" ("In Sight" 224) and where "every soul counts" (ibid. 219). While Munro's writings acknowledge that dreams and the imagination may be false comforts that readers see through, rather than mock the illusion, her work invites us, instead, to join a community based on our mutual vulnerability, one bonded by "mutual fears and desires" (Redekop 237).[25]

In sum, Munro's story play a profound role in highlighting the social construction of dementia by showing how the supposedly true stories we tell ourselves about the real world are often complicit in consolatory attempts to deny our vulnerability – epitomized by aging and dementia. Paradoxically, Munro's stories also demonstrate that fiction – which, in her hands, serves as a medium for communiqués from other countries and inner worlds to which we currently lack access – remains one of our most powerful tools for bringing us into a more ethical relationship with people coping with dementia and, more broadly, with our own vulnerability and mortality.

From the Gothic to Brecht's Epic Theatre

This is how one pictures the angel of history. His face is turned toward
the past. Where we perceive a chain of events, he sees one single catastrophe which keeps piling wreckage and hurls it in front of his feet. The
angel would like to stay, awaken the dead, and make whole what has been
smashed. But a storm is blowing from Paradise; it has got caught in his
wings with such a violence that the angel can no longer close them. The
storm irresistibly propels him into the future to which his back is turned,
while the pile of debris before him grows skyward. This storm is what
we call progress.

   Walter Benjamin, "Theses on the Philosophy of History" 257–8[1]

For good or ill, the stories and metaphors we use to represent age-
related dementia affect us personally and politically. Their effect
registers on the individual, familial, and national level. My goal in
this book has been to analyze the diverse narrative approaches to
dementia generated by scientists, the media, and writers from the
late nineteenth century to the present. I cite Walter Benjamin's evocative image of the angel of history because my book's retrospective
analysis of dementia persuaded me of the necessity of relinquishing a
narrative of progress. My methodology also reflects Benjamin's view
that the task of the historian likewise involves both letting go of historical bias and sifting among the ruins left by the storm of progress. Although it might be comforting to believe that back "then"
we were mistaken about dementia but now we know the Truth about
Alzheimer's disease, my research suggests otherwise. Instead, as I have
shown, the waxing and waning of theories about dementia illustrate shifts in the turf war between science and religion and, within

medicine, gains and losses in the ongoing battle between psychologically and somatically oriented approaches.

If, as Jay Ingram suggests in his book on Alzheimer's disease, words and thoughts can "reach across the gap and make material changes in the brain," (255) then it is advisable and perhaps even therapeutic to consider how the stories we tell about Alzheimer's and the metaphors we use within these narratives shape our view of ourselves and our loved ones as we move through the life course. Equally critical, if words and thoughts effect material changes that can make us feel better and live longer, healthier lives – acting as placeboes (from the classical Latin word *placebo*, "I shall be pleasing or acceptable" [OED])[2] – then some ways of thinking about and narrating the experience of dementia may potentially have a negative effect – what researchers investigating the negative effect of the label "mild cognitive impairment" (MCI) refer to as the "nocebo effect"[3] – (from the classical Latin word *nocēbō*, "I shall cause harm or be harmful" [OED]). In what follows, I summarize the insights from the preceding chapters' chronological approach to dementia and Alzheimer's, and, by way of concluding, highlight some of the most up-to-date, innovative, and compassionate approaches to dementia in Canada.

SECTION I: RETRIEVING THE IRONIES OF ALZHEIMER'S BURIED IN THE PAST

Reading Alzheimer's over two centuries, across several disciplinary boundaries, and comparing stories from the research bench, to the asylum bed, to newspapers, to novels exposes the similarities, differences, and productive tensions among vastly differing approaches to the illness. It also reveals fundamental and enduring uncertainties and ironies concerning Alzheimer's that are elided by our contemporary panic, which has constellated in the prevailing Gothic, biomedical model. If, as critics suggest, we have entered an "Age of Alzheimer's," then, as I have demonstrated, it is an age characterized by a host of surprises and ambiguities, starting with the basic conceptual confusion as to whether Alzheimer's is a disease at all or the natural outcome of aging. Bound up with this fundamental and persistent ambiguity is the elusive and deferred promise of a cure for the disease. Director of geriatrics at the Mount Sinai hospital in Toronto Dr Samir Sinha recently quipped: "Everyone is searching for the Fountain of Youth, but what we keep finding is the Fountain of Age."[4] Thanks to the combined influence of biomedicine, technological innovation, and changes to people's lifestyle, people are living longer than ever before. Yet there is still no cure for dementia, which affects one out of three people over the age of eighty-five.

Over a hundred years have passed since 1910, when Kraepelin first named the disease after his colleague Alois Alzheimer. Scientists still have not found the cause or the cure, but their efforts have generated a host of competing theories. As discussed in chapter four, these theories posit causes that range from the workings of a slow virus, to the toxic effect of aluminum, to faulty genetics, to a deficit of the neurotransmitter acetycholine, to excessive glucose in the brain, to vascular problems resulting from insufficient blood supply to the brain and small strokes. In addition to the hypotheses that focus on the individual and, more precisely, on the ultra-cellular level of the body, researchers have proposed psychological and public health approaches that cite the broader social effects of stress, depression, anxiety, and loneliness in modern industrialized cultures as factors contributing to dementia.

In tracing the fascinating twists and turns in the development of Alzheimer's in Canada in the preceding chapters, I have made an effort to highlight facets of this complex narrative that continue to vex researchers yet are by and large omitted from popular accounts of Alzheimer's disease. For example it is quite remarkable that, as I argued in chapter one, when the disease concept was first debated, its supposed hallmarks – the infamous plaques and tangles – were never considered discrete symptoms. To date, they have never achieved the status of credible scientific "biomarkers." From the moment Alois Alzheimer and his colleagues first observed these structures in the brains of their patients – using the newly invented technologies of the electron microscope and state-of-the art staining techniques – to the present, scientists have been forced to admit that plaques "are frustratingly absent when they should be present; they can exist in significant numbers without having any apparent effect on the brain; and they may not even be the entity that should be targeted in any Alzheimer's therapy" (Ingram 103). The same can be said of tangles, prompting researchers to acknowledge that, as I noted in chapter one, these days "it's beginning to look as if the ultimate target might be neither plaques nor tangles" (ibid. 107).

Perhaps the most notable irony that was conveniently excised from contemporary biomedical and popular models of Alzheimer's is that

Alois Alzheimer himself – the man whose name has become synonymous with the disease – disagreed with his employer, Kraepelin.
As I observed in chapter one, Alzheimer insisted in his report that
the plaques and tangles he and his colleagues observed under the
microscope did not constitute the hallmark of a new disease entity.
Instead, he maintained that they were merely the familiar symptoms
of brain aging. In his most extensive account on the illness, cited earlier, Alzheimer writes: "There is, then, no tenable reason to consider
these cases as caused by a specific disease process. They are senile
psychoses, atypical forms of senile dementia" (in *Ballenger* Self, 43).
Far from an idiosyncratic response, Alzheimer's views reflected the
prevailing attitude toward dementia in the late nineteenth and early
twentieth centuries – namely, that it was not a disease but merely a
symptom of "senility" or "dotage," as it was termed at the time, which
society viewed as an inevitable part of the life course.

Equally surprising, in its initial formulation by Kraepelin in his
eighth edition of his textbook on psychiatry, the disease referred to a
little-known, rare disorder. Early twentieth century scientists had no
interest in Alzheimer's; from 1910 to 1930, "only fourteen articles
on Alzheimer's were published in the two major American neurological journals, *Neurology* and *Annals of Neurology*" (Ingram 43).
Over seventy years later, the disease concept underwent a profound
conceptual metamorphosis and, as a result, became "the disease of
the century." Robert Katzman instigated this paradigm shift in the
late 1970s when he argued that senile dementia and Alzheimer's
disease were one and the same – on this point, he agreed with Alois
Alzheimer's original view. Unlike Alzheimer, Katzman insisted that
late-onset dementia was not part of the natural process of aging, but
instead a *bona fide* disease. The rest, as they say, is history: Alzheimer's
was transformed into a Gothic monster reputed to be anywhere from
the tenth to the third deadliest killer in the world.

My aim, however, has not been simply to reveal these fundamental
and longstanding indeterminacies, but to explore how they shape
the stories we tell about Alzheimer's. Ultimately, I argue that their
enduring presence destabilizes any singular or supposedly truthful
model by introducing ironic elements into *all* of the stories we tell
about late-onset dementia (including the story I offer here). Yet, for
the most part, the history of Alzheimer's as a disease concept – and
its attendant ironies – has been forgotten. My central contribution
to scholarly investigations of the complexities associated with the

history of Alzheimer's lies in suggesting that while the dementia, like old age, has a material basis, "the images, expectations, and experience" of dementia have been "constructed in different ways at different times and for differing people at any one time" (Thane 5).

SECTION II: ALZHEIMER'S AND THE SHIFT FROM THE ELEGY TO THE GOTHIC

In the preceding chapters I invited readers to trace the history of Alzheimer's and to consider alternatives to the prevailing biomedical model. This process highlights the array of cultural and economic factors that have contributed to the promotion of certain models and the suppression of others. Ultimately, a historical analysis of dementia supports my interpretation of the changing models of dementia within a narrative context as an overarching shift in genre from the elegy to the Gothic.

According to religious elegies, the span of a person's life, the illnesses that beset a person, and the nature of his or her death are ordained by God. The thousand-year-old Jewish prayer, popularized by Canadian poet Leonard Cohen in his song "Who by Fire," perhaps best conveys this sense of God's absolute power over the mysteries of life and death. According to this prayer, God determines "how many will pass from the earth and how many will be created; who will live and who will die; who will die at his predestined time and who before his time; who by water and who by fire, who by sword and who by beast, who by famine and who by thirst, who by upheaval, and who by plague, who by strangling and who by stoning. Who will rest and who will wander, who will live in harmony and who will be harried, who will enjoy tranquility and who will suffer, who will be impoverished and who will be enriched, who will be degraded and who will be exalted" ("Unetanneh"). As I explain in the introduction, elegy supports this view of God's omnipotence by offering "serious reflections on both the figure and death in general, to the point of granting the deceased some sort of 'apotheosis' (elevation to divine status) and the reader some form of salvation hope, nearly always Christian and usually Protestant" (Hogle 566).

In the late nineteenth century the religious view, which dovetailed with the traditional, masculine elegiac approach, was increasingly challenged by the secular discourses of science. As I noted in chapter two, leading nineteenth-century neurologists, including Charcot and Kraepelin, refused to accept the view that the power of life and death lay solely in God's hands. As I mentioned earlier, in his *Clinical Lectures on the Diseases of Old Age* (1861), Charcot proclaimed that physiology "absolutely refuses to look upon life as a mysterious and supernatural influence which acts as its caprice dictates, freeing itself from all law" (in Cole 197). At the end of the nineteenth century, scientists increasingly eschewed the consoling narratives of religion and the genre of elegy in favour of the forensic and Gothic narratives of empirical science. When science seemingly won the field to claim the territory of dementia in the 1970s, what emerged was a Gothic view that conceived of senility not as an expected part of a life course governed by God but, instead, as a mysterious crime, whose clues and solution only science could successfully parse and resolve.

The shift from the elegy to the Gothic had profound repercussions for researchers, physicians, and people suffering from dementia alike. With respect to the latter, as I observe in chapter one the fate of Auguste D. was inextricably linked to the early Gothic and gendered features of the biomedical disease model. The initial gendering of the Kraepelinian model resulted from the combination of material and ideological factors at the time. During the nineteenth century, elderly women served as the primary source of the "patient material" in the vast European hospitals and asylums such as the Salpêtrière. Moreover at the time women were viewed as more susceptible to cognitive impairment and to pathological forms of memory loss. Not surprisingly, then, the psychiatric disorders that defined the nineteenth and the twentieth centuries, hysteria and Alzheimer's disease respectively, are predicated on the view that women's bodies are prone to disease, if not inherently diseased. As a result the emergent Gothic versions of memory loss, whether in the form of hysterical forgetting or dementia, were most readily "seen" in the bodies of women. Although the "uterine" theory that anchored hysteria and cast its shadow over Alzheimer's disease had waned by the mid-twentieth century, it never entirely disappeared. For very different reasons, currently the media, scientists, and some age critics are again promoting the view that Alzheimer's must be understood as "a woman's disease."[5] The periodic gendering of Alzheimer's is only one of the many repetitions that characterize the history of this enigmatic disease.

While a full and detailed account of the implications of the shift from elegiac to Gothic approaches to Alzheimer's lies beyond the scope of my book, my analysis identifies some of the limitations associated with the diverse models used to frame dementia. The harms that attend models of age-related dementia that subsume individuals under broader categories are evident in chapter one's exploration of the fate of Auguste D. in the Municipal Asylum for the Insane and Epileptic in Frankfurt am Main, and chapter two's investigation of the experience of patients with dementia in the newly built asylums in nineteenth-century Ontario. These categories – ranging from Locke's classification of the "idiot" to the asylum "patient" – support the focus on mental and physical deficits at the expense of the person. Auguste D.'s experience of privation and isolation, followed by her death from an infection caused by bedsores, recalls Daphne de Marneffe's comments concerning Charcot's biomedical approach to the hysteria diagnosis. Her insights also hold true for Kraepelin and his researchers' approach to Alzheimer's: "Charcot's and his colleagues' firm belief in their own objectivity itself constituted a threat to that very objectivity: first, by making them unable to question their own role in constructing the picture of the disease; and second, through their inability to see their own participation in recreating the pathogenic conditions of the patients' lives – neglect, lack of empathy, and exploitation" (in Katz, *Cultural* 43). Like the early researchers, we are all in danger of ignoring the limits of our objectivity. There is no safe haven of certainty when it comes to analyzing dementia.

SECTION III: THE LIMITS OF OBJECTIVITY

The repeated cautions cited by early researchers about the limited nature of their findings remain pertinent to anyone fashioning a model of age-related dementia. As I noted in chapter one, Alzheimer's colleague Gaetano Perusini repeatedly cautioned against coming to firm conclusions, insisting instead that as "Alzheimer underscores, we must be aware of the limitations of our methods" ("Histology" 118). Equally important, as noted in chapter four, David Kay – one of the leading researchers involved in the Newcastle study – confessed that his approach to the problem largely determined his findings. Although my historical method has partly entailed shedding light on the limitations of and alternatives to various models, I remain mindful throughout the book of the temptation to adopt a Gothic model that transforms the object under investigation – in this case, dementia – into a crime or a secret, which allows for the identification of culprits and the allocation of blame. The shortcomings of this model recall Eve Kosofsky Sedgwick's insights concerning the limitations of "paranoid reading," which she argues is a "contagious" theoretical practice (126) that entails assuming "a position of terrible alertness to the dangers posed by the hateful and envious part-objects that one defensively projects into, carves out of, and ingests from the world around one" (128).[6] To her credit, Sedgwick does not dismiss paranoid readings as necessarily negative – just limited, as "paranoia knows some things well and others poorly" (130). To a great extent, paranoid readings are a natural extension of the critical enterprise. Nevertheless, I have made an effort to remain aware of my own predilection for splitting and creating hierarchies when comparing models of dementia drawn from religion, science, the media, and literature. As noted in chapter five, for instance, Munro's short story "Powers" cautions against both biomedical and literary models, specifically the masculine elegy, and shows how both rely on the potentially unethical "substitution of the ... artifact for the living being" (Zeiger 64).

Following Sedgwick's invitation to consider the utility of a non-paranoid, "reparative reading," I have tried to make space for the reader to "realize that the future may be different from the present, [and so] it is also possible for her to entertain such ... ethically crucial possibilities as that the past, in turn, could have happened differently from the way it actually did" (146). Creating a different future may involve efforts to retrieve possibilities for alternative readings of Alzheimer's that lie buried in the past – a methodological approach that echoes the Orphic journey to rescue Eurydice – a primary intertext in many of the works considered in this study. Following the lead of literary works that rely on history as an antidote to the Gothic, I have excavated past models in search of materials to aid readers in fabricating new and vital readings of the dementia. As I mentioned earlier, I was repeatedly struck by the trend among early nineteenth-century researchers and the media – a trend that persisted until the 1970s – to construct narratives about the etiology of dementia that encompassed both the physiology of the individual and the broader social environment. Late-nineteenth century models of dementia – whose legacy persisted until the ultra-cellular and genetic models eclipsed them – frequently cited the stresses associated with modern industrial life as a key factor contributing to late-onset dementia. The earliest iterations of this narrative referred to "nervous strain" and conceived of dementia as the combined result of physical, psychological, and socio-environmental factors. Viewed in the light of this theory, "hardening arteries" and "softening brains" were caused, or at the very least worsened, by the pressures of modernity. Stress-based theories of dementia were extremely popular in the 1950s and remain popular. In the 1950s, owing to the pioneering and internationally recognized work of Hungarian-born endocrinologist Hans Seyle, other European-born researchers investigating dementia in Montreal – most notably, David Rothschild and Vojtech Kral – likewise attributed dementia to the physiological and psychological influence of stress. Since the 1990s, there has been a resurgence of interest in the role of stress and anxiety; once again, what Sontag terms a "characterological predisposition" (see *AIDS* 12, 43) to jealousy, moodiness, and neuroticism is being used to explain why women are supposedly "far more likely to be diagnosed with dementia."[7]

Researchers' early view of the deleterious influence of modernization also shaped imaginative models of dementia articulated by Canadian writers including Stephen Leacock. After the Second World War, authors such as Munro and Richler continued to adopt and adapt this narrative, which linked modernization to degeneration and decline. By highlighting the burden placed on primarily female caregivers to heal or harm loved ones coping with dementia, Munro's and Richler's stories add an additional dimension to the theory that Alzheimer's is inherently a woman's disease. These works trace both the impact of modernization and the toll placed on women who were frequently left with the responsibility to care for relatives with dementia. In Munro's and Richler's respective stories, a daughter is left on her own to care for an ill mother. The daughters are forced to grapple with a brutal calculus: when each chooses self-care over caring for her mother, the mother's health declines. But when they care for their mothers, they fall ill because there is no support from other family members or the community. By underscoring the complicated relationship between "waste" and "repair," both Munro's and Richler's stories highlight that it is largely the quality of care that determines whether people with dementia thrive or decline, and thus not merely the monstrous progression of a Gothic disease. Not only do these stories highlight the burden on female caregivers, they also deconstruct models of aging and disease that posit a linear trajectory of decline. Ultimately neither story plots a causal, Gothic relationship between modernity and dementia or between dementia and death. Instead, they invite readers to ponder the broader social policies that, since the nineteenth century, have pitted one generation against the next.[8]

As I argue in the early chapters, a historical understanding of Alzheimer's illustrates that intergenerational conflict and the hard choices families must make, which are poignantly depicted in the fictions analyzed, are not solely the result of a dementing illness. Instead these circumstances arose in part as a result of the Canadian government's decision – prompted by the recession at the end of the nineteenth century – to cut costs by phasing out community support for vulnerable, aged individuals. In turn, the government's policy impacted decisions made by asylum superintendents. The latter were understandably trying to gain legitimacy by enhancing cure rates – a goal they achieved in an era of fiscal restraint by refusing to care for "chronic cases," many of whom were aged individuals suffering from dementia. As a result of the combined effects of these space-saving and cost-cutting measures, the onus increasingly fell on families – and primarily on women – to cope on their own with relatives suffering from dementia. As my analysis of Richler's and Munro's fiction in chapter three illustrates, the repercussions of this budgetary decision were exacerbated during the Depression. In the late 1960s government claw-backs to health care again played an important role in the deinstitutionalization movement, the focus of chapter four and portrayed in Alice Munro's "Powers," analyzed in chapter five.

To be sure, not all healthcare policy or organizations responding to the needs of people with dementia in Canada were driven by a bureaucratic, top-down impetus to cut costs. As I argue in chapter six, the Alzheimer Society of Canada was in fact the brainchild of two researchers – Dr D. McLachlan and Dr A. Dalton – affiliated with the University of Toronto. They wanted to support families caring for a loved one with dementia and to obtain brain tissue for their research. Another intriguing facet of the history of Alzheimer's in Canada which has been forgotten is that all Alzheimer societies in the Western world can trace their origins to an event that took place in Toronto in 1977 (Chang 2). The "event" that took place sprang from an extraordinary gesture of compassion: Dr McLachlan approached Lori Dessau, a social worker supporting the families of children with Down syndrome, and asked her to set up a similar network for families looking after loved ones with Alzheimer's. As these examples and many others demonstrate, contextual information – including institutional and medical history, interviews with key players in the early Alzheimer's movement – and literary models are crucial to developing a nuanced understanding of Alzheimer's in

Canada. Whereas the biological models of dementia, with which we are most familiar, focus on the individual body, historical and imaginative texts shed light on the economic, political, and social milieu that play an equally crucial role in shaping society's view of Alzheimer's.

Recently Sandra Black, a leading Alzheimer's researcher in Toronto, stated that "Alzheimer's is a creepy disease that literally creeps through one's brain over a lifetime."[9] I cite her comments to emphasize that Gothic narratives have all but eclipsed alternative approaches. On one level, in using the word "creeps" Black was objectively describing a disease process. But her prior use of the word "creepy" as an adjective metaphorically envelopes the disease within the Gothic, aligning the disease with a villain that advances or comes on "slowly, stealthily, or by imperceptible degrees; to insinuate ... [itself] *into*; to come *in* or *up* unobserved; to steal insensibly *upon* or *over*" (OED). In our post-9/11 era, our current conception of "the war against Alzheimer's" likens the disease to an agent of bioterrorism, whose invisibility and stealth resonates with Western culture's fears of "sleeper cells" and other "pathological" elements hiding in the individual, familial, and national body.[10]

SECTION IV: ALTERNATIVES TO THE GOTHIC

Gothic narratives portray an evil victimizer stalking a helpless victim: a pathological disease "creeps" imperceptibly through the victim's brain slowly over decades. If the Gothic model is understood as the Truth, it affirms the view that nothing can be done expect to wait for researchers to discover a cure (be it a pill or a vaccine) that will vanquish our mortal enemy. By contrast, non-Gothic models of Alzheimer's offer some agency to individuals because they promote the view that a socially oriented, public health approach to Alzheimer's may, in fact, offer the most powerful ways of preventing dementia. Although these models necessitate relinquishing the fantasy that humans can maintain eternal youth, they nevertheless identify steps that people can take to protect themselves against dementia. For instance, scientists repeatedly cite the statistically powerful, protective benefits of higher education – a benefit that no drug has been able to match. According to Ingram, "literally dozens of studies have established that the further you go with your schooling, the lower your risk of Alzheimer's. Those who stop at or before grade 8 have about double the risk of those who complete high school, who in turn are at greater risk than those who complete university and so on" (143). Another unexpected, albeit related finding is that bilingualism likewise protects against Alzheimer's disease (ibid. 145).

Both protective benefits of education and the age-old conundrum associated with the disease's connection to plaques and tangles were strikingly evident in the famous Nun Study conducted in the 1990s when Dr David Snowdon and a research group studied the Sisters of Notre Dame. Not surprisingly, the Nun Study confirmed the longstanding anomalies associated with Alzheimer's pathological hallmarks. When scientists examined the brains of "alert, happy, attentive, smart" women, they found them to be full of plaques and tangles, "especially in the hippocampus and part of the cerebral cortex: classic signs of Alzheimer's disease" (ibid. 114). Individuals with this type of pathology "should have been demented," yet they were not (114). More important was the team's discovery that the severity of the women's dementia was correlated to their capacity to organize and convey complex words and thoughts. This new revelation was made possible due to the fact that, prior to taking their vows as young women, the would-be nuns were required to write a brief essay about themselves. When the researchers scanned these essays for their complexity, what they termed "idea density," they found that without exception, the nuns who scored the lowest suffered from dementia later in life. Equally surprising is the demonstrated protective influence of the character trait best described as "conscientiousness" – a trait that is partly attributed to nature, but may also be developed and nurtured.[11] My point in citing these non-biological factors lies in highlighting the very different models of Alzheimer's in circulation, and, equally important, the roles and agency they attribute to the characters within their discrete narratives.

Historical accounts and contemporary research into dementia increasingly suggest that cognitive decline is, in part, the result of natural aging and a lack of nurturing ranging from physical abuse (brain trauma) to psychological abuse and social marginalization (low levels of education, poor nutrition, anxiety, loneliness, and depression). Viewed in this light, the illness, which accrues over decades, may not be a Gothic monster after all. Instead it may well be an accurate reflection of the accumulation of psychological and physiological insults or traumas to the mind and body over a person's lifetime. As trauma theorist Bessel van der Kolk argues in regards to the registering of psychological trauma physiologically: "the body keeps the score." Rather than view Alzheimer's as a "singular dramatic illness," late-onset dementia might be better understood "as a reflection or accumulation of effects of a life lived, not well or poorly, but in full and in particular."[12]

SECTION V: TURNING TO PAST MODELS OF DEMENTIA – BENJAMIN'S ANGEL OF HISTORY

My book increasingly turns to literature precisely because fiction often explicitly or implicitly adopts a non-biomedical, historical approach to dementia. Literary works also frequently consider the effects of language and metaphor on our understanding of illness. As I stated earlier, for good or ill the stories we tell about dementia affect us all. Although religious, psychodynamic, and sociological explanations of Alzheimer's were by and large abandoned by the scientific community in the latter half of the twentieth century, Canadian writers continued to seek inspiration and consolation from prior models. In Margaret Laurence's *The Stone Angel*, for instance, the traditional English elegy offers a powerful form of consolation in the face of illness and death. Traces of earlier religious, elegiac, and philosophical models of consolation are also evident in Michael Ignatieff's *Scar Tissue*, a novel that powerfully illustrates contemporary society's "melancholic" orientation to dementia. The narrator's melancholy springs from his sense of the failure of both religious and scientific narratives to redeem the losses experienced by people with dementia and their families. His melancholy also results from, or, at the very least, is exacerbated by the fracturing of rhetorical conventions and narrative genres. As he explains: "No one knows any more what should be said and unsaid, what should be respected and kept in silence. No one knows any more what proprieties should attend a person's dying" (168). Rather than view the deconstruction of the master narratives of religion and science as a wholly tragic turn of events, this type of fracturing can also prompt one to adopt an archeological approach to dementia, as my close readings of the historical materials and literary works in the previous chapters suggest.

In contrast to *Scar Tissue*'s narrator, who bemoans the loss of master narratives and adopts a tragic view of events, I argue that one can glean valuable insights from the ruins of the past. My own critical penchant for sifting among historical fragments, as noted in the introduction, draws on Foucault's "genealogical method." As I explain, this method enables me to ask why certain terms, approaches, and "informed opinions took on the status of truth at specific historical junctures, while others were marginalized or disparaged" (Katz, *Cultural* 73). While also echoing Robert Kroetsch's emphasis on the value of "unhiding the hidden," my methodology owes a greater debt to Benjamin's theory of the fragment.

In his brief epigrammatic essays known as the "Theses on the Philosophy of History" (1940), Benjamin writes: "nothing that has ever happened should be regarded as lost for history" (254). Although he remains optimistic about the possibility of understanding history, Benjamin's innovative, archeological approach does not entail recreating a seamless narrative. Equally important, Benjamin realized that the historian's understanding of the past is inevitably coloured by her experiences in the present. Rather than lament this situation or view it as evidence of the contamination of a potentially pure, scientific endeavour to know the Truth of History, Benjamin viewed the subjective element as essential to the historian's imaginative matrix. To articulate the past historically," writes Benjamin, "does not mean to recognize it 'the way it really was.' It means to seize hold of a memory as it flashes up at a moment of danger" (255). For Benjamin, the historian's efforts to "grasp the constellation which his own era has formed with a definite earlier one" (263) are improvised, self-consciously aesthetic, and desperate. Benjamin likens the historian to an artificer who "seizes" images of the past and assembles a collage or "constellation" from its fragments (263). Far from offering the reassurance of traditional narratives, this process challenges prior models and ideally generates a shock. As he explains: "Where thinking suddenly stops in a configuration pregnant with tensions, it gives that configuration a shock" (262).

In addition to outlining a methodology predicated on the shock effect, Benjamin cautions against celebrating a nation's progress or praising its cultural achievements. Instead he enjoins historians to view these "cultural treasures" with detachment. As he explains: "There is no document of civilization which is not at the same time a document of barbarism. And just as such a document is not free of barbarism, barbarism taints also the manner in which it was transmitted from one owner to another. A historical materialist therefore dissociates himself from it as far as possible. He regards it as his task to brush history against the grain" (256). I cite Benjamin's insights concerning the tension between civilization and barbarism, the practice of reading "history against the grain," and the value of creating a collage from fragments of narrative that has the potential to shock the reader because his views capture my experience of trying to come to grips with the story of Alzheimer's – a fragmented historical narrative bristling with complexities, contradictions, and ironies – during a historical moment when the Gothic model prevails. Benjamin's awareness that barbarism is the secret sharer of civilization resonates with many of the historical incidents identified in the preceding chapters. A similar irony underlies the fact that Auguste D. died from an infection caused by bedsores whereas her brain cells were preserved with the utmost care and have recently attained the status of a cultural treasure. The twinning of barbarism and civility is likewise apparent in the decision on the part of nineteenth-century asylum superintendents to discharge vulnerable, demented, elderly individuals because they were lowering the cure rates of the newly built institutions. One of the darkest ironies we have forgotten is that our current panic about dementia and our use of apocalyptic metaphors, which repeatedly refer to the "tidal wave of dementia coming our way,"[13] are merely the most recent iterations of an earlier panic concerning the menace of the "feeble-minded" in the first half of the twentieth century.

In 1940, when Benjamin wrote the "Theses," he was living in exile in France. As a German Jew, he was forced to flee Paris when the Nazis threatened the city. He headed for a well-known passage between France and Spain, and had made plans to catch a boat to the US. Due to his heart problems, however, the mountain pass between France and Spain proved too difficult for Benjamin to traverse swiftly. This setback, combined with the news that he would need a visa to leave France, caused him to despair. Faced with the prospect of being sent to a concentration camp he took his own life in the middle of the night. He was forty-eight years old. On discovering his lifeless body the next morning, officials were so shaken that they allowed the other members of his party to travel across the border into Spain.

I cite this biographical information because, for me, Benjamin's philosophy offers an innovative and imaginative approach to the ruins of history. His experience as a German prior to the First World War also highlights what is potentially at stake in conversations about dementia that implicitly or explicitly touch on whose lives are worth living and, conversely whose lives are not. Benjamin lived and died in the grip of a political regime that, like no other before it or since, highlights the potential dangers associated with our current panic concerning "defective" or "feeble-minded" individuals. As I argued in the penultimate and final chapters, one of the most ethically troubling and elided ironies reflected in contemporary society's panic about dementia is its connection to the late-nineteenth and early twentieth century international eugenics movement that culminated in the Nazi death camps. In Caroline Adderson's *A History of Forgetting* and Alice Munro's short stories "The Dance of the Happy Shades" and "In Sight of the Lake" these connections are rendered explicit, leading to the shocking (for some) recognition that our current terror of Alzheimer's is not new. Recalling prior efforts to rid the nation of "undesirables," "burdens," and "waste" is crucial in our current historical moment. On Friday, 6 February 2015, the Supreme Court of Canada charged the government to legalize physician-assisted suicide for people suffering from grievous and irremediable medical conditions, including age-related dementia and Alzheimer's disease. These new laws are coming into effect as I write this last chapter. I am neither for or opposed to the law; my concern is that the largely unspoken and unacknowledged history associated with cognitive impairment coupled with the more recent myths and dread that surrounds Alzheimer's is increasingly prompting people with late-onset dementia to view themselves solely as a burden. Owing to the power of these myths, it is unclear whether Canadian society people with dementia are able to choose to live or die of their own free will.

SECTION VI: DEMENTIA AND THE AIDS CRISIS

Despite the limitations that attend a "paranoid" reading, like other age studies critics, I argue that it is important to consider how society's panic in the face of dementia in the present may have lethal consequences. Gullette worries, for example, that the Gothic model – which has been adopted by a host of celebrated writers and filmmakers – may lead people to believe that when faced with dementia, suicide and euthanasia are the only rational and socially responsible choices. She cites Tony Kushner's recent play *The Intelligent Homosexual's Guide to Capitalism and Socialism with a Key to the Scriptures* (2009) as a particularly troubling depiction of dementia. The play features a seventy-two-year-old widower who brings his adult children together to tell them he is going to kill himself because he has Alzheimer's. As Gullette points out, two decades earlier, Kushner rallied around homosexuals during the AIDS crisis. With his earlier play *Angels in America*, Gullette says, Kushner came to the rescue of people who were killing themselves because they had AIDS, which at the time was the most feared disease in the country ("Politics" 8). Now, "with Alzheimer's not AIDS the most feared disease in the country," Kushner writes *The Intelligent Homosexual's Guide*. Far from being instructed on how best to survive adversity, the elderly protagonist, who has just been diagnosed with a dread disease, finds himself "abandoned, holding a bag of lethal drugs given to him by a sympathizer" (8). Reading the text somewhat problematically as a guide to best practices, Gullette argues that from this play the audience learns, should Alzheimer's strike, not how to live with courage but how to die in a "failsafe way" (ibid.).

The analogy Gullette draws between the AIDS crisis in the 1980s and our current panicked response to Alzheimer's recalls both *Memory Board* and *A History of Forgetting*, which, as I note, drew similar comparisons decades earlier. As Gullette astutely observes, homophobia, "a capacious prejudice, once had disease-terror built into it. Now it is ageism" (9) – and, I would add, late-onset dementia. "It is possible," Gullette asks, "in our frightened world to internalize this bias and not notice that MCI is the new HIV, the last word in death sentences" (9).[14] Recalling the initial association between Alzheimer's and women drawn by nineteenth-century clinicians, Gullette points out that nowadays in both art and life the majority of the current victims of this "death sentence" are women. Yet, as she asserts, Alzheimer's is a woman's disease not because of an essential connection between women's physiology and disease, but because women live longer; hence, "more women will live to be 80 or 90, getting poorer as they age" (3). For these demographic and economic reasons, Alzheimer's is also a woman's fear: "Violence selects the weak" (3).

Gullette highlights narratives that seemingly sanction the murder of elderly women with cognitive impairment and suggests that society is becoming accustomed to viewing vulnerable women as disposable burdens. Her insights recall the troubling scene in *Scar Tissue* where the narrator contemplates smothering his mother as a means of resolving his challenges with coping with her dementia. Whereas some readers may be tempted to side with the exasperated male caregivers, Gullette warns against this type of misguided empathy.

Instead, she insists that both fictive and real-life plots which advocate suicide and euthanasia – and courts that show leniency to men who kill elderly women suffering from dementia, using the phrase "mercy killing" to obscure the transgressive violence of "murder" – reveal our society's lack of basic knowledge about both MCI and Alzheimer's. Researchers concur, for example, that much MCI "never becomes AD. It can take two decades to turn into AD. As many people go back to their own normal state as go on to develop AD" (Gullette 6). With respect to Alzheimer's, as many people over centuries have insisted, the experience of dementia need not and often does not entail a monstrous erasure of personhood. It is immoral to persuade people with dementia and their caregivers that death is preferable to living with dementia.

SECTION VII: NEW APPROACHES TO DEMENTIA IN CANADIAN CULTURE

If, as I have suggested, every model of Alzheimer's is contingent and constructed, then the onus is on readers to find words and images – perhaps even fragments of a story – they can live with. Generating an alternative narrative may involve unraveling prior texts and using their threads to weave a different story. In the remainder of this chapter, I want briefly to consider four recent interventions by Canadian artists and researchers – David Chariandy's *Soucouyant* (2007), John Mighton's *Half Life* (2005), Aynsley Moorhouse's *Sounds of Forgetting* (2011), and Pia Kontos's research with elder-clowns in locked dementia wards (2015). Their work constitutes some of the most innovative approaches to and understandings of dementia I have encountered in the course of my research.

Soucouyant perhaps best illustrates Benjamin's tactic of brushing history against the grain in its deconstruction of prior models of dementia to arrive at a new understanding of the illness. In my essay "Purging the World of the Whore and the Horror: Gothic and Apocalyptic Portrayals of Dementia in Canadian Fiction" (2015), I trace a long-standing pattern in Canadian writing that entails conflating the figure of the old woman with what society deems shameful and evil, revelling in the latter's "fall," and banishing the elderly from the new world to pave the way for its ideal, youthful citizens. This pattern, I argue, can be discerned in Sheila Watson's modernist classic

The Double Hook (1959), Michael Ignatieff's *Scar Tissue* (2006), and David Chariandy's *Soucouyant* (2007).[15] While the presence of this apocalyptic motif in the US, a nation that explicitly viewed itself as the New Jerusalem, is not entirely unexpected, I argue that a similar mechanism can also be traced in Canadian literature from the mid-twentieth century to the present.

A recent satirical iteration of this pattern can be found, for example, in Margaret Atwood's story "Torching the Dusties," the final tale in her collection *Stone Mattress* (2014). The story offers an account of two nursing home residents, Wilma and Tobias, who are initially trapped inside Ambrosia Manor by a violent mob – an anti-elderly vigilante movement called "Our Turn." Members of the group, which has branches throughout the world and operates with the tacit approval of the state, wear baby masks and set fire to nursing homes, "torching the dusties" – a reference to "the dustballs under the bed" (256). Brandishing signs that read: "TIMES UP. TORCH THE DUST-IES. HURRY UP PLEASE ITS TIME" (262), and chanting "*Time to Go. Fast Not Slow. Burn Baby Burn. It's Our Turn*" (265), they surround Ambrosia Manor.[16] After secretly escaping from the home, Wilma and Tobias watch in horror as the baby-faced protesters use oil drums and explosives to light it on fire. Wilma recognizes that neither the firefighters nor the police arrive on the scene to rescue the trapped inhabitants, many of whom suffer from physical and cognitive disabilities. Watching the flames engulf the home, Tobias tries to reassure Wilma by suggesting that perhaps their friends who remain trapped in the building will "jump out of the windows" (268). "'No,' says Wilma. 'They won't'" (268). Recalling Gullette's concerns about internalized ageism, Wilma admits to herself, "She wouldn't if it was her. She would just give up" (268).

My first encounter with this apocalyptic pattern in Canadian literature occurred when I read Watson's *The Double Hook*. Whereas Watson's novel relies on the fragmented poetic techniques characteristic of literary modernism to trace the agonistic struggle between a wandering mother and her son, as I argued in chapter seven, *Scar Tissue* offers a realist portrait of a middle-aged philosophy professor's struggle to find meaning in his mother's illness – an illness diagnosed as Alzheimer's and relentlessly portrayed as a pathological maternal legacy. In keeping with *The Double Hook*, *Scar Tissue* features the deadly fall of an elderly parent (in this case, the narrator's father), followed by the purgation of the supposedly tainted maternal home. *Scar Tissue* also contains both Gothic tropes and the apocalyptic impulse to rectify original sin.

In contrast to *The Double Hook*'s and *Scar Tissue*'s adherence to Gothic and apocalyptic plots, *Soucouyant* draws on Caribbean mythology to deconstruct both genres' tendency to associate transgressive and demented women with evil and thereby justify the latter's violent expulsion from the new world. *Soucouyant* tells the story of a young man in the 1980s who returns to his mother's home in Scarborough, Ontario, after a two-year absence. Rather than portray the mother's dementia as a pathological maternal legacy that calls for apocalyptic purification, the narrative suggests that her illness was partly instigated and certainly exacerbated by the traumatic dispersal of native Trinidadians by Allied military forces during the Second World War and the subsequent scattering of these peoples across North America. In its graphic depictions of the fires that rained down from the sky and the Allied troops' sexual exploitation of the local women, *Soucouyant* politicizes and deconstructs apocalypse's portrayal of the death of the Whore of Babylon and the eradication of the old world in favour of a New Jerusalem reserved for the male elect.

The familiar Gothic destruction of the mother occurs in *Soucouyant* when Adele wanders and falls to her death in the house she shares with her son. Although not pushed to her death like the old lady in *The Double Hook*, her death, like the father's death in *Scar Tissue* (which is triggered by the stress associated with caring for his wife), is the direct result of dementia, which, as in *Scar Tissue*, is portrayed in excruciating detail. In *Soucouyant*, the narrator remains haunted not by his mother's illness, but by the mythic, Caribbean tale of an evil female spirit who disguises herself as a woman by day, and by night, slips out of her skin and transforms herself into a ball of fire. Moving from house to house, the soucouyant feasts on the blood of its neighbours. The uncanny presence of ancestral spirits together with apocalyptic attempts to exorcise these spirits in these novels demonstrates how dementia functions in the modern, Canadian nation-state as a trope of dreadful otherness that must be expelled. *Soucouyant*, however, relies on the trope of dementia to destabilize normative temporalities and to afford possibilities for a doubling back to repressed histories and origins. These alternative histories include knowledge of matriarchal and non-Christian spiritual traditions and knowledge, and non-individualistic and non-hierarchal relationships predicated on dyadic states epitomized by an unbroken mother-son bond.

Using fragments from his mother's intermittent tales of the soucouyant, Chariandy's narrator eventually pieces together the story of his mother's and grandmother's traumatic past in Trinidad during the Second World War. In contrast to *The Double Hook*'s and *Scar Tissue*'s portrayals of a universal Oedipal battle restricted to two generations within a single family, *Soucouyant* demonstrates that the family's struggle is inextricably tied to the earlier political violence and trauma instigated by the Allied occupation of Trinidad during the Second World War. Elusive shards of Adele's traumatic memory gesture further into the past, to the African diaspora caused by slavery and the Indian diaspora triggered by indentured labour, adding further layers to the text's complex palimpsest of cultural memory. The reappearance of oppressed groups in cultural memory serves as the novel's means of insisting on the presence of elided and alternative histories – alternatives to the Canadian nation-state's Freudian Oedipal plot of generational supersession.

Whereas *The Double Hook* portrays intergenerational tension resolved by matricide, and *Scar Tissue* ends with the narrator's apocalyptic fantasy of joining the elect and passing through the gates of truth, *Soucouyant* represents the burning of women – the narrator's mother and grandmother – as the text's central, unspeakable trauma. In Adele's mind, as in her son's, the horrific fire is fused with the dream-like memory of glimpsing a soucouyant. Yet, as Adele's son explains, "it's not really about a soucouyant. It's about an accident. It's about what happened in her birthplace during World War II. It's a way of telling without really telling" (66).

Initially, in keeping with the Gothic story, the boy viewed his grandmother as "a monster": "Someone with a hide, red-cracked eyes, and blistered hands. Someone who would claw her stiffened thumb across her eyes and try to smile through the ruin of her mouth" (116). His mother, whose skull was seared during the fire, lost her hair and wears a wig. At one point, when she is too ill to remember to conceal her defacement, she appears without her wig, and her son views her as a monster. Toward the conclusion, however, readers learn how these supposed monsters were created.

Adele and her mother were forced from their home in the 1940s, when the Allies seized Trinidad. Unable to feed herself or her daughter, Adele's mother prostituted herself to American soldiers and, at age five, Adele locks eyes with a soldier having sex with her mother, who later teaches Adele how to use his lighter. When the mother returns home and discovers that the soldier has consorted with Adele and brought her gifts, she is enraged and vents her anger on her child. Rejecting her mother, Adele shouts: 'You disgusting ... You a whore ... You not my mother. You *horror*. All *horror*!" (189). Afterward, Adele runs away to the Army base, but her mother follows. After a soldier douses Adele's mother with gasoline, Adele is overcome by the fumes, and believes that she and her mother "will forever stink of something shat from the bowels of the earth and cooked in hell. They will never be clean again" (192).

Invoking apocalypse's Manichean divisions between the clean and the unclean, the elect and the non-elect, this episode restages the infamous burning of the Whore. In a "miraculous achievement of agility and determination, Adele flicks the lighter," setting both her mother and herself on fire (192), so that in Chariandy's retelling of the soucouyant story, the monster does not willingly transform into a fireball; instead, the apocalyptic fires unleashed on the island by the Americans literally efface its most vulnerable inhabitants. Equally important, according to the narrative, the trauma associated with this event contributes to Adele's dementing illness. As the narrator explains, his mother wasn't "simply forgetting"; her past was also coming back to her: "a word would slip from her mind and pronounce itself upon her lips" (22). At one point, she says the word "Chaguaramas," and it triggers a memory of how she and her mother were burned: "She loss she skin at the military base in Chaguaramas. She wore a dress of fire before it go ruin her. I wore a hat of orange light, a sheet of pain, yes, on my head and neck" (24). Rather than portray dementia as an isolated biomedical disease, *Soucouyant* represents pathological forgetting within the larger social context of the gendered and racialized, traumatic history of the Afro-Indian diaspora.

Thus in contrast to *The Double Hook* and *Scar Tissue*, which insist on the malignancy of the maternal legacy, *Soucouyant* affirms that both destruction and the capacity to heal are part of this complex inheritance. Recalling *Scar Tissue*'s uncanny maternal doubling, in *Soucouyant*, the figure of the abject old woman multiplies and includes the narrator's mother, Adele, his nameless grandmother, and an old lady who acts as a healer in the community. We are told that the "old lady" had "long memories and the proper names for things ...

Most of all, the old woman could heal, a skill she had inherited from a long line of knowledgeable women" (182). From his very different vantage point, Chariandy's narrator mimics the old lady by looking backward into the past. In contrast to *Scar Tissue*, *Soucouyant* turns to the past to find a "way out of a Freudian world limited to two generations, one from which older women are missing" (Woodward, "Generational" 150). Whereas the purgative rituals in Watson's and Ignatieff's novels entrench the patriarchal and Freudian model of the family composed of two warring generations, the fires in Chariandy's novel illuminate an alternative model based on three generations – a model that affirms "a long line of knowledgeable women" and establishes a heritage that, in Woodward's terms, is "based not on a struggle for domination but on ... care" ("Generational" 151), demonstrated when Adele's son responds to his mother's confusion by imaginatively taking their part and retelling their story. In this way Chariandy's narrator helps his community to imaginatively "undo" the legacy of violence (193).

In contrast to *The Double Hook* and *Scar Tissue*, *Soucouyant* deconstructs the fall of the old woman and, in so doing, offers an alternative to the apocalyptic promise of a new world reserved for a male elect – as reflected in its concluding counter-image. The narrator recollects walking as a child "along a shore of hot rocks and trash. My grandmother stumbling and reaching, without thinking, for Mother's hand. Each reaching for the other and then holding hands the rest of the way" (196). As the narrator explains: "I remember being awed by this. It was all so incredibly ordinary. They were just a mother and daughter" (196). In view of the dominance of the apocalyptic and modernist plots of aging and dementia, which view women as vehicles of a degeneration linked with evil and sinful transgression – all whores, all horror – *Soucouyant*'s reliance on the trope of dementia to offer an alternative image of intergenerational matriarchal kinship, a secular revelation, is nothing short of miraculous.

SECTION VIII: THE WORKINGS OF TRANSFERENCE IN JOHN MIGHTON'S *HALF LIFE*

As *Soucouyant* and many similar examples cited in this book illustrate, age-related dementia is not merely an isolated, individual, biological experience. Canadian literature repeatedly demonstrates that the challenges posed by dementia constitute, yet ultimately also exceed, what might best be described as a family affair. The latter phrase is apt because, as the texts under consideration repeatedly illustrate, the children of individuals suffering from cognitive decline become the custodians of their parents' lives and the bearers of the latter's memories. Yet as John Mighton's play *Half Life* (2005) illustrates, the problem of dementia is both a family and a national affair.[17] In keeping with *A History of Forgetting*, *Memory Board*, and *Soucouyant*, Mighton's play draws an analogy between our current war on dementia and the Second World War. Set in a nursing home for veterans and their families, where many of the residents are celebrated for their heroic participation in the war, *Half Life* installs and subverts our understanding of roles played by various participants in our current war on dementia. Mighton's play portrays the amorous relationship between two residents of the nursing home – Patrick, a brilliant mathematician who worked with Special Services as a code breaker during the war, and Clara, a woman with dementia of the Alzheimer's type. In addition to tracing Patrick and Clara's affair, the play focuses on how this relationship affects their respective divorced and middle-aged daughter and son. Clara claims to have met Patrick during the war, but her son Donald, who has only second-hand knowledge of his parents' wartime experiences, can neither verify nor discredit her memory of their encounter. Donald's relationship to his parents' wartime past recalls Marianne Hirsch's observations in her essay "The Generation of Postmemory." Hirsch coined the term "postmemory" to describe the relationship that "the generation after those who witnessed cultural or collective trauma bears to the experience of those who came before, experiences that they 'remember' only by means of the stories, images, and behaviours among which they grew up" (106). As she explains, the "formative events of the twentieth century have crucially informed our biographies, threatening sometimes to overshadow and overwhelm our own lives. But we did not see them, suffer through them, experience their impact directly" (106). Postmemory's "connection to the past is thus not actually mediated by recall but by imaginative investment, projection, and creation" (107). In keeping with Hirsch's research on the conjunctions between the family and memory, *Half Life* emphasizes the effect of transference on individual and collective remembrance, and suggests that we know our own history and that of others only in fragments coloured by transference.

Whereas Hirsch emphasizes the roles of projection and photography, I argue that Mighton's play highlights the psychological operations of transference to interrogate society's unquestioned valorization of masculinity and heroism and the creation of a category of elect, male citizens. Rather than install the image of the female parent suffering from dementia as a Gothic monster and cast her among the non-elect, *Half Life* suggests, instead, that society's seemingly benign practice of institutionalizing and marginalizing individuals suffering from mental and physical decline constitutes a socially sanctioned ethical transgression. Put differently, *Half Life* demonstrates that in waging a war against dementia, due to the unconscious workings of transference, benevolent caregivers unwittingly find themselves playing the role of Gothic victimizers.

None of Freud's epochal discoveries, argues Aaron Esman, has proved more heuristically productive or more clinically valuable than his account of transference: the demonstration that humans "regularly and inevitably repeat with the analyst and with other important figures in their current lives patterns of relationship, of fantasy, and of conflict with the crucial figures in their childhood – primarily their parents" (1). Owing to its origins in the unconscious, Freud felt that transference narrows the scope and efficacy of the ego because it instigates the "transfer of powers from the subject to the Other" (Lacan 486). In the grip of transference, the individual's unconscious – the Other within – holds sway. In Freud's initial remarks regarding transference, he stresses its powerfully deceptive features. The patient, he asserts, makes "a false connection" to the person of the analyst when "an affect became conscious which is related to memories which are still unconscious" (*Fragment* 139). According to Freud, the patient in the grip of transference inevitably "acts it out before us," rather than consciously "reporting it" (Freud, "An Outline" 174–6).

As a play *Half Life* literally "acts out" the workings of transference, whose operations explicitly define its central question – namely the veracity of Clara's insistence, after encountering Patrick at the nursing home presumably for the first time, that she met him earlier, during the war, and that she has loved him ever since. Rather than unconsciously bringing to bear the early emotions associated with a parental relationship on an entirely new relationship, Clara consciously insists that the past and present objects of her affection are identical, and she names them both Patrick. Her son, Donald, maintains that Clara's memory is unreliable and that his mother – like a patient in full transference – is deceived. Yet Donald's denial of his mother's memory of Patrick serves to shore up an idealized image of his father. In Donald's fantasy, his mother eternally adored her husband – and by extension Donald himself, as their cherished son. In keeping with the affectively and temporally disruptive nature of transference, *Half Life* explores how our understanding of the past influences and fractures our experience of the present: were Patrick and Clara lovers many years before or is this a recent fiction – what Freud might term "a compulsion and a deception"? (Freud, *Studies* 230). Rather than focus solely on Clara, the play emphasizes that no one's memory, including that of the audience, is free from the operations of transference and projection and, by extension, from the ethical implications of acting in the half-light of its shadows. Due to the effects of transference, virtually all of the characters in the play and the audience see through the proverbial "glass darkly" (I Corinthians 13:12).

The operations of transference structure both the experiences and responses of the patients in the nursing home to the staff and vice versa. The ethical complications arising out of the ambiguities associated with memory and postmemory are starkly rendered because Donald must decide whether or not to credit and honour Clara's memory – which Patrick never contradicts – and her passionate attachment to Patrick. Due to Donald's need to affirm his fantasy of his parents' supposed eternal fidelity, he is tempted to discredit his mother's story of having met and fallen in love with Patrick during the war. But dismissing Clara's story of Patrick to shore up Donald's preferred story constitutes a potentially unethical act of appropriation and revision. At bottom, his dilemma raises a fundamental question posed by Hirsch: "How can we best carry stories forward without appropriating them?" (104).

What is perhaps most striking is how *Half Life* links individual and cultural transference phenomena to the workings of national memory and postmemory. The play repeatedly juxtaposes Donald's obsessions with his mother's fidelity and his father's heroism to the communal investment in these roles as manifested in public rituals such as marriage and Remembrance Day. By portraying the agonistic struggle between individuals such as Donald, whose memories serve and reflect personally and culturally iconic interests, and individuals such as Clara and Patrick, whose memories transform and decay, and who resist the discourses of heroism and fidelity, and by literally juxtaposing Alzheimer's disease with Remembrance Day, *Half Life* interrogates our construction of and investment in personal, familial, and national memory. At one point, during the Remembrance Day service in the church at the nursing home, the congregation sings Isaac Watt's famous hymn that paraphrases Psalm 90:

> A thousand ages in thy sight
> Are like an evening gone;
> Short as the watch that ends the night
> Before the rising sun. (ll. 17–20)

Drawing on a text written in 1719, which refers to God's capacity to fathom time in its entirety – "a thousand ages" as a "single evening" – *Half Life* poignantly illustrates the limitations of human perception and memory, which remains imperfect and fragmented. Later, Donald and the Reverend explicitly discuss God's role as a preserver of memory. As the Reverend says, "A Russian novelist – I believe it was Dostoevsky – said that if there is no God then everything is permitted. But I think it's even worse than that. Because if there is no God, then everything will be forgotten" (69). Donald, the champion of secular science, agrees, but insists there is "no point inventing an omniscient God to console yourself … You can't have consciousness without constant loss" (69). Without religious consolation, however, Donald is left to contend with the brute fact of his mother's death and the losses it entails. As he confesses to the Reverend, "unfortunately, she's dying. And when she's dead, no one will ever think of me the way she did again … Not even God" (69). His comments recall the similar heartfelt plaint uttered by *Scar Tissue*'s narrator.

In *Half Life*, the threat of late-onset dementia highlights the shift from religious, elegiac modes of consolation to the Gothic. The play's depiction of dementia also forcibly recalls John Locke's powerful contribution to Western society's understanding of the relationship between memory and human identity. As noted earlier, in *An Essay Concerning Human Understanding* Locke famously distinguishes between human identity, which corresponds to substance and is dependent on bodily or physical continuity, and personal identity, the identity of the self, which is a function of the continuity of consciousness. For Locke, personal identity is predicated on remembering one's own actions and the ability to narrate past experiences in the present (see Whitehead 53–8). As Ian Hacking puts it, for Locke "the person is constituted not by a biography but by a remembered biography" (81).

Whereas scholars, myself included, have focused primarily on Locke's valorization of memory, *Half Life* sheds light on Locke's often-elided account of the challenges to memory posed by forgetting, interruption, and passionate eruptions of turbulent emotions. As Locke maintains, consciousness itself is susceptible to "being interrupted always by forgetfulness" (302). According to him, memory is inherently entropic: "there seems to be a constant decay of all our ideas, even of those which are struck deepest, and in the minds the most retentive" (149). Whether interrupted by sleep, forgetfulness, or an inability to attend to all of a given memory at one time, for Locke consciousness is always already interrupted. This awareness prompted Locke to question how such moments of oblivion can be accounted for in an understanding of the self. Ultimately Locke determined that remembering and forgetting provide the foundation for human identity. In addition to remarking on the inevitability of interruption and, hence, forgetting, Locke also recognized that memory is not solely the product of voluntary cognitive activity since memories and remembering are activated and disrupted by passion. Memories, Locke writes, are "roused and tumbled out of their dark cells" by "some turbulent and tempestuous passion" (150). In contrast to that of Aristotle, Locke's conception of memory is, as Anne Whitehead observes, "non-intentional and seems to initiate a chaotic, if not threatening chain of activity which releases memories from the 'dark cells' within which they have hitherto been secured and confined" (55). The disruptive effects of interruption and passion, elided features of Locke's writings on memory and identity, are foregrounded in *Half Life*, and are signalled from the start by the play's title, since the term "half-life" measures exponential decay (*OED*). Viewed in this light, the title of Mighton's play implicitly posits decay as integral to identity, and suggests that forms of decay including forgetting are the property of all matter.

In *Half Life* this insight is repressed and projected onto the bodies of the elderly residents. Worse, the "bare" lives of elderly people, filled with meaningless, childish games and puzzles, are separated from the lives of the active members of society, and ruthlessly contained in the nursing home. I use the term *ruthless* because, as Joanne Faulkner, citing Giorgio Agamben, maintains, the disavowal and misrecognition that secures the category of the human entails that there is an aspect of the self that "is akin to meat, and accordingly is available for others' use" (74). The self "akin to meat," in essence the corporeal self, renders humans vulnerable to exploitation and harm. As Faulkner states, this form of bare life haunts political relationships "as a threat of violence" (74) – a threat that is realized in the unethical treatment of the residents at the nursing home, who are the targets of theft as well as physical and possibly sexual abuse. This type of danger is precisely what Gullette fears and Atwood envisions in "Torching the Dusties."

The banality of the transgressions against the residents in *Half Life* demonstrates further that evil individuals are not restricted to historical or foreign enemies such as the Japanese during the Second World War. Instead, ostensibly well-meaning, responsible citizens – reverends, nurses, sons, and daughters who uphold the values of the nation-state – are revealed as contemporary doubles of the historical villains who starve and imprison inmates. It is significant in this regard that on several occasions, Anna and Patrick explicitly voice their concerns that their parents are starving (3, 74). At one point, the Reverend makes a direct comparison between prisoners of war in the Second World War and the residents of the nursing home (47), but no one attends to his analogy and he himself does not understand his complicity in the residents' imprisonment. After Patrick attempts to escape, the staff put him in a straitjacket. By the end of the play, Clara and Patrick have been forcibly separated, and Patrick is confined to the locked ward. At one point, Donald even assumes the role of the interrogator of a prisoner of war when Patrick is captured after trying to escape the home. In this perverse interrogation scene, which links familial and national wars, the prisoner is willing to talk but his words threaten his interrogator, who therefore refuses to listen.

Despite the fact that virtually all of the characters' memories and motivations remain opaque, *Half Life* repeatedly stresses the material consequences of the analogies and the labels that we use to determine people's identities. Donald's beliefs about his mother and his role as caregiver are thus not merely abstract philosophical problems requiring more profound contemplation. Instead, as the play repeatedly illustrates, Donald must act – and he does, for good or ill. On both thematic and formal levels, *Half Life* engages in the ethical work of highlighting both the necessity of acting (pun intended) and the limits of our ability to comprehend the Other – limits that are, not surprisingly, foregrounded by a host of interruptions.

On several occasions, Tammy interrupts Donald's conversations with Anna and the Reverend. The latter repeatedly interrupts Patrick and Clara's privacy. In the scene cited earlier in which Tammy and the Reverend treat the couple like puppets, forcing them to dance, Agnes interrupts them further. "Would you mind keeping the noise down in here?" she says. "I'm trying to sleep" (55). Her comment is significant because, as noted earlier, sleep is one of the central interruptions of consciousness that Locke identifies in his writing. Taken together, the interruptions prompt the characters to forget what happened and embark on new trains of thought and action. The repeated interruptions might also cause some audience members to forget information and events that occurred prior to the interruption. Thus, in addition to portraying the inescapable workings of transference, *Half Life*'s formal structure implicates us in the challenges associated with remembering and forgetting.

Rather than viewing the tactic of interruption solely as a trap that demonstrates our compromised ability to remember – shattering the myth of the autonomous, fully functioning citizen – the technique can also be interpreted as an attempt to demonstrate the pitfalls associated with our attempt to master the Other – both the external Other and the Other within. With respect to the former, by strategically introducing obstacles to communication, *Half Life* frustrates the hermeneutical impulse to cross barriers and merge self and other, particularly when this impulse is directed at vulnerable or marginalized groups. The various obstructions, including the repeated use of curtains that preclude our vision and the instances of interruption, prompt readers to relinquish "the exorbitant (and unethical) but usually unspoken assumption that we should know others enough to speak for them" (Sommer 206).

What makes *Half Life* remarkable is its ability to use fragmentation as a tactic to suspend revelation while exposing the relationship between individual transferences and more widespread analogies that shape our understanding of human identity. At the core of the play lies a familiar, haunting question posed so memorably by Plato, who likewise used the language of projected shadows: is it possible that what we believe to be true about someone or about a group of people (in this case, senior citizens) are merely shadows that prevent us from grasping the complexity and wonder of the world and its diverse inhabitants? What if the metaphors – human, child, animal, and machine – that we have inherited and that currently structure our thinking do not help us to make sense of ourselves or the changes that we experience throughout the life course, particularly in old age?

Half Life does not inscribe new and better metaphors or more accurate postmemories that we can project onto the bodies of senior citizens; nor does it attempt to resolve the challenges posed by transference. As Joanne Faulkner suggests, "the moment of human 'salvation' is not its recuperation to divinity or to its proper place, but rather an embrace of abandonment or displacement" (79). Ending as it does with an anti-revelation – Clara, obscured behind a curtain, alone in bed, falling asleep – *Half Life* bids us to confront and accept interruption and decay as integral to our humanity, and to risk ourselves in this emptiness: the suspension of the relation between human and non-human – the moment of interruption when the subject transfers its powers to the Other.

SECTION IX: BRECHTIAN ALIENATION AND EPIC THEATRE AS AN ANTIDOTE TO THE DECLINE SCRIPT

Both *Soucouyant* and *Half Life* represent an important trend in Canadian fiction that involves deconstructing the narrative of dementia as a singular, Gothic narrative of monstrous decline. To a great extent, *Half Life*'s use of interruption and its emphasis on shards of conversation recall Benajmin's preference for the fragment over familiar, seamless narratives. Recently, theatre scholar and age critic Elinor Fuchs proposed Bertolt Brecht's idea of an "alienated" theatre as an aesthetic model for age studies because it forcibly resists the tragic Aristotelian model of decline. Brecht, a friend and colleague of Benjamin, defined a theatre of "Verfremdung" while the two men were living in Paris in exile from Germany. In keeping with Benjamin's valorization of "detachment," in Brecht's new style of epic theatre "the spectator was no longer in any way allowed to submit to an experience uncritically by means of simple empathy with the characters ... The production put [the subject matter and the incidents] through a process of alienation: the alienation that is necessary to all understanding. When something seems 'the most obvious thing in the world,' it means that any attempt to understand the world has been given up" (*Brecht on Theatre* xxx). As I have shown in the preceding chapters, stepping back and releasing our hold on a singular model of dementia, which seems like "the most obvious thing in the world," may allow us to see what the prevailing Gothic model elided.

Viewed in terms of the trope of irony, specifically the image of the "duck/rabbit," Brecht's mode of epic theatre invites the audience to refrain from tracing the outline of the duck so that they can see the image of the rabbit, which was there all along. In his essay "The Short Organum for the Theatre" of 1948, Brecht elaborated on his notion of the V-effekt and its capacity to interrupt a unified image: "The bourgeois theatre's performances always aim at smoothing over contradictions, at creating false harmony, at idealization … Conditions are reported as if they could not be otherwise; characters are drawn as … incapable by definition of being divided, [as] cast in one block … None of this is like reality, so a realistic theatre must give it up" (*Brecht on Theatre* 277). In keeping with Benjamin's preference for improvisation based on fragments, Brecht's epic theatre likewise championed a process that enabled people to view phenomena from different epistemological perspectives and to tolerate the resultant tensions and ambiguities. This type of theatre represents a powerful alternative to what Fuchs, drawing on Gullette, terms the "Decline Script." Comparing aspects of Aristotelian tragic and Brechtian epic theatrical conventions laid out in a chart, Fuchs observes that the "Epic Theatre side of the chart lifts the heavy hand of fate from the performance of theatre (and by analogy of Aging) along with the heavy emotion that goes with it" ("Rehearsing"). Citing phrases from the chart that describe epic theatre – "'each scene for itself,' human life 'as a process,' the human subject as both 'alterable' and 'able to alter'" – Fuchs observes that they are all "compatible with the greater individualism, variation, and flexibility" ("Rehearsing") associated with critical, humanistic approaches to models of aging and, I would add, of dementia.

SECTION X: AYNSLEY MOORHOUSE'S SOUNDSCAPE OF DEMENTIA

A similar aesthetic process of working with fragments to deconstruct the Gothic script is evident in Aynsley Moorhouse's recent sound art compositions. Moorhouse's sound pieces are both artistically and ethically innovative largely because they abandon text-based and visual representation altogether. The shift from visual to aural representation is historically and politically significant in the case of dementia since, as we have seen, at the beginning of the twentieth century the "feeble-minded," like Charcot's infamous hysterics, were understood through stigmata that were supposedly "seen" and, as a result, rendered iconic via the empirical technology of the photograph (Brave and Slyva 35–6).

In *The Sounds of Forgetting* (2011), Moorhouse creates a soundscape of "a mind suffering from dementia that immerses the listener in a disorienting chaos of memories, thoughts, and experiences" (1). Moorhouse's raw materials were two recordings of jazz standards, approximately four hours of her recorded conversations with her father, Dr John Moorhouse, from October 2009 and December 2010, and two tapes of dictations from his medical practice (1). One of the tapes was the last recording of his career, in which he states that he is "retiring from patient care" (1). The latter was recorded in 2005, when her father was seventy-nine, soon after he began showing signs of dementia. As Moorhouse explains in her prefatory artist's statement, her goal was to create a simulation of her father's mind "while creating a through-line that would represent a movement from a life guided by intellect to one guided by perception" (1). The resulting collage of fragments constitutes a sonic transcoding of Brechtian epic theatre. Moorhouse's initial aim, however, was far more akin to Aristotle's notion of tragedy. As Fuchs explains, for Aristotle, "Tragedy is 'superior to the Epic.' The contest between the two – the tragic, or dramatic, and epic forms – is won on idealist grounds, the overwhelming ideal being Unity. Epic lacks unity. In fact, it could provide the 'subject matter for several tragedies.' It is an additive form, focused on one thing after another. Its near relation to history is a compounding flaw" ("Rehearsing"). Initially, Moorhouse hoped to create a unified work of art, "a memory theater that would preserve her father's cherished memories, highlighted by sound images associated with each memory" (2). In her view, this unrealized and unrealizable project, "would have provided the listener with an aural tour of his mind" (2). Yet, as she explains, circumstances forced her to abandon this initial goal: "I soon discovered, these memories were not available to him on the days of our interviews, and what I got instead was a recording of my father's current experience of the world, with very little reference to the past. I was struck by his readiness to 'live for the moment' and to, for the most part, fatalistically accept the loss of his memory. I

made the decision to explore his new phenomenological way of living" (2). Although many memories were unavailable, in the final section of *The Sounds of Forgetting*, her father begins to sing two songs
that they sang together when she was growing up. As Moorhouse
explains: "He has never forgotten the words or the tunes of songs
he knew in his youth, and if I play a pop song from the 1950s or
1960s, he often has a very visceral reaction to the music, at times
appearing to be almost transported. When asked what he remembers when hearing one of these songs, he says that he feels emotions from the past but cannot recall a particular time or place" (4).
Citing Leonard B. Meyer's view, Moorhouse observes further that
"unlike a closed, non-referential mathematical system, music is said
to communicate emotional and aesthetic meanings as well as purely
intellectual ones" (4). In the case of her own work, Moorhouse suggests that the music in the final section "speaks to my father's emotions and to his body but not to his intellect" (4). At the end of the
piece, her father stops singing, and one of the final sounds is hands
clapping, which for Moorhouse represents a "shift to the primacy
of the body" (4). According to Moorhouse, the sound of her father's hands clapping affirms his agency and connection to the world
around him: "The availability of the 'past and future' is limited, but
my father can receive references to them from the stories of those
around him, as he does in the middle section of my piece, and he
can become connected to other people through universal actions
such as hand clapping, as he does at the end. He becomes an active
part of the world around him and not just a passive observer" (4).
Her insistence on the shift from passivity to activity foregrounds
her father's presence and recalls my earlier discussion of the implications of different models of dementia. As we saw in Munro's "In
Sight of the Lake," which likewise depends on an alternative reading
of dementia, it is possible to shift from the Gothic to an awareness
of multiple and sometimes contradictory narratives.

SECTION XI: "SEND IN THE CLOWNS": ELDER-CLOWNING IN A DEMENTIA UNIT

Moorhouse's relational, arts-based approach, which underscores her
father's agency, shares important features of a study conducted by
Pia Kontos and a team of researchers at the University of Toronto,
which took place from 2012–14 in Ontario. Kontos's study

introduced and evaluated a twelve-week elder-clown program involving twenty-three residents of a locked dementia unit in a long-term care facility (1). Researchers hired four elder-clowns who "had been professionally trained at recognized Canadian clown organizations" (5). The program "consisted of twice weekly clown duo resident visits (approximately 10 minutes per visit)" (5). Their analysis was based on videotaped clown-resident interactions, and elder-clowns' videotaped reflections, and post-intervention interviews.

In her reflections on the program, Kontos observes that Hippocrates (470 BC–350 BC) "was famously claimed to have used troupes of clowns and musicians to enhance healing" (2). While clowns have been used in Canada in children's hospitals, elder-clowns were only recently introduced to engage residents in long-term care settings in the 1990s. To date, however, clown theory has focused almost exclusively on individual clown practitioner strategies and techniques such as humour, empathy, and improvisation, as well as expressive tools including song, dance, and musical instruments. This focus, however, has neglected what the residents may "bring to the interaction, including their own ways of being, provoking and performing" (4).

Kontos explains that clown interactions, known as "play," rely on key elements including "verbal, physical and musical interactions that incorporate fantasy, surprise, inversion, physical comedy and story telling" (3). Citing B. Warren and P. Spitzer, Kontos notes that in the health-care setting, "plays additionally include reminiscence techniques, music and song structures, and ... bedside magic" (3). As one of the elder-clowns explained, "In an ideal clown scenario, you build what's called 'more.' 'More and more,' and you keep going with the play and ideas which can result in humour or incredible emotional states one way or the other [like] sadness, joy, excitement" (8). Another clown, Kate/Zazzi, added that clowns also rely on the improvisation technique of "yes, and" to deepen the connection between themselves and the residents: "There are [clown] principles ... that are ... in line with improv principles, "Yes, and-ing." So if someone makes an offer, you "yes-and" it, so you accept the offer, and you add to it. So when [residents] would say a word, we would delight in it, take it on board, and then repeat it and give [them] back that same thing or add to it, or do something musical to support it" (8). As Kontos states, however, the "fundamental goal of clowning is to achieve a state known as 'presence'" (4). As I noted in the introduction, this notion constitutes a central aspect of the female elegy identified by Zeiger (32). In theatre, however, "presence refers to making spontaneously fictional propositions real and immediate for the spectator, as well as an actor's manipulation of engagement with physical space and the audience to create a heightened 'now' between actors and audience" (Power in Kontos 4). Kontos's emphasis on presence recalls Moorhouse's intimate interaction with her father in *The Sounds of Forgetting* and is in keeping with R. de Grann's view that clown presence is achieved through a "dialogic inter-action." The clown develops a special intimacy with an individual or group audience that "results, ideally, in a mutuality or '*communitas*'" (in ibid.).

The residents who participated in Kontos' study engaged in what researchers term "reciprocal play." After hearing Kontos talk about the program and watching excerpts from the taped interviews, I was struck by the clowns' willingness and ability to enter the often surreal world of dementia. Drawing on the insights of J. Davidson, Kontos explains that clowns "have always played with breaking up reality, and have no problem with existing in both worlds at once: real and pretense" (Davidson in ibid. 11). As Kontos argues, imaginative possibility "is particularly valuable in the context of dementia where boundaries shift between time, place, and person, and become more fluid and less defined and where speech patterns may be slow, broken, or incoherent" (12). From Kontos's detailed notes on the clown-resident interactions, it is evident that the plays provided room for both joy and sadness. Her insights resonate with Margaret Laurence's portrayal of Hagar, specifically her imaginative and emotionally cathartic experience of play in the cannery scene. In the case of Kontos's study, the researchers report that "emotions such as grief and sadness were found to be a central component of the experiences of residents. This stands in contrast to most of the existing research on grief in relation to dementia, which focuses on caregiving spouses, troublingly termed 'crypto-widows' due to the losses of intimacy and companionship that renders them 'married in name but not in fact'" (13). Rather than reproduce a monologic Gothic script, which, as I have argued, has become the standard dementia narrative, Kontos developed a model that – in keeping with Benjamin's emphasis on the fragment – entails weaving a narrative from fleeting interactions. Moreover, instead of relying solely on experts, these constructions constitute "imaginary co-constructions" (14). As Kontos explains and as many of the texts under consideration illustrate, this type of "relational presence is an important corrective to the hierarchical positioning of persons with dementia as passive recipients of services" (15) – uncanny bodies devoid of personhood and relegated to the black hole of the social imaginary.

Both Moorhouse's emphasis on sound as a medium for healing and Kontos's research into the therapeutic and imaginative possibilities associated with elder-clowns recall the similarly musical and playful negotiation between the worlds of fantasy and reality in "Dance of the Happy Shades," which in Munro's fiction likewise entails blurring the boundary between the two. As I observed in relation to "Dance of the Happy Shades," what initially appears as "seemingly fixed, socially sanctioned rhythms of life can and do change; and the ironies or jokes that arise from these changes illuminate the arbitrary and often exclusionary, implicit rules that each generation relies on to determine notions of normalcy and their antithesis" (ch. 9). Like "Dance of the Happy Shades," Moorhouse's and Kontos's aesthetics rely on sound and improvisational techniques to retrieve the humanity of people previously consigned to the land of the dead.

In closing, I want to return briefly to Benjamin's image of the angel of history, whose face is turned toward the past. Having been graced with the companionship of my parents and my husband's parents, all of whom are navigating old age, I can deeply empathize with the desire to make whole what has been smashed. Looking back on the process of writing my book, I am struck by the fact that I spent the past five years sifting through a myriad of stories and speaking to hard-working and compassionate scientists, clinicians, social scientists, artists, students, and caregivers who like me are trying to solve the riddle of Alzheimer's. In the end, however, my book neither resolves the mystery of Alzheimer's nor redeems the painful losses that can attend the experience of late-onset dementia. Instead, I have subjected the prevailing biological model of Alzheimer's disease to what Brecht would term "a process of alienation," so that our tragic view of dementia, which nowadays seems like "the most obvious thing in the world" (xxx), can be seen from an alternative perspective as one narrative approach among others – many of which have been forgotten. Although I do not share Benjamin's paranoid view that progress is the enemy, nevertheless I must admit that the Gothic and the related impulse toward splitting retains its appeal. The Gothic continues to beckon because it offers the consolation of clearly demarcated villains and victims. Ultimately, however, it cannot defend against the understanding furnished by Brecht's V-effekt that there is no cure for the evils of forgetting, decay, and loss – evils that are, paradoxically, integral to our humanity. Rather than enable me to "master" dementia, then, my research has ushered me into a larger community of vulnerability and risk. Perhaps it is fitting that Redekop's insights in *Mothers and Other Clowns* – concerning Munro's short stories – hold true for my experience in writing this book: "False comforts are seen through, but there is no true comfort simply in debunking the false ones. The comfort, rather, comes from our sense of participating in a community that has mutual fears and desires" (237).

Notes

INTRODUCTION

1 Philosopher Ian Hacking observed that fiction rather than medicine is responsible for introducing new disease concepts. Our understanding of pathological memory loss and altered states of consciousness is the direct "consequence of how the literary imagination has formed the language in which we speak of people be they real or imagined" (*Rewriting* 233).

2 As I explain in detail in chapter one, when it was first named, Alzheimer's disease referred to a rare dementing illness that affected people in their fifties. As a result, it did not gain widespread attention.

3 Stephen Post cites Thomas Lewis in "Alzheimer [sic] Disease in a Hypercognitive Society." As early as 1983, Canadian Arthur Dalton, psychologist and president of the Alzheimer Society of Canada, presciently announced that Alzheimer's "will soon be labelled the 'disease of the century'" (Hollobon, "Is the Boat Being Missed," 5).

4 As age critic Margaret Morgonroth Gullette argues, "Our era is like the 1980s in relation to HIV-AIDS, and not only in terms of scientific ignorance, rumors, bad jokes. It's another era of stigmatizing the victims" (*Agewise* 193).

5 The survey results were quoted in Greenberg's "Just Remember This," 10.

6 See, for example, Shenk's bestselling *The Forgetting* and, more recently, Ingram's *The End of Memory*, 35.

7 Recently, the *Toronto Star* published the following table in an article entitled "Dementia: A Private Tragedy Looms as a Public Catastrophe Worldwide" that includes the following table:

DEMENTIA BY THE NUMBERS

7.7 million – approximate new dementia cases every year; about one new case every four seconds.

444 million – the number of hours a Canadian spent caring for a relative with dementia in 2011 representing $11 billion in lost income.

1.4 million – the estimated number of Canadians who will be living with dementia. In twenty years, costing the Canadian economy $3 billion (Cdn.) a year. Left unchecked costs could grow to $293 billion by 2040.

50,000 – the number of Canadians age fifty and younger who had dementia in 2008.

+300% – in Asia the number of dementia cases is expected to triple in the next thirty-five years. In Latin America and Africa cases are expected to quadruple.

604 billion – estimated cost (U.S.) in 2010 for dementia care worldwide. By 2030 that cost will grow to an estimated $1.2 trillion. (Yang)

8 See Ingram chapter 12, "Is The Epidemic Slowing?" (155–66) in which he observes that reports are beginning to emerge suggesting that in "some countries and with certain patient groups Alzheimer's disease or more broadly, dementia is declining" (155). Recently, studies from Britain announced the analyses from three regions in England "showed 25 percent less dementia than had been expected" (Matthews et al.).

9 See Marchione, "U.S. Alzheimer's Rate Seems to Be Dropping," D3.

10 As age critics observe, there is a lack of connection between disability studies and age studies due in part to disability studies' early alliance with "the transformative and liberation politics of the 1960s new left movements" in the 1960s (Chivers "Barrier" 307; see also Neufeldt). These changes affected not only people with disabilities but also the linkages between youth and elderly people coping with disability. As Higgs and Gilleard observe, in the case of disability organizations, the historical alliance with the youth movements of the 1960s "rendered suspect any close alliance with the old" ("Frailty" 482).

11 See Rudy's essay "What Does It Mean to Be Neurotypical?"

12 Personal email 11 Sept. 2015.

13 As Sontag explains, her goal is not "to confer meaning, which is the traditional purpose of literary endeavor, but to deprive something of

meaning to apply that quixotic, highly polemical strategy, 'against interpretation,' to the real world this time. To the body" (*AIDS* 14).

14 See Thane, Cole, Achenbaum, Ballenger, Basting, Gullette, and Whitehouse, to name only a few. Canadian age studies critics who focus on narrative include DeFalco, Chivers, and Charise.

15 In her pioneering essay "Estragement," Fuchs argues that the decline narrative traces its origins to classical theatre: "We, we theater people!, invented peak-and-decline. We (with Aristotle) mapped it in classical plot structure – in reversals, recog, and suffering. We (with Sophocles) memorialized it in the riddle of the Sphinx and her 'three legs at night.' We codified it in Freytag's Pyramid (Freytag, "Dramatic Structure"). And then, after two or so millennia, we scrapped it for the life course structures of Epic Theatre" (72).

16 As Jerrold Hogle explains, the elegy as most writers use it "is descended from a firmly poetic, sometimes ritualistic, Greco-Roman model, linked for centuries to Theocritus, Bion, Moschus, and Virgil at their most 'pastoral'" ("Elegy" 566). It was subsequently turned by early modern English writers from Spenser to Milton, all steeped in such traditions, into an "elaborately worked formal and lyrical poem lamenting the deaths of a friend or public figure" (Kennedy 147). In a highly stylized rural simplicity, the early modern elegy offers "serious reflections on both the figure and death in general, to the point of granting the deceased some sort of 'apotheosis' (elevation to divine status) and the reader some form of salvation or hope, nearly always Christian and usually Protestant" (Hogle "Elegy" 566). Nowadays, readers are likely most familiar with the elegies recited at funerals, which derive from their classical ancestors – funeral songs and poetic laments for the dead.

17 As Canadian age studies scholar Amelia DeFalco argues in *Uncanny Subjects*, the result is that "the field of cultural studies repeatedly overlooks the structuring force of what age critic Kathleen Woodward calls 'gerontophobia' (*Discontents* 193) in western culture" (DeFalco xv).

18 My consultants for the historical facet of my research are Professor Edward Shorter, a social historian of medicine and clinical scientist at the University of Toronto, and Professor David Wright, who is currently Canada Research Chair in the History of Health Policy at McGill. In writing this book, I also worked closely with Professor Wright's student, Renee Saucier – a medical historian – to ensure the accuracy of my work.

19 Drapetomania was "a supposed mental illness described by American physician Samuel A. Cartwright in 1851 that caused black slaves to flee captivity. Today, drapetomania is considered an example of pseudoscience," in keeping with the hysteria diagnosis ("Drapetomania"). I am grateful to Peter Whitehouse for many things, including drawing my attention to this "disorder" (see *Myth* xiii).

20 Alzheimer Society, "Normal Aging."

21 Berrios, "Dementia" (2010), 5.

22 Berrios, "Dementia" (2005), 5.

23 Berrios, "Dementia" (2010), 7.

24 Berrios, "Dementia during the Seventeenth and Eighteenth Centuries," 833.

25 Berrios, "Dementia" (2010), 14.

26 Ibid.

27 Ibid., 7.

28 Ibid., 14.

29 Berrios, *History of Mental Symptoms*, 172, 200.

30 "Alzheimer's Disease," *The Oxford Companion to the Mind*.

31 Hachinski, "Shifts in Thinking about Dementia," 2172–3.

32 "Alzheimer's Disease" in *Black's Medical Dictionary*.

33 Ibid.

34 "Alzheimer's Disease" in *Dorland's Illustrated Medical Dictionary*.

35 Ibid.

36 Lyman, "Bringing the Social Back In," 340–56.

37 Peters and Katz, "Voices from the Field," 285.

38 Ibid.

39 Heinik, "VA Kral," 314.

40 Peters and Katz, "Interview with Dr. Ronald Petersen," 305.

41 See "Canadians Concerned" *Toronto Star*, 19 April 2011, A12.

42 Quotation in Cronk, "Down Syndrome," In *The Cambridge Historical Dictionary of Disease*. See also Wright, *Downs*, 7–9.

43 Ibid.

44 Kwentus, "Alzheimer's Disease" in *The Cambridge Historical Dictionary of Disease*.

45 Alzheimer's Association, "Down Syndrome and Alzheimer's Disease"; "Down's Syndrome" in *Black's Medical Dictionary*; similarly see Kwentus, "Alzheimer's Disease" in *The Cambridge Historical Dictionary of Disease*.

46 "Parkinson's Disease" in *Mosby's Dictionary of Medicine, Nursing & Health Professions.*

47 Alzheimer's Association, "Parkinson's Disease Dementia."

48 Alzheimer's Society UK, "Rarer Causes of Dementia."

49 With respect to the clinical accuracy of the text, throughout the process of conceiving of and writing my book, I have consulted with internationally recognized specialists in geriatrics as well as dementia researchers and clinicians including Dr Sandra Black (director, Hurvitz Brain Sciences Program at Sunnybrook Research Institute), Dr Peter Whitehouse (professor of neurology, Case Western University), Dr Gary Naglie (chief of medicine, Baycrest), Dr David Conn (vice-president, education and director, Centre for Education, Baycrest), Dr Jason Karlawish (professor of medicine, medical ethics and health policy, University of Pennsylvania), Dr Tiffany Chow (senior scientist, Rotman Research Institute, behavioural neurology, Department of Medicine, Baycrest), and Dr Michael Gordon (head of geriatrics and internal medicine, Baycrest).

50 My project does not offer a sustained analysis of nursing care narratives, although they constitute an extremely important genre in their own right, which is the focus of excellent studies by age critics including Ulla Kriebernegg, Patricia Life, and Sally Chivers.

51 See Aldred Neufeldt's "Growth and Evolution of Disability Advocacy in Canada," 11–32.

52 As Wendy Roy asserts, "Canadian fiction has for more than two decades grappled with important literary, theoretical and social questions related to language, selfhood, narration and Alzheimer's disease in a way that challenges if not entirely counteracting often damaging and inaccurate Western popular cultural representations of these subjects" (58). Since my book traces the shift from the elegy to the Gothic, I do not focus on certain well-known examples of dementia narratives including Ethel Wilson's *The Innocent Traveller* (1949), Richard Wright's *Sunset Manor* (1990), Anne Carson's "The Anthropology of Water" in *Plainwater* (1995), Mordecai Richler's *Barney's Version* (1997), Carol Bruneau's *Purple for Sky* (2000), Sandra Sabatini's *The One with the News* (2000), Kyo Maclear's *The Letter Opener* (2007), or Joan Barfoot's *Exit Lines* (2008). Please see the appendix for a more complete list.

53 Whereas the US and Britain became preoccupied with mental illness and the anti-institution movement in the 1960s, in Canada the literary fascination with mental illness was sparked a decade earlier. During

the 1950s, Sheila Watson, the foremother of modernist fiction, was
leading the vanguard by exploring the world of people with mental illness in short stories such as "Brother Oedipus" (1954) and "Antigone"
(1959). Watson herself grew up on the grounds of the Public Hospital
for the Insane in New Westminister, BC, where her father, Dr Charles
Edward Doherty, was superintendent. "I was born and raised inside
the walls of a madhouse," Oedipus explains, in the eponymous story
(Watson, *Five* 63). Watson's compassionate and avant-garde portrayals
of marginalized individuals in her short stories and in her celebrated
novel *The Double Hook* (1959) had a powerful influence on the
next generation of writers. Watson's respectful approach to non-
neurotypical and eccentric individuals is echoed, for example, in novels by Timothy Findley such as *The Last of the Crazy People* (1967),
The Wars (1977), *Headhunter* (1993), and *Pilgrim* (1999).

Throughout the 1960s and 1970s, modern Canadian writers continued to explore the experiences of mental illness and altered states
of consciousness, and they were powerfully affected by the work of
the iconoclastic psychiatrist R.D. Laing, who published the best-seller
The Divided Self: An Existential Study in Sanity and Madness (1960),
when he was twenty-eight years old. Laing went on to spearhead the
anti-asylum movement in Britain. Atwood launched her career by
publishing *The Edible Woman* (1969) and *Surfacing* (1972) to great
acclaim. On the west coast, Audrey Thomas portrayed postpartum
depression and psychosis in novels such as *Mrs Blood* (1970). During
this period, owing to Laing's influence, schizophrenia was popularized by the media. Michael Ondaatje immortalized the life of Buddy
Bolden, the jazz musician with schizophrenia who died in an asylum,
in *Coming through Slaughter* (1976).

54 For example, the penultimate story in her collection *Beggar Maid*,
"Spelling" offers a poignant portrait of age-related dementia through
the eyes of the protagonist, Rose. Once a consummate story teller and
gossip, Rose's step-mother, Flo, becomes delusional and demented,
gradually losing her power to speak; she ends her life in the County
Home, confined to a crib. See DeFalco's discussion of "Spelling" in
Uncanny Aging, 83–7.

55 See Cohen's *No Aging in India*; see also Jacklin et al., "Informal
Dementia Caregiving among Indigenous Communities," 106–20.
See also Jacklin et al., "The Emergence of Dementia," e39–44. See
also Jacklin and Warry "Forgetting and Forgotten," 13–21. See also
Kobayashi and Smith "Making Sense of Alzheimer's Disease," 213–25.

56 Nash, "The New Science of Alzheimer's."

57 For information about the female elegy and women elegists, see
    Zeiger's *Beyond Consolation*.

58 In her recent article concerning legislation about assisted dying in
    the United States, age studies scholar Margaret Morganroth Gullette
    writes:

    > Around the world in the Age of Longevity, apocalyptic demography
    > (Gee & Gutman, 2000) tries to make aging-past-earning seem like
    > an economic crisis. In the United States, political forces combine
    > with opinion-makers to make sick old people seem superfluous.
    > Major media publish articles about expensive dying that should
    > alarm people of any age thinking ahead to whether they too might
    > be considered "burdens" by their adult children or by society or
    > both ... Given the virulent spread of ageism and ableism, any bill
    > "relative to death with dignity" will coincide with pressure to
    > refuse Medicare treatment that might prolong our lives. There is
    > evidence that the public language of "burden" is spreading from
    > Alzheimer's (the "zombie" illness, sometimes called "a living death")
    > to cover Parkinson's, amyotrophic lateral sclerosis (ALS), and other
    > illnesses called "degenerative" or "terminal," as well as cancers –
    > even though people often live for a long time with them, as with
    > Alzheimer's, pursuing their interests and pleasures and being cared
    > for with patience and affection. ("Why" 118–19)

59 Discussing the relationship between elegy and revenge tragedies, Peter
    Sacks invokes Francis Bacon's statement that "Revenge conquers
    Death" (in Sacks 67). In contrast to the work of mourning facilitated
    by the elegy, in the case of revenge tragedies – and, I would add, in
    certain Gothic texts – the individual attempts, instead, to cancel "out
    his sense of violation and passivity" (ibid.). According to Sacks, the
    sufferer refuses elegiac consolation and seeks revenge instead when
    the "need for consolation or redress is obstructed by his loss of faith
    in the power of art's reply"; included in the term art are "the linguistic
    mediations of justice and the law" (64).

60 Edgar Allan Poe is known, for example, as a consummate writer of
    Gothic tales and as the father of the detective novel.

61 Sigmund Freud's distinction between mourning and melancholia
    may be helpful here, as biomedical accounts favour the melancholic
    compulsion to repeat in the hope of mastery. However, as Freud
    observes, the melancholic individual repeats *instead of* remembering.
    In its repeated efforts to cure age-related dementia – the disease of

forgetting – biomedicine forgets (refuses to "remember") that all humans must die.

62 Echoing Dylan Thomas, Ellen Bater entitled her article "Alzheimer's: 'We Will Rage against the Hell of It,'" 9.

63 See Sontag's book on AIDS, which explicitly sets out to retire military metaphors, 11, 94–5; see also Whitehouse and George, "War."

64 As noted earlier, although these stigmata supposedly attest to the presence of "evil," they are also found in the brains of "normal" individuals. Researchers such as George Perry of the University of Texas suggest that the beta-amyloid deposits which form the plaques "may reflect a normal protective response to inflammation," which Perry views as the primary cause of the disease (in Groopman 41). Despite the controversy, contemporary neurologists recently heralded the rediscovery of Alzheimer's perfectly preserved specimens of Auguste D.'s brains with their plaques and tangles.

65 See "Alzheimer's Sleuths Chase Clue Hidden in Protein," A3; see also Taylor, "On the Trail of the Mind Killer," A26.

66 Carol Brayne is professor of public health medicine at the University of Cambridge. She gave the keynote address entitled "The Relationship between Public Health, Population Perspectives, and the Concept of MCI" at Critical Intersections at Trent University on 8 May 2015. She presented current data from studies she conducted that prove MCI is decreasing due to public health initiatives.

67 An article in the *Globe and Mail* published in 1927, for example, is entitled "Improvement in Diet Will Delay Senility," 1. In addition to addressing diet and the need to eat "sufficient vitamins and minerals" (see "Simple Living," *Globe and Mail*, 25 November 1940, 11), prior to the Gothic view of Alzheimer's, experts also focused on "sleep" (see "Growing Senile? Suggest Sleep As Elixir," *Globe and Mail*, 20 May 1957, 15) and acquiring second and third languages in childhood (see "Penfield," *Globe and Mail*, 8 June 1960, 17). Compare these perspectives to contemporary headlines, which again observe that "Developing Alzheimer's Linked to Lifestyle More than Genetics" (André Picard, *Globe and Mail*, 3 September 2004, 12) and pose familiar questions: "Alzheimer's: Should Prevention Rather Than Cure Be the Focus?" (*Vancouver Sun*, 24 November 2011, A14).

68 My research illustrates, for example, that the first reference to dementia in 1947 concerned "dementia praecox," which is now known as schizophrenia. Subsequent references likewise focused on "dementia praecox" until the early 1970s, when the term "dementia" was

invoked for the first time in a discussion of drug trials on elderly people. See "Drug an Aid to Elderly Patients Who Were Vegetables, MD Says" (*Globe and Mail*, 7 January 1971, W3); it is worth noting that six years later, these same drugs were described as "quackery" (*Globe and Mail* 10 October 1977, 25). By contrast the term "senility" appeared more frequently in the nineteenth and first half of the twentieth centuries, but it was used either as an honorific or as a medical term denoting an *inevitable* facet of aging. However, prior to deinstitutionalization, in the early 1960s, psychiatrists began criticizing the term "senility" and "attacked what they said was a tendency to label mental deviations in the aged as senility and too great a readiness to put such persons in mental hospitals" (*Globe and Mail*, 17 May 1963, 13).

69 The dearth of materials, coupled with accounts of cognitive decline found in personal letters by people such as Catharine Parr Traill, suggests that in earlier periods of Canadian history, people adopted alternative frameworks in which to interpret aging and dementia. Put differently, the sporadic literary references to dementia before the 1960s support my research findings that the medical diagnosis of dementia as we now understand it (as applicable to elderly individuals and, by and large, irreversible) was constructed in the late 1970s.

70 Dr Barry Greenberg, director of strategy at the Toronto Dementia Research Alliance, was cited recently in an article where he stated that "Dementia is still getting less than AIDS or cancer, yet ... *the tsunami is coming*, and, if we don't deal with it, our kids will have to" (Greenberg in Sherman "Dementia – a Fight," E1).

71 Currently, age critics such as Gullette are worried that by aligning the baby-boom generation with the "Alzheimer's generation," and by encouraging both the US and Canada to support euthanasia, society is encouraging elderly people with cognitive impairments to commit suicide. She fears that "gerontocide" may become a "more insidiously widespread medical practice" (*Agewise* 31).

CHAPTER ONE

1 A number of valuable scholarly works explore the history and controversial status of the evolution of Alzheimer's as a disease concept, ranging from Cohen's *No Aging in India* (1998), to Ballenger's *Self, Senility, and Alzheimer's Disease in Modern America* (2006), to Lock's *The Alzheimer Conundrum* (2013). Yet these well-researched accounts

have not impacted contemporary discussions, which tend to unequivocally accept the contemporary biomedical model.

2 Germany serves as a key point of departure in my study for several
reasons. First, in the late nineteenth century German clinicians and
researchers were at the forefront of laboratory medicine and pathological anatomy. Their efforts, in turn, signalled a more pervasive shift
away from bedside medicine to the hospital clinic and the laboratory
bench. Second, during this period North American scientists regularly
visited Germany and implemented the new discoveries and approaches
on their return home (see Ackerknecht 170; Duffin 55; and Roelcke
et al. 1–11). Finally, as the fictions considered in my book illustrate,
German and North American members of the international eugenics
movements staged crucial debates concerning the status and fate of
individuals designated as "feeble-minded." These early debates serve
as the foundation for current discussions about the status and fate of
elderly people coping with dementia.

3 As one of the leading psychiatrists who introduced a comprehensive,
usable classification system, Kraepelin is often seen as the "father" of
scientific psychiatry. He endeavoured to place psychiatry on a scientific basis, as a medical science grounded in research and the collection of clinical data. He divided diseases into those with exogenous
and endogenous causes and sought to establish the neuropathological
bases of mental diseases in contrast to Freud's psychological approach.
(See Shorter's *Historical Dictionary of Psychiatry*.)

4 In constructing his theory of hysteria in the 1870s, Charcot concluded
that a series of motor and sensory abnormalities – anaesthesias, hyper-
athesias, paralyses, and contractures – were the most important manifestations of hysteria. Most observers have stressed hyperemotional
behaviours. (See Micale.)

5 Albert Londe's photographic images of hysterics appeared in three
volumes called *Iconographies* (Gilman et al. 352).

6 See Mitchinson's *Body Failure*, ch. 10.

7 For a detailed history and clinical picture of hysteria, see Micale's
Approaching Hysteria: Disease and Its Interpretations (1995).

8 I have chosen to anonymize her name for ethical reasons.

9 According to the dominant biomedical paradigm, the formation
of amyloid plaques and neurofibrillary tangles are believed to contribute to the degradation of the neurons (nerve cells) in the brain
and give rise to the symptoms associated with Alzheimer's disease –
namely, problems with recall. As I argue in this chapter, however, the

association between the organic changes in the brain and the symptoms of memory loss is not clear-cut. I should also add that during the
historical period under consideration, the discovery of plaques and
tangles was predicated on advances in cellular staining techniques,
microscopy, the development of photography, and the increasing reliance on post-mortem diagnosis to demonstrate the organic locus of
disease. Again, as noted earlier, Germany was at the forefront of this
new trend of pathological anatomy and, as a corollary, a new brand of
medicine that was intent on locating the lesion in the brain.

10 As Jay Ingram observes: "Over the course of fifteen to twenty years
after infection, the disease spreads to the brain and results in loss of
tissue in the frontal and temporal lobes and a dementia-like syndrome
called "general paresis," "paralysis of the insane" or "paralytic dementia." Syphilis first appeared in significant numbers after the Napoleonic
Wars and I've seen estimates that suggest it was responsible for at least
half of all cases of so-called insanity throughout the nineteenth and
early twentieth centuries. However, syphilis-induced dementia wasn't
actually distinguished from other dementias until 1874" (41). For
my purposes, it is significant "that syphilis-induced dementia wasn't
actually distinguished from other dementias until 1874" (41). Equally
important, as Ingram maintains: "Syphilis was usually associated with
damage to the blood vessels of the brain; that connection – blood vessels and dementia – held sway long after syphilitic dementia had been
made irrelevant by antibiotics. This persistent belief helped establish
the now mostly outmoded idea that dementia results from 'hardening
of the arteries'" (42).

11 The ongoing fixation on Auguste D.'s brain is strikingly evident in
David Shenk's recent account of the journey of her "brain, brainstem,
and spinal cord" (23). As Shenk explains, her body parts were likely
wrapped in formalin-soaked towels, and packed carefully in a wooden
crate, before being shipped by locomotive 190 miles from Frankfurt
to Munich (23). "Imagine, now," Shenk writes, "that lifeless brain on a
passenger trail. A coconut-sized clump of grooved gelatinous flesh; an
intricate network of prewired and self-adapting mechanisms perfected
over more than a billion years of natural selections; powered by dual
chemical and electrical systems, a machine as vulnerable as it is complex" (23). In this gruesomely objectifying passage, Auguste's brain is
likened both to a fruit fit for consumption and to a machine.

12 In her translation of Perusini's report, Bick translates this as "desolate"
expression (Perusini, "Histology" 83).

13 As Ingram observes, contemporary researchers have determined that
    Auguste suffered from an extremely rare form of early onset demen-
    tia caused by a genetic mutation: "Auguste's brain was subjected to
    genetic analysis and was shown to have a mutation of the gene called
    'presenilin,' which creates a biochemical domino effect resulting
    in early-onset Alzheimer's. Hers was a unique mutation – no other
    human with the same alteration has ever been found" (32).

14 The phrase "moral treatment" came into vogue late in the eighteenth
    century and was used by Vincenzo Chiaguri and Philippe Pinel in their
    respective textbooks. In his 1801 work, Pinel outlined "the general
    precepts to follow in psychological treatment" (*le traitement moral*).
    As Edward Shorter observes: "In the well-founded hope of returning
    to society individuals who seemed lost," Pinel recommended gain-
    ing the confidence of his patients by talking to them and treating
    them fairly, organizing fixed daily schedules of asylum life, involving
    patients in work of various kinds, giving them timely and appetizing
    meals, and other steps directed toward a well-run and orderly mental
    hospital. Given that many of the patients suffered from "a lesion of
    their psychological faculties … a psychological approach rather than
    sheer physical confinement seemed the best way of imposing "ener-
    getic and long-lasting impressions on all of their external senses"
    (see "Pinel" in Shorter's *A Historical Dictionary of Psychiatry*).

15 Sandra Black cited this information in her lecture "Understanding
    Alzheimer's Disease," University of Toronto at Scarborough,
    12 February 2015.

16 As Bick explains: "The close collaboration between Germany's
    vigorous chemical industry and their renowned academic centers was
    responsible for the prominence of German science in the early part
    of the twentieth century. Indeed, Nissl and his friend Alois Alzheimer
    could not have studied the nervous system as they did without the
    aniline dyes synthesized by the German industrial dye chemists"
    (Katzman and Bick 237).

17 As a university student, for example, Alzheimer enjoyed some wild
    adventures: he was left with a dueling scar to the left side of his face
    (Maurer and Maurer 32), and the penal register of 14 Feb. 1887 "con-
    tains evidence that he had the occasional run-in with the law" (34).
    After university, Alzheimer went on "to earn some money by acting
    as a physician cum travel companion. He accepted a post as physi-
    cian to a lady suffering from a mental disorder with whom he traveled
    for five months" (37). Alzheimer's skill as a psychiatrist also played a

role in his initial encounters with his future wife. In the early 1890s, Alzheimer treated "the prosperous merchant Otto Geisenheimer, who was suffering from encephalomalacia, or softening of the brain, a form of progressive paralysis" (48). At that time "it was still unknown that this was a form of late syphilis" (48). Otto was married to a Jewish woman, Cecilie Simonette Nathalie Wallerstein. After Otto died from syphilis in 1892, Alzheimer began courting Cecilie, and they were married in 1894. Cecilie, however, died in 1901 at an early age – she was 41. Although her death was tragic, Alzheimer enjoyed "absolute financial independence as a result of the bequest left to him by his wife" (Finsterwalder in Maurer and Maurer 12). As Alzheimer's grandson, Dr Rupert Finsterwalder, explains, "By waiving his salary from the Clinic of Nervous Diseases at the Munich University and by paying the salaries of the laboratory staff himself, my grandfather no doubt achieved great scientific independence. Only this way was he probably largely able to hold his own against scientific teachings contrary to his own" (in Maurer and Maurer 12). Alzheimer's independence and his position as a senior physician in Frankfurt also enabled him to open an institution in Köppern Taunus. The asylum in Taunus was "conceived of as a treatment centre for alcoholics" (ibid. 67).

18 Although nowadays few people equate schizophrenia with dementia, cognitive decline remains one of its primary outcomes. As another dementing illness, it offers yet another example of the prevalence of dementia in the broader spectrum of human experience, which society would prefer to label and limit to the non-elect or the not-me. Individually and as a society we prefer to imagine ourselves as wholly sane, meaning that we perceive reality accurately (we observe rather than invent or imagine), consistently, and linearly (without gaps, omissions, or episodes of forgetting). This model of "sanity" provides the foundation for Western medicine.

19 Currently, 72 per cent of patients with Alzheimer's disease are women; yet this disproportionately high rate is likely due to several factors. For one, women live longer than men. Secondly, women are over twice as likely as men to suffer from depression, a factor associated with the development of dementia. For more information on women and Alzheimer's, see MacDonald, "A Need for Change."

20 As Eric J. Engstrom argues, "one of the most glaring deficits of laboratory research was its spectacular failure to deliver on promises of a system of disease classification based upon organic etiology" (*Clinical* 127). The lack of diagnostic consensus, numerous ephemeral and

abandoned diagnoses, and dramatic revisions to diagnostic boundaries (as evidenced, for example, by approaches to dementia praecox/schizophrenia) were not restricted to the development of Alzheimer's disease.

21 Kraepelin's coining of the term "senium praecox," in essence, premature senility, recalls the term "dementia praecox," initially used by Arnold Pick in 1891 to describe what we now term schizophrenia.

22 For contemporary information on these persistent and confusing findings, see Ingram's outline of two contemporary studies: "The Nun Study" (1990) and the subsequent "Rush University Medical Center in Chicago Study" (113–23).

23 When Alzheimer presented his paper on Auguste D., two other papers on the subject of psychosomatic symptoms that were read captivated both the crowd's and the local press's attention. As Alzheimer's biographers explain, C.G. Jung was "among those in the auditorium" and the "then nascent discipline of psychoanalysis took the prize instead" (Maurer and Maurer 100).

CHAPTER TWO

1 See Katz "Alarmist Demography."

2 Although the media repeatedly blames seniors for overusing health care services, research suggests that the increasing costs are, in fact, driven by two key elements: the pharmaceutical industry – which has steadily increased the price of drugs and blocked the production of generics – and physicians, who until recently, controlled over 80 per cent of health care costs (Chappell et al. 429–30). Until the 1990s, physicians were not restricted by limits on how much they could earn and on how much they could utilize hospital services. The latter represents the most significant health care cost. In the case of seniors, physicians are even more prone to over-servicing since the medical conditions associated with old age are frequently nonspecific and chronic. While biomedicine cannot offer a cure for most of the ills associated with old age, nevertheless there is always something that a physician can check, increasing the likelihood of over-servicing seniors. To date, physicians remain the gatekeepers to drugs, tests, and appointments with specialists. Increased physician servicing and the cost of drugs have taxed the health care system, but there is no solid "evidence that seniors are better off for it" (Chappell et al. 416).

3 An article by J.V. McAree entitled "Mentally Deficient Still Multiplying," published in 1939, states that "since there appear to be no

immediate need for worrying about the war, suppose we turn our thought to something that is worthy worrying about. We refer to the growth of mental illness and deficiency in our population" (6).

4 In an article entitled "Life Expectancy Rising: Maladies of Elderly Said Major Problem," the anonymous author draws on the findings of Dr A.H. Sellers, director of the Medical Statistics Division of the provincial Health Department of Ontario. Referring to the work of Dr Sellers, the author explains that "the diseases which account for the majority of deaths in the older age groups are chronic or degenerative rather than acute or infectious" (4). He goes on to observe that "concerted efforts to reduce them have been started. He [Sellers] said it is inevitable that in the future the causes of invalidism at older ages will be reduced" (4). In 1943, Josephine Lowman published an article entitled "Why Grow Old: Medical Aid Holds Back Age Onset." As she explains: "Now, for the first time, medicine is turning its energies more toward the questions of longevity, and prolonging the active youthful years of men and women. Already great progress has been made and long vistas of new knowledge are opening up before consecrated scientists. They are learning about vitamins, more about our glandular setup and much more about proper nutrition. They are beginning to understand the psychological factors which enter into health and aging. They now know more about the effects of emotions and thoughts on health and youth" (10). In light of medicine's triumph, Lowman confidently suggests that it is "not inconceivable that senility at 80 may some day seem as unnecessary as it is today at 40. I only hope the scientists work fast in their laboratories so it may come in time for you and me" (10).

5 As I explain in chapter four, its return was coincident with the transformation of Alzheimer's into a single entity. In 1976, neuroscientist and founder of the national Alzheimer's Association in the US Robert Katzman convincingly argued that that presenile dementia (understood to be a rare form of dementia affecting those under sixty-five) and senile dementia (associated with a host of afflictions affecting the elderly) were, in fact, a single disease – Alzheimer's.

6 In 2006, articles warned that the "Baby-Boom Generation Could Be the Alzheimer's Generation" (see also "Alzheimer's Generation," A16).

7 In 1992, Mike Funston of the *Toronto Star* called Alzheimer's a "Ticking Time Bomb" (L6). In the 1990s, terms like "emergency" and other martial metaphors became commonplace in media reports about dementia. In 2009, the *Toronto Star* ran an article by Lauran

Neergaard entitled "Report Sounds Alarm for the Worldwide Alzheimer's 'Emergency'" (21 September 2009, A2). In 2013, David Sherman wrote an article entitled "Dementia: A Fight We Can't Afford to Lose" (12 August 2013, E1). In this article, Sherman refers to Dr Barry Greenberg, director of strategy at the nascent Toronto Dementia Research Alliance, as "the point man in Canada's efforts to deal with a disease the economic fallout of which he believes will topple economies" (E1). Sherman also cites Greenberg's apocalyptic warning that "Dementia is still getting less than AIDS or Cancer" although "the tsunami is coming" (E1). I found only one article, published in 1982, entitled "Is There Any Need to Fear Old Age?" that contradicts the prevailing apocalyptic demography (Angela Dunn, *Globe and Mail*, 11 February 1982, T1).

8 In her study of the elderly poor incarcerated in the Wellington Country House of Industry (1877–1907), Stormie Stewart likewise observes that during this period, "unpalatable relief was considered wise even for the infirm aged since it would prompt individuals to make adequate provision for the old age and families to care for their aged members" (421).

9 Admittedly, the parallel Montigny draws between the 1890s and our own era is not entirely symmetrical, most obviously because in the 1890s the number of elderly people was relatively modest. In addition, the government of Ontario was not wealthy. Equally important, the government's decisions as to where to direct funds was motivated by the perceived acuteness of need rather than ageism, which became increasingly prevalent after the First World War.

10 The discrepancy between the figures, according to Reaume, suggests that "other asylum superintendents did not apply this diagnosis as often as Clarke did when he was at Toronto, even though dementia praecox remained the dominant diagnosis in Ontario's mental hospitals" (17).

11 My deepest thanks to Misao Dean for directing me to this invaluable reference.

12 In a letter to her friend Ellen Dunlop, Catharine offers a detailed account of Susanna's newfound obsession with dolls: "Do you know my dear that my sister who used to rail against dolls and call them hideous idols and find fault with mothers for giving little children dolls to play with has a great wax doll dressed like a baby and this she nurses and caresses – and believes it is her own living babe and cannot bear it out of her sight – puts it to sleep and talks to it and has it

placed in a chair that she may look at it or has it fed and laid to sleep. This is to me the saddest sight for it shews the entire change that has come over her fine intellect. She is a child again in very truth … Some times she gets strange fits of terror about robbers, and is difficult to pacify" (Ballstadt, Hopkins, and Peterman 284–5).

13 After Susanna's death, Catharine wrote to her niece, Annie Atwood, and offered another account of Susanna's confusion:

> On Sunday Easter – there had been a new church bell put up close to Adelaide St and the first tolling of it for church had greatly dis-turbed her poor brain. She exhibited great signs of uneasiness and fancied it was tolling for the execution of some murderer who was to be hanged for cutting off her – your Aunt's [Susanna's] head – for you must know my dear Annie that the poor Aunt's head was all in a deranged state lately she was the victim of all sorts of terrible delusions – The nurse who never leaves her only for a few minutes found her charge out of bed kneeling by a chair praying that this man might not be hung for killing her or she lost her own *identity* at times. (Ballstadt, Hopkins, and Peterman 286)

14 In her letter to Annie Atwood, her niece, Catharine explains that she found consolation for her sister's travails and her death in religion: "The total loss of [Susanna's] … faculties had indeed reconciled us to the final close of her life on earth consoled by the hope that it was the entrance by death of the frail body to a higher state of life where no death has power – for The Lord in whom she believed had overcome the sharpness of death having purchased by His life and sufferings on the Cross, eternal life for all believers" (Ballstadt, Hopkins, and Peterman 286).

15 Historians also note that "a tremendous shift in caring for the indigent elderly" can be discerned if one compares the beginning to the end of the nineteenth century. As Sharon Anne Cook explains, "typical of earlier forms of aid was the 1817 Society for the Relief of Strangers, where the only criterion for receiving aid was poverty" (25). This out-relief fund (the term "out-relief" refers to the fact that they were not housed in an institution) was supported "by subscription from the 'charitable and well-disposed' townspeople of York" and "dispensed without the complication of a residential asylum" (25). By the 1880s, however, "out-relief had been abandoned in favour of housing the indigent in institutions segregated by age, sex, and class" (25). Equally critical, the classification and understanding of inmates was also changing: "no longer viewed as temporarily incapacitated, the elderly

destitute were accepted as a progressively degenerating underclass in society and beyond much improvement" (25).

16 The institution classified those aged fifty-five and over as "elderly" (421).

17 When it opened, thirty people were inmates. Over a thirty-year period beginning in 1877, more than 1,000 admissions were recorded (419). Until 1898, however, children were a significant presence in the poorhouse, accounting for 22 per cent of all admissions (421). Also competing with the elderly for space during the first two decades of the Wellington Country House of Industry's operation were "deserted wives and unwed mothers" (421).

18 As Stewart observes, "mentally or severely physically handicapped young inmates continued to be committed throughout the period … but their numbers were always low. The insane, as opposed to the 'weak-minded,' were not considered fit subjects for the poorhouse and they were committed elsewhere" (433).

19 Theorists have attempted to account for these vast changes in traditional retirement patterns associated with the Industrial Revolution by invoking a range of terms including the "deconceptualization of retirement," "partial retirement," "reverse retirement," "spells of retirement," and "unretirement" (Chappell et al. 320).

20 See the following texts for a critique of apocalyptic demography: National Academy on an Aging Society's *Demography is Not Destiny*; Mulan's *The Imaginary Time Bomb*; and Gee and Gutman, eds, *The Overselling of Population Aging*.

21 As Titmuss wrote:

> Viewed historically, it is difficult to understand why the gradual emergence in Britain of a more balanced age structure should be regarded as a "problem of ageing." What we have to our credit as humanists and good husbanders is a great reduction in premature death since the nineteenth century; as a result, we have derived many benefits from our growing ability to survive through the working span of life. Much of the inefficiency and waste of early death has been eliminated by an increase in the expectation of life at birth of the working classes to a point that now approaches close to that achieved by more prosperous classes … I believe that the present alarm is unjustified; that the demographic changes which are under way and are foreseeable have been exaggerated and that unless saner views prevail harm may be done to the public welfare. (in Thane 349)

22 Admittedly, institutional care "never replaced community and community care" (Bartlett and Wright viii). Although "research has signaled
   a vast history of 'community' or non-institutional care of the insane"
   – and, I would add, the dependent elderly in Canada – it is in the process of being written (ibid. 4). The decision to restrict my investigation
   to the provincial rather than the national level is based on the fact
   that "welfare, poor relief, and institutional care were by the British
   North America Act of 1867 deemed to fall within provincial jurisdic-
   tion" (Montigny, *Foisted* 14). Since each province was responsible for
   providing these services, in what follows I likewise restrict my analysis
   to the provincial level. Equally important, Ontario was the largest
   English-speaking province in Canada by population. Owing to its
   population density, detailed records of asylum practices and scholarly
   analyses of these practices are readily available. In addition to limiting the geographic scope to Ontario, I chose the temporal framework
   of the end of the nineteenth century to the present because the late
   nineteenth century marks the beginning in Canada of government and
   medical responsibility for providing care, protection, and primitive
   therapeutic treatment to people suffering from mental illness.

23 "The medical dissection of the bodies of paupers was common practice" (Stewart 430). Recognizing that it "caused undue misery to
   elderly inmates," the Inspector of the Wellington poorhouse "refused
   to send the bodies of inmates to medical schools in Toronto" contra-
   vening "the wishes of the provincial government" (430).

24 To appreciate the shift from a religious to a modern account of dementia, it is useful to compare Nightingale's description of her mother's
   experience of dementia to Lytton Strachey's account of Nightingale's
   own experience of cognitive decline:

   When old age actually came, something curious happened.
   Destiny, having waited very patiently, played a queer trick on Miss
   Nightingale. The benevolence and public spirit of that long life had
   only been equalled by its acerbity. Her virtue had dwelt in hard-
   ness, and she had poured forth her unstinted usefulness with a bitter
   smile upon her lips. And now the sarcastic years brought the proud
   woman her punishment. She was not to die as she had lived. The
   sting was to be taken out of her; she was to be made soft; she was
   to be reduced to compliance and complacency. The change came
   gradually, but at last it was unmistakable. The terrible commander
   who had driven Sidney Herbert to his death, to whom Mr. Jowett
   had applied the words of Homer, *amoton memaniia* – raging

insatiably – now accepted small compliments with gratitude, and indulged in sentimental friendships with young girls. The author of "Notes on Nursing" – that classical compendium of the besetting sins of the sisterhood, drawn up with the detailed acrimony, the vindictive relish, of a Swift – now spent long hours in composing sympathetic Addresses to Probationers, whom she petted and wept over in turn. And, at the same time, there appeared a corresponding alteration in her physical mood. The thin, angular woman, with her haughty eye and her acrid mouth, had vanished; and in her place was the rounded, bulky form of a fat old lady, smiling all day long. Then something else became visible. The brain which had been steeled at Scutari was indeed, literally, growing soft. Senility – an ever more and more amiable senility – descended. Towards the end, consciousness itself grew lost in a roseate haze, and melted into nothingness. (111–12)

25 One hundred and thirty-one years after Nightingale's mother's death, in 2011 to be precise – after decades of Gothic descriptions of Alzheimer's disease referring to "the agony," "the scourge," "the nightmare," and "the living hell" – the Canadian media began publishing personal accounts that, like Nightingale's, cited positive aspects associated with dementia. Two articles by two different authors were published in the *Globe and Mail* with the same title: "The Unexpected Gifts of Alzheimer's." In the first, Patricia Calder writes of her stern, overbearing father whose dementia "opened his heart" (L8). In the second, published the following year, Robin Leckie explains how receiving a diagnosis forced him "to slow down, to delight in [his] ... family, [and] to be grateful for the beauty around ... [him] (L8).

26 In this passage, Montigny cites Thomas Brown's "Living with God's Afflicted: A History of the Provincial Lunatic Asylum at Toronto, 1838–1911," PhD diss., Queen's University, 1980, 24.

27 Thanks to the efforts of clinicians and researchers such as Martin Roth, scientists and clinicians now distinguish between affective psychosis (manic-depressive moods), senile psychosis (now termed Alzheimer's disease), paraphrenia (late-onset schizophrenia), acute confusion (clouded and delirious states), and multi-infarct or arterio-sclerotic psychosis. Prior to Roth's work in the 1950s, however, these conditions were viewed as a single category; when they were manifested in elderly individuals, for the most part they went untreated.

28 Lehmann was cited later in an article published in the *Globe and Mail* in 1979 entitled "Grade 1 Is Not Too Early to Find Out about Drugs."

The author, Kathleen Rex, draws on Lehmann's expertise to trace the dramatic changes associated with the administration of drugs: "The use of drugs over the past 150 years has progressed form those used to treat pain to bromides for anxiety. Next came the amphetamines in the 1930s and 1940s to alter emotional states. In the 1950s the anti-anxiety drugs were developed to allay stress" (11). Rex goes on to cite Lehmann's view that "in our sick, over-stressed society, we cannot survive without drugs" (11). She explains that back "in the days when most people lived tranquil, rural lives, there was no need for drugs. In this day of pressure and jet lag, it just isn't possible, he [Lehmann] said" (11). Rex includes Lehmann's admission that he couldn't function in his fast-paced profession, if he "didn't take the odd Valium" (11).

29 Had Auguste D. lived in Ontario, she most certainly would have been committed – not because of her cognitive impairment, but because she showed menacing symptoms of jealousy. As Canadian medical historians observe, "pathological jealousy was one of the most dangerous mental symptoms since there was a likelihood that it could lead to the murder of a spouse or another individual" (Warsh 70).

30 The belief that people do not respect their elders as they did in "the past" has itself "a very ancient history" (Thane 39). As Thane argues, in Hesiod's classical characterization of history as a succession of stages of decline from a perfect Golden Age, for example, "he described his own age, the fifth as an Age of Iron, so degenerate that 'men will not pay their parents the due reward for their rearing'" (in ibid.).

CHAPTER THREE

1 As scholars of nineteenth-century print culture appreciate, researching media accounts during this period entails poring over single-spaced print sources and microfiche. To complicate matters further, library holdings of these materials are neither complete nor always legible. For this chapter, my research assistants and I surveyed library holdings of four different newspapers over the following time spans: the *Toronto Telegram* 1860–1900, the *Christian Guardian* 1860–1900, the *Globe* 1844–2015 and the *Daily Mail* 1872–86. We looked at all promising articles but searched for three key terms: dementia, senility, and Alzheimer's. Due to the limited scope of my research (no other publications or magazines were consulted), this chapter in no way

claims to provide an exhaustive account of the media's response to
aging, old age, and dementia.

2 In her email to the group, Dr Andrea Cabajsky admitted that after
undertaking a "mental inventory of the English- and French-Canadian
novels that were published between 1800 and 1914," she could not
"think of any that address age-related dementia." Reflecting on the
dearth of material concerning dementia in this period, Carole Gerson
stated: "I find it interesting that this long list of scholars is coming up
with few examples of age related dementia in early Canadian writing, and those that have been named thus far carry a decidedly gothic
flavour."

3 As Misao Dean explained, the dearth of references was likely due to
the fact that "hale and hearty" older characters were required by the
plots in the fiction of this period. Jody Mason likewise observed that
Adeline Whiteoak in the *Jalna* series (who is one hundred in the first
novel, *Jalna*) does not experience dementia; instead, she is notable for
commanding "a central role in the plot of the series." Intrigued by the
Gothic flavour of the portrayals of dementia, Carole Gerson observed
that in the short stories by English-Canadian writers such as Duncan
Campbell Scott and Susie Francis Harrison, Francophone people
from Quebec are portrayed as insane or demented. Rather than view
these portrayals as instances of dementia, Gerson felt that it was more
appropriate to characterize them as examples of "gothic eccentricity."
On a related note, Jennifer Henderson maintained that the Gothic and
exoticist flavour of nineteenth-century characters who are insane and
aging underscores "the problems with projecting a medical category
back in time." She went on to argue that the decidedly Gothic flavour
of insane/demented characters in Scott's and Harrison's stories might
signal the workings of an alternative "discursive/knowledge" framework in which "the 'otherness' of dementia is interpreted … and constituted very differently."

4 See "Death: Marion Poole," 49.

5 The numbers in table 1 reflect several social changes: first, as noted
earlier, a diagnosis of Alzheimer's disease became widely popular
in the late 1970s, when it was transformed from a rare dementing
"pre-senile" illness affecting people in their 40s and 50s – in contrast
to "senile dementia" affecting people in their 60s – to a single disease entity. Second, deinstitutionalization occurred in the late 1960s,
sending many mentally ill and elderly demented people into the
streets. People were suddenly and literally faced with the challenge of

dementia. Third, the first baby boomers (1946–64) turned sixty-five in 2011; in the late 1980s and 1990s, this cohort began looking after their parents and facing their own status as aging Canadians. Finally, online publications have added tremendous depth to materials available: previously only the *Globe and Mail* was available online from the 1840s. The majority of online databases begin in the late 1970s and early 1980s.

6　According to aging and modernization theory, four interrelated aspects of modernization are central to aging (Chappell et al. 49). One aspect is the development of health technology, which led to improvements in sanitation and nutrition as well as curative and surgical medicine and eventually increased life expectancy (49). A second element is economic modernization, which increased the number of specialized jobs, particularly in cities; typically, young people filled these positions as they were more likely to have the training and were more geographically mobile. This resulted in an inversion of status, with younger people obtaining more lucrative jobs and older people remaining in jobs that tended to become obsolete. The latter created a pressure toward retirement (49). The third, related feature is urbanization, which likewise lowered the status of the aged because, as younger people migrated to urban areas, elderly people became geographically separated from their children and grandchildren, and the former became more peripheral to the family. Finally, increases in education associated with modernization also lowered the status of the aged. Whereas in earlier historical periods, older individuals were viewed as repositories of knowledge, increases in education diminished this role; "during the industrial revolution in Canada, the younger generation gained more knowledge and skills than their parents had" (49).

7　As noted in chapter two, Catherine Parr Traill likewise found solace in religion in the face of her sister Susanna Moodie's dementing illness and death.

8　In 1961, Bruce MacDonald published an article in the same vein in the *Globe and Mail* entitled "Will Senility Kill Canada's Senate? With the Stubbornness of Age, The Upper House Faces Demands to Clear Out Its Deadwood" (29 April 1961, A7).

9　As the author writes: "So whatever may be Mr Ryerson's fitness for a long practiced profession, to commence a new sphere of action at his age, and with the associations that his former calling will ever and anon call up, renders it almost a certainty that his political enterprise will result in but little satisfaction to himself or benefit to his country" (120).

10 In view of the hostility directed at politicians who showed signs of cognitive decline in the nineteenth century, it is worth noting that by the 1990s, Canadian society was seemingly more tolerant of dementia among its leadership. In 1992, for example, the *Globe and Mail* published an article entitled "Alzheimer's Sidelines New Brunswick MP: Maurice Dionne Won't Seek Re-election." As the article explains, when Dionne informed Liberal leader Jean Chrétien, and offered to step down, as Dionne recalls the latter was quite adamant "that he didn't want me to resign." Instead Chrétien "referred Mr Dionne to his brother, a Montreal physician, who put the MP in touch with a specialist conducting research into the disease" (A4).

11 As noted in chapter two, the doctor informed Catharine Parr Traill that her sister Susanna died from "softening of the brain" (288).

12 As noted in the first chapter, the link between blood vessels and dementia was established primarily due to the workings of syphilis (see Ingram 42). Although cardiovascular problems have been linked to Alzheimer's disease, physicians in the past argued convincingly that "cerebral arteriosclerosis was the primary cause of [later-life] dementia" (Lock 37). Both medical professionals and the media recognized that strokes and heart attacks contributed to senility. These historical views are significant for at least two reasons: first, well-respected Alzheimer's researchers including Sandra Black and Mark Smith are probing the links between damage to blood vessels and dementia. Second, the emphasis on blood vessels offers a sharp contrast to the contemporary Gothic approach promoted by the media, which maintains that a single dementing illness is responsible for the impending "tsunami" of demented senior citizens – formerly baby boomers – who will overwhelm the economic resources of the nation-state. Although the contemporary media has fuelled the panic concerning Alzheimer's disease, Statistics Canada confirms that, in keeping with historical opinion, heart disease and cancer remain "the main causes of death for seniors" (Turcotte and Schellenberg 44). Whereas the Gothic approach calls for a consolidated effort to mobilize resources to find a pharmacological cure for a "disease," earlier approaches were, in fact, more compatible with bio-psychosocial approaches that promote healthy aging by addressing risk factors such as diet, exercise, and education.

13 Cole argues that this negative image prevailed because the veneration of aged individuals was "ill-suited" to North American societies,

where individuals were "less and less willing to submerge their identities or constrain their activities within the communal confines of family, church, and town" (56). His views, which reflect the tenacious belief that in the past families were the mainstay of older people, have recently come under fire. Evidence suggests that most elderly individuals were self-sufficient and, equally important, that care between the generations was not one way, but was more often reciprocal (see Thane).

14 Nascher also complained that the elderly were "useless" and "a burden to themselves, their family and to the community at large" (v–vi). Earlier, Thomas Jefferson (1743–1826) had expressed the milder view that the generations should not encroach on each other: "There is a ripeness of time for death, regarding others as well as ourselves, when it is reasonable we should drop off, and make room for another growth. When we have lived our generation out, we should not wish to encroach on another" (in Cole 106–97). Nascher's far more contemptuous comments paved the way for contemporary ageist views. On 29 March 1984, for example, Governor Richard D. Lamm of Colorado stated bluntly that sick, old people had an obligation to "die and get out of the way" (ibid. 169).

15 The shift from rest to activity as a curative process evident in the articles cited above reflects the more general move away from late nineteenth century "rest cures," which were promoted in Europe and North America from 1873–1925 (see Stiles). In light of recent findings that bilingualism protects the brain from dementia, it is also worth noting Penfield's advice that "Children should start learning second and third languages early in the first 10 years of their life" ("Penfield" 17).

16 As the Alzheimer's Association website explains: "The brain changes caused by Parkinson's disease begin in a region that plays a key role in movement. As Parkinson's brain changes gradually spread, they often begin to affect mental functions, including memory and the ability to pay attention, make sound judgments and plan the steps needed to complete a task" ("Parkinson's"). According to the website, Parkinson's disease dementia constitutes "a decline in thinking and reasoning that develops in someone diagnosed with Parkinson's disease at least a year earlier."

The website lists the common symptoms as follows:
- Changes in memory, concentration and judgment
- Trouble interpreting visual information

- Muffled speech
- Visual hallucinations
- Delusions, especially paranoid ideas
- Depression
- Irritability and anxiety
- Sleep disturbances, including excessive daytime drowsiness and rapid eye movement (REM) sleep disorder

The website also states that an "estimated 50 to 80 percent of those with Parkinson's eventually experience dementia as their disease progresses. The average time from onset of Parkinson's to developing dementia is about 10 years." With respect to diagnosis, the website explains that "as with other types of dementia there is no single test – or any combination of tests – that conclusively determines that a person has Parkinson's disease dementia."

17 See Chappell et al., 49–50.

18 Rather than assume, in keeping with the previous generation, that everyone who lived long enough would become ill and bent with years as punishment for Adam's sin, after 1830 Victorians increasingly insisted that everyone could be healthy and self-reliant in old age. This shift occurred for a number of reasons, including the waning influence of religion and growing insight into the material and biological origins of diseases affecting aged individuals (see Chappell et al. 219). Anything short of this ideal was viewed as a sign of individual moral failure. As noted earlier, in the Victorian era "the declining body in old age, a constant reminder of the limits of physical self-control, came to signify dependence, disease, failure and sin" (Cole 91). Yet as Cole observes, the quest for perfect health "saddled many middle-class Americans with feelings of failure and shame in the face of physical decline" (95).

19 Munro's portrayal of her mother's plight recalls my discussion in chapter one of the fate of Auguste D. Following her incarceration in the Frankfurt asylum, Auguste D. became a medical curiosity and was also deemed unintelligible. In keeping with my analysis of Auguste D.'s experience in the asylum, Munro's narrative challenges the traditional Gothic's and elegy's effacement of women's experience by emphasizing the elusive voice of a woman suffering from a dementing illness. In this way, "The Peace of Utrecht" illustrates fiction's capacity to restore a demented woman's effaced subjectivity and thereby render the Gothic monster human, and goes against the grain of science's Gothic tendency to reduce individuals to artifacts.

20 The theory of waste and repair has repercussions that exceed Munro's narrative. Applied retrospectively, it transforms chapter one's account of Auguste D.'s appalling decline and death in the Frankfurt asylum from a simplistic story about the inevitable termination of a disease process into one that also speaks to the more complex ethical failure to recognize a woman's fundamental humanity and to provide the conditions, however modest or limited, to allow for repair or, to borrow Auguste D.'s words, to put herself "in order." It is striking, in this regard, that each time a request was made to transfer Auguste and release her from his hospital, Alzheimer refused it because, as Engstrom observes, Alzheimer was bent on studying Auguste's brain.

21 The mother's experience in hospital recalls Ivan Illich's observation that the depersonalization of diagnosis and therapy has turned malpractice from an ethical problem into a technical problem, where, "within the complex technological medical environment of the hospital, negligence becomes 'random human error' or 'system breakdown'; callousness becomes 'scientific detachment'; and incompetence becomes 'a lack of specialized equipment'" (in Chappell et al. 417).

22 This symbolic gesture echoes both Henry James's *The Golden Bowl* (1904) and Ecclesiastes 12:6–7, which urges the young to turn to God before they, too, grow old and frail: "Or ever the silver cord be loosed, or the golden bowl be broken, or the pitcher be broken at the fountain, or the wheel broken at the cistern. Then shall the dust return to the earth as it was: and the spirit shall return unto God who gave it." For a scholarly analysis of this episode see Redekop, x–xii.

23 The concluding scene also portrays the modern rupture of traditional, Victorian ideals of female domesticity and maternal care that resonated through prior generations, providing a vivid image of waste beyond repair. In the text's final lines, Helen futilely enjoins Maddy to seize her freedom and leave Jubilee, saying, "Take your life, Maddy. Take it" (210). Ironically, Helen's choice of phrase, with its two diametrically opposed meanings, uncannily recalls Aunt Annie's earlier outrage at the prevailing, albeit implicit, view that the elderly, particularly when stricken by illness, should meekly take their lives (acquiesce to their own deaths).

24 Although Munro's story does not foreground the broader political context, both Thane's research on Britain and Canadian historians' analyses of Upper Canada reveal that the Ontario government's policies concerning the dependent elderly, enacted in the late nineteenth century, exacerbated the difficulties families faced in caring for loved

ones suffering from mental illness. As Montigny observes, "family situation played a large role in determining whether an aged person was deemed eligible for asylum treatment" ("Foisted" 820–1). As it turns out, asylum superintendents were far "more willing to accept a person as insane if he or she had no relatives" (ibid. 820). As early as 1860, the unpaid labour of family members was a vital and necessary component of the government's plan to reduce the costs associated with caring for the dependent elderly. In keeping with Thane's observation concerning women's role as caregivers, Montigny likewise points out that in Canada, care "by community" – the foundation of the government's plan – "means that the provision of primary care falls not on the community as a whole but on specific groups and individuals, usually female family members" (ibid. 141).

25 As noted in the introduction, to ensure the clinical accuracy of my book I consulted with internationally recognized specialists in geriatrics as well as dementia researchers and clinicians including Dr Sandra Black (director, Hurvitz Brain Sciences Program at Sunnybrook Research Institute), Dr Peter Whitehouse (professor of neurology, Case Western University), Dr Gary Naglie (chief of medicine, Baycrest), Dr David Conn (vice-president, education and director, Centre for Education, Baycrest), Dr Jason Karlawish (professor of medicine, medical ethics and health policy, University of Pennsylvania), Dr Tiffany Chow (senior scientist, Rotman Research Institute, behavioural neurology, Department of Medicine, Baycrest), and Dr Michael Gordon (head of geriatrics and internal medicine, Baycrest).

Although some readers might view Hagar as suffering from delusions only when she is drunk at Shadow Point, a careful reading of the text offers strong evidence that she is experiencing dementia. The following is a list of her symptoms – in the order of their appearance in the text – that I sent to my team of experts to determine whether I was correct in asserting that she has dementia:

1 Hagar has recently become disinhibited – she finds herself crying when, in the past she prided herself on remaining stoic in the face of emotional and physical pain. She is shocked to find herself crying frequently in public.

2 Hagar forgets events that happened recently. For example, she forgets that her caregiver – her daughter-in-law, Doris – made her tea and that Hagar dumped it down the sink. She remembers neither the tea nor dumping it down the sink.

3 Hagar forgets that she transferred ownership of her home to her son, Marvin. She also made arrangements for her furniture to be dispersed, but cannot remember who will get what.

4 Doris asserts and Hagar admits that Hagar is no longer physically or mentally capable of looking after the house; this is done by her son and her daughter-in-law.

5 Hagar confesses that she finds it increasingly difficult to remain tactful; as noted above, she has become disinhibited and says what comes to mind.

6 Hagar has trouble maintaining focus during conversations. At one point, she thinks she is talking to her children about who owns the house, but finds that, to her shock, the conversation is, in fact, about whether she should move to a nursing home.

7 Hagar has no clear sense of time. In one episode, she sits on a log, lost in thought, and, when night falls, she is shocked to discover that she has been sitting on the same log from morning to evening.

8 She asks Doris if her granddaughter, Tina, will be joining the family for dinner, only to be told that her granddaughter no longer lives with them.

9 Hagar "forgets" months of incontinence at night. She cannot believe it when her daughter-in-law informs her that the latter has been washing her sheets every night for months. "How could I not have noticed," Hagar asks.

10 Hagar does not realize that, at times, she is not thinking, but, in fact, speaking aloud.

11 Doris reports that Hagar frequently forgets agreeing to things such as whether to go on outings. As a result, Hagar is surprised and/or angry when her children take her places in accordance with her forgotten agreement.

12 Hagar is convinced she sees her husband, Bram, when she visits the nursing home, forgetting that Bram has been dead for decades.

13 Hagar is impulsive: upon hearing that her children want to put her in a home, she runs away to an abandoned cannery; when she arrives at her destination, Shadow Point, by bus, she cannot precisely remember why she fled there.

Although Peter Whitehouse cautioned that his insurance does not cover the diagnosis of fictional characters, he and the other physicians whom I consulted on this matter concurred with my reading that she does, indeed, exhibit characteristic signs of dementia; Karlawash felt strongly that her symptoms suggested Alzheimer's disease. I also asked my clinical consultants whether her additional symptoms – which suggest cancer of the stomach and/or liver – complicate the dementia diagnosis. Both Naglie and Conn agreed that this was an important factor that muddled a straightforward diagnosis of dementia; however, Michael Gordon observed that since 35 per cent of people over eighty-five experience dementia, the latter is frequently the background condition for other concurrent illnesses; he explained that he has seen this time and time again on his unit. To conclude, based on my discussions with respected clinicians I maintain with confidence that Hagar is experiencing dementia.

26 The Hebrew name Hagar means "one who flees" or "one who seeks refuge." Genesis 16:1–16 relates how Sarah, Abraham's wife, was unable to bear children, so she sent her Egyptian servant Hagar to Abraham, and they conceived a child. Jealous of her servant, Sarah treated her harshly, and Hagar fled into the wilderness. There, she was found by an angel of the Lord who met her by a fountain of water. The angel commanded Hagar to return to Sarah and assured Hagar that he [the angel] would multiply her seed, and that she would bear the son whom she had recently conceived, and that his name would be Ishmael.

27 For a discussion of the relationship between femininity and weakness in *The Stone Angel*, see Riegel, 25.

28 Contemplating in her mind's eye the stone angel that adorns her mother's grave, the elderly Hagar wonders if "she stands there yet, in memory of her who relinquished her feeble ghost, as I gained my stubborn one" (3). As this assertion demonstrates, Hagar constructs her identity based on the contrast between her mother's supposed feebleness – a term used to describe defective minds and bodies – and her own stubborn vitality, which critics have also termed her "survivorship" (Riegel 11, 23). Hagar also links the stone angel with her father's pride and desire for material gain. As she says, her father bought her mother's angel "in pride to mark her bones and proclaim his dynasty, as he fancied, forever and a day" (3). In *The Stone Angel*, as Hinz and Teunissen argue, "memorial statuary serves to mock rather than satisfy spiritual yearnings by reason of its solidity" (478). In *Look Homeward, Angel* (1929), Thomas Wolfe's American elegy, the stone angel, due to its solidity or reification, is characterized as a "fearful, awful unnatural monster"; by contrast, narrative remembrance is endowed with the capacity to bring the dead back to life (Hinz and Teunissen 479).

29 The request to wear the clothes of the dead and the emphasis on textiles recalls a similar request in Munro's "The Peace of Utrecht." Like Helen, Hagar refuses to don the clothes of her deceased mother. This is not surprising since both women identify themselves in contrast to their mothers as strong, independent, modern women.

30 Throughout *The Stone Angel*, references are made to stillborn children (12) and Hagar repeatedly likens the dying to children, emphasizing her initial trauma and suggesting that she was emotionally dead due to her mother's death in childbirth. When her husband Bram lies dying, for example, in his delirium, he calls out for Hagar. When she goes to his room, Hagar finds him lying "curled up and fragile in the big bed where we'd coupled" (183). As she confesses, "it made me sick to think I'd lain with him, for now he looked like an ancient child" (183). The horrific conflation of birth and death persists when Hagar places her hand on his forehead, and finds "the skin and hair faintly damp, as the children's used to be in the airless, summer nights" (183).

31 The references to moribund births and imprisonment in *The Stone Angel* allude to the epigraph to Thomas Wolfe's novel *Look Homeward, Angel*, which explicitly refers to life as a prison that begins in the womb: "*In her dark womb we did not know our mother's face; from the prison of her flesh we have come into the unspeakable and incommunicable prison of this earth.*" As Wolfe's epigraph clarifies, works by modernist writers share a misogynist view of death-as-mother. It is worth noting in this regard that prior elegists, most notably Walt Whitman, envisioned death as a soothing maternal figure. Whitman's "When Lilacs Last in the Dooryard Bloom'd" (1865) offers a powerful example of this tendency to view death as both female and welcome. This contrast between earlier and later elegiac responses marks a turning away from an acceptance of death to a more modern raging against the dying of the light.

Given *The Stone Angel*'s tendency to reinstall the traditional religious elegiac approach to loss and death, the novel's allusions to Whitman are significant. Hagar reminds readers, for example, that her lilac silk dress is her favourite and that it is "the exact same shade as the lilacs that used to grow beside the gray front porch of the Shipley place [Bram's home]" (29). As she explains, "the lilacs grew with no care given them and in the early summer they hung like bunches of mild mauve grapes from branches with leaves like dark green hearts, and the scent of them was so bold and sweet you could smell nothing else, a seasonal mercy" (29). In Whitman's poem, in addition to the central association between lilacs and death, the narrator learns of the release provided by death in the song entitled "Death Carol" sung by the hermit thrush, whose first stanza beckons Death:

> *Come lovely and soothing Death*
> *Undulate round the world, serenely arriving, arriving,*
> *In the day, in the night, to all, to each,*
> *Sooner or later, delicate Death.* (ll. 135–8)

Later, the thrush sings of "the body gratefully nestling close to thee," portraying death as a loving maternal embrace that brings mother and infant closer (l. 159). Although, to my knowledge, Laurence was not consciously writing in response to Whitman, for the purposes of my argument it is significant that both the sense of release and the image of "nestling" close to the mother are subverted in Laurence's image of the chicks' hideous abandonment at the dump, echoing Hagar's own sense of abandonment at birth. Yet the locus of the dump expands the personal nature of loss since in many of Laurence's Manawaka novels, the dump serves as the site of waste specifically associated with modernity and a new-found materialism that commodifies life itself and, in the process, deems certain lives – on the basis of class, race, and age – valuable, and others, useless or, to borrow a word from the passage cited above, "unsaleable."

32   "Oh, my lost men," she exclaims, "No, I will not think of that. What a disgrace to be seen crying" (6). Equating tears with femininity, childishness, and animality, Hagar disavows those bodily responses and deems them abject: "I perceive the tears, my own they must be although they have sprung so unbidden I feel they are like the incontinent wetness of the infirm" (31). Shortly after this, Hagar feels a stab of pain, a sign of her undiagnosed illness: "I cannot speak, for the pain under my ribs returns now, all of a stab. Lungs, is it? Heart? This pain is hot, hot as August rain or the tears of children" (35). When she hears her own passionate, "torn voice," she does not even recognize it; instead, she assumes that it comes from an animal: "Can it be mine?" she asks. "A series of yelps, like an injured dog" (31).

33   In Milton's famous elegy, "Lycidas," for example, in the speaker's opening statement, the phrase "once more" highlights the repeated gesture of mourning the dead:

> Yet once more, O ye laurels, and once more
> Ye myrtles brown, with ivy never sere,
> I come to pluck your berries harsh and crude,
> And with forc'd fingers rude

Shatter your leaves before the mellowing year.
Bitter constraint and sad occasion dear
Compels me to disturb your season due;
For Lycidas is dead, dead ere his prime[.] (ll. 1–8)

As Riegel observes, in the opening phrase, Milton's elegist "invokes the repetitive nature of elegy, that the process or mourning entered into by the composition of the poem is one that has occurred before and will, presumably, occur again" (144). As Kennedy explains, "death and mourning are too painful to be confronted directly and can only be approached through the words of others, through pre-existent stories ... The story of our grief must always be someone else's first before it can be ours" (15). Kennedy argues further that "the use of pre-existent stories and others' griefs highlights elegy as a self-conscious literary performance" (15). His emphasis on the performa-tive structure of elegy sheds light on the nature of the lesson that Hagar missed when, as a child, she found herself unable to "play the role" of her dead mother; simply put, lacking a compassionate parent, with only an emotionally reserved father as a role model, she never learned the *art* of consolation, which entails responding to another person empathetically, immersing oneself completely in the other's psychodrama, and identifying with the abject. With no opportunity to learn this lesson in the art of necromancy – the art of raising and com-muning with the dead – Hagar remains unable to offer consolation to herself or to others, until she meets Lees at the cannery and sees him perform this ritual on her behalf.

34 After hearing about Murray's loss, Hagar initially dismisses his suf-fering, "He thinks he's discovered pain, like a new drug. I could tell him a thing or two. But when I try to think what it is I'd impart, it's gone. It's only been wind that swelled me for an instant with my accumulated wisdom and burst like a belch" (234). The references to the "wind that swelled" Hagar in this passage allude to Edmund Spenser's portrayal of the giant Orgolio, the personification of pride in *The Faerie Queene* (1590). After he is defeated by the poem's true Christian hero, Prince Arthur, Orgolio, whose name comes from the Italian word for pride, deflates, suggesting that his impressive size was merely due to being puffed up like a balloon full of air. Hagar, whose pride similarly deflates, recognizes that she has nothing to offer Lees.

35 Hagar finds herself in desperate need of consolation because, like most survivors, she feels responsible for the death of her loved ones. In John's case, Hagar feels as if she instigated his death because, on the

night he died, they had an argument. Hagar berated John for engaging
in pre-marital sex with his girlfriend, Arlene, in Hagar's home. That
same night, John fled his mother's house and took Arlene to a dance.
On their way home, on a dare, John drove home on a train trestle.
When their car was struck by an unscheduled train, he and Arlene
died instantly.

36 Margaret Laurence set five of her works in the fictional town of
Manawaka, located in Manitoba. The series consist of *The Stone
Angel, A Jest of God, The Fire Dwellers, A Bird in the House,* and
The Diviners.

CHAPTER FOUR

1 Selye began researching the effects of stress in the 1930s. He developed the stress model, known as the "General Adaption Syndrome,"
in 1936 while working at McGill. From 1946 until the mid-1970s
Selye served as the director of the Institute of Experimental Medicine
and Surgery at the Université de Montréal. During his career he
authored thirty-three books and over 1,600 articles, the majority of
which addressed the workings of stress, which Selye insisted could
be "physical, chemical or psychologic [sic] in nature" (Szabo et al.
474). He is frequently credited with saying: "Every stress leaves an
indelible scar, and the organism pays for its survival by becoming
a little older."

2 Kral is perhaps best known for developing the concept of "benign
senescent forgetfulness" – also known as age-associated memory
impairment – which he distinguished from pathological forms of
dementia (Rae-Grant, *Psychiatry* 11).

3 Research on correlation between stress and Alzheimer's disease persists. In 2013 two articles in the Canadian media focused on the links
between stress and Alzheimer's disease. The first, "Mid-life Stress
Linked to Alzheimer's" by Makiko Kitamura, cites the results of a
Swedish study spanning forty years, which found that stress in middle
age may contribute to the development of Alzheimer's disease later in
life: "Psychological stress was associated with a 21-per-cent-greater
risk of developing Alzheimer's disease, according to a study of
800 Swedish women born between 1914 and 1930 who underwent
neuropsychiatric tests periodically between 1968 and 2005" (E7). The
second article by Laura Donnelly entitled "Psyche May Impact Risks
for Dementia; Women: Link between Anxiety, Alzheimer's," published

in Vancouver, cites a different study that traced a link between "neurotic" women and dementia:

> Women who are jealous, moody and worried in middle age are twice as likely to develop Alzheimer's disease … A study that tracked 800 women over four decades found that those who were scored highly for neuroticism and stress in personality tests were far more likely to be diagnosed with dementia. At the start of the research, participants underwent personality tests that assessed them against a 'neuroticism scale,' scoring them after examining traits such as anxiety, guilt, distress and sociability. The term neuroticism is used to describe those who are easily distressed and display personality traits such as worrying, jealousy or moodiness, and are more likely to express anger, guilt, envy, anxiety or depression. The women had an average age of 46 at the start of the University of Gothenburg study. After 38 years, 19 per cent had developed dementia. Those who scored most highly for neuroticism and reported high levels of stress – in their work, health or family situation – when they were first tested were twice as likely to end up being diagnosed with Alzheimer's as those with low scores, the research found. (B9)

The following year two articles conveyed the findings of a Canadian study performed at Baycrest that showed a clear link between anxiety and Alzheimer's disease. As Adriana Barton reports: "In patients with mild, moderate or severe anxiety, Alzheimer's risk increased by 33 per cent, 78 per cent and 135 per cent, respectively, the researchers found. The Baycrest study, published online in the American Journal of Geriatric Psychiatry, is the first to identify anxiety as a potential risk marker for Alzheimer's disease in adults diagnosed with mild cognitive impairment" (L7). Barton cites Dr Linda Mah, a psychiatrist at the University of Toronto and principal investigator on the study, who "explained that people with anxiety disorders have higher levels of the stress hormone cortisol, which has been shown to damage the hippocampus, a brain structure important for memory processing and emotion" (L7).

4 The Somatikers drew their inspiration, in part, from phrenologists of the late eighteenth century who advanced the "idea of localization of 'faculties' in different parts of the cortex of the human brain" (Lock 48). Phrenology was the first system "to anchor psychological qualities and behavior in localized regions of the cerebral cortex" (Vidal 16). In the second half of the nineteenth century localization theory received

added support from Paul Broca's and Carle Wernicke's experimental and anatomo-clinical research.

5 As the editors of the *The Principles and Practice of Geriatric Psychiatry* explain: "the concept of 'senile or involutional psychoses,' which featured so prominently in Kraepelin's early classification, included presenile delusional insanity, senile dementia, late catatonia, and involutonional melancholia" (Abou-Sale et al. 592)

6 Although lesions in the presenile Alzheimer's disease brain and in senile dementia were similar in their regional distributions, he concluded that "the number of lesions was often greater in presenile cases and the progression of dementia and involvement of language were most severe in the younger cases" (in Katzman and Bick 5).

7 In 1956 Selye published his immensely popular book *The Stress of Life* (New York: McGraw-Hill). Researchers and the Canadian media frequently cited Selye's insights. One of the feature articles in the *Globe and Mail*, an interview with Selye by Zena Cherry published in 1966, summarizes Selye's theory of stress as follows: "At all times, the body strives to maintain equilibrium. In the main, the balancing job is done by the pituitary and the two adrenal glands. Whenever the body is confronted with a challenge, it is the task of these glands to meet it. But if the challenge is continuous, the glands are worked too hard and thrown out of chemical kilter. The apparent cause of illness is often an infection, an intoxication, nervous exhaustion or merely old age. Actually continued stress seems more frequently to be the real cause" (12).

8 Currently, researchers suggest that factors affecting dementia include "neuroticism (especially anxiety) and loneliness" (Ingram 125). As Jay Ingram observes: "Here the picture becomes both clearer and more complex. For instance, emotional neglect and/or parental intimidation and abuse experienced by children are associated with neuroticism: Does that imply that some cases of Alzheimer's disease were triggered by such issues when the individual was less than ten years old? Putting all this research together shows that something about the young brain (maybe even the very young brain) and the individual's experiences may result in unhealthy aging and possible dementia" (125).

9 See "The Homemaker," which insists that "senility seldom occurs in people who have work, companionship and an adequate noon meal" (13).

10 An article by David Spurgeon published in 1962 cites a similar observation by GP, Dr Peter Kinsey: "Some folk in their 80s can be more

alert than those in their 40s and can recover from illness relatively easily ... The desire to recover, the desire to live is important ... Everybody ages at a different rate and they need to be told there is no need to feel old, act old, and look old just because they are over 70" (6).

11 In the 1960s and 1970s the rise of senility was explicitly correlated with the experience of stress of "rejection" and the depression that attends "the losses that occur in aging: Retirement from a job [and] impoverished social life" (Hollobon, "Depression" 11). See also Jo Carson's article "The Elderly Deserve a Better Break from Doctors" in which she observes that "A person often writes himself off" and that there are many illnesses among the elderly triggered by the stress associated with "forced retirement, loss of control over one's life situation, which create frustration, rejection and social dislocation with a sense of isolation" (13).

12 In 1951, an article cited Dr E.W. McHenry, Professor of Health Nutrition at the University of Toronto. McHenry urged the federal government to offer funds geared to the study of health problems of elderly persons. "As it stands now," McHenry explains, "a great deal is known about children, but almost nothing about such questions as why one person begins to show signs of senility at 50 and another at 70" ("Physicians Urge" 2). In 1963, the media featured an article about two Canadian psychiatrists who attacked the tendency to ignore the health problems of elderly individuals. Dr Marvin Miller, psychiatric consultant to Baycrest Hospital criticizes the "senility label," arguing that it is "a wastebasket term used to label any deviation in an older person from former behaviours" ("Senility Label" 13). He maintains that there is "an unfortunate tendency among the public and even among professions treating older persons to view deterioration among the aged as inevitable" (13). Jo Carson likewise insists that "too often there is the tendency to see the aged person's problems and deficits without looking at his assets," and she cites the chief of psychogeriatric services at Queen Street Mental Health Centre, Dr Kingsley Ratnanather's view that "too many old people have been written off with a diagnosis of 'senile dementia.' At the centre we make no such assumption. A patient's illness is regarded as reversible and treatable" (in J. Carson 13).

13 Before they concluded that their hypothesis was incorrect, however, in 1963 McLachlan visited Robert Terry's lab. Terry was too busy to speak with him, so he asked his assistant, Wisniewski, to take McLachlan on a tour. During their discussion, McLachlan asked

Wisniewski how they induced the tangles into the animal model. As Wisniewski explains: I, in my young scientist naïveté, told him everything about the way we did it. He made detailed notes about it. After some time, Terry came to the laboratory, and McLachlan asked him whether he could get the protocol on how to induce the neurofibrillary changes. To my great surprise, Bob [Robert Terry] told him that we were applying for an NIH grant and therefore, at this time, we could not give the recipe. Don [McLachlan] without blinking an eye, said he understood this and that once we got the grant, he would contact us again" (in Katzman and Bick 134). Ingram devotes an entire chapter to the failed aluminum hypothesis – a "lovely example of how a scientific idea can rise – and then fall" (6). As he explains, the aluminum scare in the 1980s and 1990s constitutes a particularly fraught, Canadian contribution to the myriad theories concerning the etiology of Alzheimer's.

14 The connection between Alzheimer's and Down syndrome was not well publicized in the Canadian media; only twelve articles appeared on the topic from 1985–2000.

15 See Black, "On the Trail of the Alzheimer's Gene"; see also Krivel, "U of T Scientist."

16 In the first article detailing the cholinergic hypothesis published in the media, "The Doctor Game: Charting Maze of Alzheimer's," Gifford-Jones writes that "Doctors now believe that Alzheimer's Disease may be due to an imbalance of the transmitter system in the brain. The brain is like a complex electrical circuit, with neurons functioning as wires. Unlike electrical wires, brain neurons are not attached to one another. A gap called a synapse separates them. To pass along a message, a neuron releases a chemical messenger called a neurotransmitter. The chemical stimulates the next neuron and translates the message so it can be passed along. Research indicates that patients with Alzheimer's Disease have a deficiency of neurotransmitters, which manufacture the chemical acetylcholine" (CL.4).

17 See Picard "Developing Alzheimer's Linked to Lifestyle." In addition to citing health risks, the media also emphasized the positive effects of education and bilingualism. They were essentially repeating the findings of studies promoted in the early 1990s, which noted education profoundly cut the risk of Alzheimer's (see Kotulak, "Education Cuts," C3; see also "People with 10 Years," A12). In 1960, as noted earlier, Wilder Penfield advocated acquiring a second language to ward against senility. He argued that children "should start learning a

second and third languages early in the first 10 years of their life ... Three languages were just as easy to learn then as one" ("Penfield Says" 17).

18 In 1972–73 the cost of maintaining a patient in a psychiatric hospital was $7,670, as compared to $4,562.50 in a nursing home and $2,372.50 in a residential home.

19 As Simmons explains, given the composition of the committee, it is not surprising that everything was viewed from a psychiatric perspective and the medical model provided the framework for analysis (91).

CHAPTER FIVE

1 Metonymy is a figure of speech consisting of the use of the name of one thing for that of another of which it is an attribute or with which it is associated (as "crown" in place of a royal person).

2 Although it is Tessa who experiences the deleterious effects of both institutionalization and deinstitutionalization, and is mourned in Ollie's elegiac narrative, by juxtaposing Tessa's fate with that of Nancy "Powers" suggests that during the 1920s and 1930s in rural Ontario towns virtually all women experienced a measure of subjugation and erasure. Formally, the erasure of Nancy's status as a subject and her ensuing silence are encoded in the text via the abrupt termination of her first-person diary entries and the subsequent shift to third person narration in the story's remaining sections. Moreover, Nancy's parting words in her diary indicate that, even as a young woman, she is rapidly losing faith in her belief that she is destined to have an adventurous life. As she writes: "Good-bye Diary at least for the present. I used to have a feeling something really unusual would occur in my life, and it would be important to have recorded everything. Was that just a feeling?" (283). I mention Nancy's experience because structurally "Powers" draws a parallel between the effacement of Nancy's subjectivity and agency within the institution of marriage and Ollie's exploitation of Tessa, as well as her fate within an insane asylum.

3 In light of Rothschild's promotion of detachment, outlined in the previous chapter, it is surprising that throughout his life Wilf is a highly solitary and self-reliant individual, and Nancy is the opposite; nevertheless Wilf is the one who succumbs to dementia.

4 Eleanor Cook helpfully explains that elegists "try to commemorate, and even immortalize the dead. They can't help acknowledging their

survival directly or indirectly"; in her view, Ollie's narrative is "'false elegiac' rather than elegiac. It's a lie."

CHAPTER SIX

1 For more information about this topic, please see DeFalco's *Imagining Care*.

2 In contacting Andrew for information, I was doing what historians do when there are gaps in textual sources. I first met with Andrew on Tuesday, 25 January 2011. Following that, we conversed via email and then met again on Saturday, 25 June 2014 for a final discussion of this chapter. This meeting prompted another email exchange. In my notes, I state the source (both the form and the date) of the information gleaned from Andrew.

3 The material in this section concerning Andrew's religious faith was outlined in an email 22 July 2014.

4 Andrew told me this story when we first met on 25 January 2011, at my request, and he repeated it to me in his email on 17 June 2014.

5 Ibid.

6 Ibid.

7 Andrew wrote this script from the Bible (Luke 2:30–2) in his email of 22 June 2014.

8 Email 26 January, 2011.

9 My contact with Lori Dessau, née Kociol, began on June 2011, when I sent her a description of my project and asked if she would be able to speak with me. I then interviewed her on 8 July 2011 at her office in Hamilton, ON.

10 Now an international organization operating in forty countries and on every continent, L'Arche was launched in 1964 by Jean Vanier, the son of Canadian governor general Georges Vanier and Pauline Vanier. Responding to the deplorable state of local institutions, Vanier invited two men with disabilities to stay in his home in the town of Trosly-Breuil, France (see L'Arche Canada, "Our History").

11 In 1995, Dorothy Lipovenko published an article in the *Globe and Mail* entitled "Alzheimer's a Risk for Down's Adults," which highlights the problems facing people over forty with Down syndrome. As Lipovenko explains: "Today [1995], there are 42,000 Canadians with Down's and, according to the Canadian Down Syndrome Society, life spans began improving 25 years ago, dramatically so in the late 1980s. In 1965, half the children with Down's did not survive past their

fifth birthday. Now, more than half will reach 50" (A1). Lipovenko
cites the view of Barbara Gilchrist, supervisor of Camsell House in
Richmond, BC – a residence for Down's adults with dementia or those
expected to be stricken by it – that because of people with Down's
syndrome's increasing life span, Alzheimer's "is a long-term concern
that we have to deal with ... a big time-concern" (A1).

12 On Lori's suggestion, I contacted Dalton twice in 2011 and 2013, but
each time, he declined to be interviewed; unfortunately, McLachlan
was ill and also unavailable.

13 Bessner is featured in Dorothy Lipovenko's article "Alzheimer
Group Counsels Families with Senile Member" (*Globe and Mail*,
17 January 1981, 17). In her article, Lipovenko also cites McLachlan,
who explains that he was personally "motivated to set up the society because 'there's a tremendous need for public awareness about
Alzheimer's disease and its effect on families ... We want to give support to families by sharing information on how to handle patients
with this condition'" (17).

CHAPTER SEVEN

1 The list of toxic substances said to contribute to the risk of Alzheimer's
includes the following: aluminum, tea, smoking, iron, acid rain, mercury, dental fillings, zinc, power tools (due to electromagnetic fields
– EMFs), microbes, E. coli, salmonella, obesity, meat, power lines, fast
food, algae toxin, defective genes, copper, anxiety, and DDT. Certain
diseases are also cited as possible instigators of Alzheimer's, including
diabetes, small strokes, gum disease, and glaucoma.

2 Potential treatments listed, some of which were studied by researchers, include nicotine, ginseng, ginkgo, anti-inflammatories, estrogen,
testosterone, vitamin B12, vitamin C, vitamin E, vitamin D, melatonin,
wine, green vegetables, nuts, lithium, drugs used for athlete's foot, fish/
fish oil, daffodil root, Gila monster spit, sage, bee propolis, folic acid,
sleep, celery, tofu, caffeine, marijuana, anti-depressants, mustard, curry
powder, magnetic waves, drugs for cholesterol, juice, pond scum, stem
cells, coconut oil, cellphones (good EMFs), deep brain stimulation
(DBS), and insulin spray.

3 This list is based on my survey of Canadian media articles found
on the *Globe and Mail* online database (1840s to 2016) and the
Canadian Newspaper Database from 1970 to 2015.

4 Lederman, "A New Life," R3.

5   Embarked on a spiritual pilgrimage on the Camino de Santiago in
    Galicia, Spain, the narrator recalls the summer her father "began to
    lose his mind" (216). She adopts a familiar medical image to convey
    his transformation: "He was falling away from himself in shreds, the
    inside became visible like bones hanging black and loose in the glare
    of an X ray" (216). Before setting off on her pilgrimage, she visits her
    father. Using a detached, clinical tone, she explains that he "lives in a
    hospital because he has lost the use of some of the parts of his body
    and of his mind" (117). Incorporating scientific terms, she explains
    further that all his life, her father was "a silent man. But dementia has
    released some spring inside him, he babbles constantly, in a language
    neurologists call 'word salad'" (118). Rather than embrace a scientific
    paradigm, the narrator seeks to gain answers from ancient religious
    rituals. As she says, "pilgrims were people in scientific exile" (131).

6   The series of linked stories are told from the point of view of fam-
    ily members, professional carers, and Ambrose, an elderly man with
    Alzheimer's. Toward the conclusion, the third-person narrator unchar-
    acteristically offers a glimpse of a utopian future in which Alzheimer's
    is treatable: "We know that Ambrose has Alzheimer's and after he
    dies we'll find out that it's indeed familial Alzheimer's and after Peggy
    his wife dies, but before Alice his daughter dies, we'll find out, we
    the world at large, that the DNA can be manipulated in utero so that
    the disease becomes marginally treatable" (105).

7   Moore's novel traces the efforts of Noel Burun – a hypermnesic syn-
    aesthete, whose memory is flawless and who sees bursts of colour
    associated with the words people speak – to find a cure for his
    mother's Alzheimer's. Tinkering at home with various combinations of
    pharmaceutical and natural ingredients, Noel and his friends eventu-
    ally discover the cure and restore his mother's health.

8   For example, after Ambrose dies, his daughter Connie dreams of
    witnessing his resurrection: "This is what I want: I want to claim
    Ambrose's body from the authorities. With my tears, these tears I live
    with, I would wash his feet and dry them tenderly with my hair. I want
    to lay him in a vault, roll a stone in front of it, and mourn him daily.
    When some days have passed, I want to take some scented oil from
    the shelf over the bathtub, and visit that vault on a misty, quiet morn-
    ing. I want to be terrified to see the stone rolled back and light blaze
    within the tomb. I want two angels wearing lightning to tell me he is
    risen. I want to be the one with the news" (107). The narrative does
    not end with Connie's dream of religious consolation. Instead it closes

with Peggy's perspective. In the final scene, she contemplates the real-life figure of John Bailey, husband of the late Iris Murdoch, the British writer and philosopher who died from Alzheimer's. Peggy muses, in particular on the "graceless picture" portrayed by John who, at one point, resorted to pulling off Iris's clothing (139). Nevertheless, she admits that John's unflagging and selfless care for Iris constituted a protracted gesture of "stunning grace" (135).

9　This episode in *Scar Tissue* is drawn from Michael's autobiographical essay "August in My Father's House."

10　In an essay entitled "Every Moment of Absent-Mindedness Terrifies Me," which appeared in the *Globe and Mail* on 2 February 2015, a fifty-three-year-old woman named Debbie Hopson poignantly wrote about the impact of learning from an Alzheimer's specialist that her genetic makeup resulted in an 80 per cent chance of her developing the disease. As she confesses: "What I didn't anticipate was that knowing I will probably get the disease would put a burden on me to live the rest of my life as consciously, as fully and as in-the-moment as possible." She goes on to admit that if she had the chance to do things over again, she isn't sure she would want the information.

11　In speaking of this episode, Andrew offered his perspective on this event. He maintained that his mother never ordered him to destroy her work; nor was there a feeling of despair in the act or a sense of covering up her life's work. As he explained: "Alison made light of it, we made it an activity that was fun: I mixed up the colours myself so that they came out as my favourite colour (as an eight year old boy) *caca d'oie* (goose shit). She told me to cover all the partially completed canvasses in exactly the same way, much the same way as I had learned to prime the canvasses and boards with white paint. It was just a job that needed to be done to help Mum with her painting. It wasn't till years later, when I realized that she had never painted again after that moment, that I fully understood what she had got me to do for her, something that she couldn't bring herself to do" ("Message," 17 June 2014).

CHAPTER EIGHT

1　The term "eugenics" was coined by Francis Galton (1882–1911) to denote the science of improving the mental and physical qualities of future generations.

2　The distinguished zoologist Lankester argued for degeneration on the basis of the Darwinian concept of evolution. He suggested that evolutionary trends can lead to degeneration as well as to advance (he cites the loss of limbs in some lizards as an example of degeneration). The corollary of this argument, largely based on animals, was that the same degenerative processes can appear in man.

3 Locating selfhood in touch has been the focus of a great deal of research by social scientists. See for example, Kontos "Embodied Selfhood."

4 These terms are used in William Cullens's *Lectures on the Institutions of Medicine, Part I, Physiology* (London: 1772) in Andrews 94–5. Dementia is a composite term (*de*, down, from; *mens*, mind) as is Amentia (*a*, without; *mens*, mind). Cullen ranked "all forms of mental disablement and distinguished them by 'an imbecility of mental judgment in which men neither perceive, nor remember the relation of things as "Amentia."'" (Jackson 94).

5 Leading the way for later, empirically minded physicians such as Kraepelin and Charcot, Locke's ideas formed an important component of the Enlightenment that swept through Europe during the seventeenth and eighteenth centuries. As Wright explains: "This intellectual movement, at its most fundamental level, proposed new and radical ideas about the relationship between 'man' and his world. Following from Locke, leading thinkers of the Enlightenment affirmed that human experience, rather than clerical authority, was the foundation of human understanding. Those drawn to the central tenets of the Enlightenment believed that the universe was fundamentally rational and knowable, and that its mysteries could be unveiled through observation and experimentation" (32).

6 As Wright observes, Churchill was by no means alone amongst politicians and intellectuals threatened by the social implications of the apparent rise of cognitive impairment. H.G. Wells, who had attended several lectures of Francis Galton, openly advocated the "sterilization of failures" (in Wright 84). George Bernard Shaw, the novelist and playwright, who also lectured occasionally for the Eugenics Education Society, was reported in the *Daily Express* as quipping that "a great many people would have to be put out of existence simply because it wastes other people's time to look after them" (ibid.).

7 As Hannah Zeilig observes:
    The danger of flooding has long been associated with dementia. A 1982 U.K. report was entitled: "The Rising Tide: Developing Services for Mental Illness in Old Age" (Arie & Jolley, 1983). Rising tides continue to inform the language of contemporary politicians

when discussing dementia. Thus, the U.K. Prime Minister (David Cameron) referred to the need for Britain to change its attitude to the "rising tide of people suffering with dementia" (26 May, 2012). The "silent tsunami" of dementia has also been a dominant watery image in many news stories. There are reports of the "slow-moving tsunami" (an oxymoron: tsunamis are not slow moving) and the "wave" of dementia (26 April, 2012). In both cases, there is a sense of an unstoppable force of nature coupled with quiet stealth. Indeed, the silence is particularly sinister suggesting something that we cannot anticipate (insistent references to "the silent epidemic" of Alzheimer's were also noted by Gubrium [1986, 34]). The notion of floods is also curiously biblical. (260)

8 This translation can be found at http://lyricstranslate.com/en/heureuse-happy.html and was consulted on Wed. 28 Jan. 2015.

9 Christian's physical distinctiveness is particularly salient given that the "cause of eugenics was in part propelled by the visual aversion to 'the unfit' giving rise to legal support for segregating them from society, as well as preventing their future propagation" (Brave and Slyva 36).

10 The references to Grace's tongue washing Malcolm's hand recall the biblical figure of Pontius Pilate, who washed his hands to show that he was innocent of the decision to shed Christ's blood (see Matthew 27:24).

CHAPTER NINE

1 See Sedgwick, *The Coherence of Gothic Conventions*.

2 In the narrative, the compassion shown to those with dementia parallels Diana's and Constance's compassion for a young man with AIDS.

3 It is worth noting in regard to the problem of persecution that Rule, an outspoken activist and lesbian, "immigrated to Canada in 1956 because of McCarthyism; gays and lesbians were suspected of being communists; homosexuality was still a criminal offence; intellectual repression was the norm" (Farrant n.p.).

4 The title, "Dance of the Happy Shades," refers to a song from *Orphée et Eurydice* (1762), an opera written by the German composer Christoph Willibald Gluck.

5 My references to both the story's historical and the literary contexts are drawn from Trevor Berrett and Betsy Pelz's discussion from the following website: http://mookseandgripes.com/reviews/2013/04/11/alice-munro-dance-of-the-happy-shades/. 25 March, 2015.

6 As noted in my account of the rise of the Alzheimer Society of Canada in chapter 4, Down syndrome predisposes people coping with this genetic disorder to dementia, a fact that provided a key insight into the genetic basis of early onset Alzheimer's in the late 1970s and early 1980s.

7 In Munro's story "Walking on Water" (1974) for example, the elderly protagonist Mr Lougheed observes how the disjunction between past and present generates ironies and, at times, parodies. Listening to the music played by the younger generation, "he would hear an absolutely clear, and familiar, unmolested line of music. And he knew what would happen, how this would be mocked and twisted around, blown up, blasted out of all recognition. There were similar jokes everywhere" (67). Mr. Lougheed wonders further if he should opt for the defense mechanism adopted by the majority of his generation – forgetting – but he remains too curious about the new world of the younger generation to pretend that life is static and devoid of irony.

8 As Bewell argues, this type of identification was progressive in Wordsworth's day (54); I would argue further that it remained progressive, albeit to a lesser extent in the 1960s when Munro wrote "Dance of the Happy Shades." Nowadays, of course, portraying people with disabilities like Rain Man – "the autistic savant in Armani descending the escalator to win big at Vegas" – is broadly critiqued by disability studies theorists (Riley 84).

9 See Kroetsch, "Unhiding the Hidden."

10 Moses Znaimer, founder of Zoomer Media, defines a Zoomer as follows: "The demographic of active people aged 45 plus; 'Zoomers.' Zoomers; noun. Derived from "'Boomers With Zip!' People age 45 plus who enjoy life to the fullest." See Revie, "A Boomer is a Zoomer."

11 Sarah Powell offered the insights in her seminar presentation "'I Can't Be Sure': Illness and Selfhood in Sarah Polley's *Away from Her*" in my graduate class, ENG 5040, 7 March, 2014.

12 As DeFalco states, "It is Grant who now occupies the role of 'reluctant witness'" (*Uncanny* 79).

13 My reading of the enduring ambiguity of Munro's conclusion recalls Coral Ann Howells's observation that Grant's "not a chance" is "an echo of his old duplicitous reassurances," emphasizing the indeterminacy of the closing scene (77).

14 There are two extant versions; the short story published in *The New Yorker* in 1999 and the final version published in Munro's collection in 2001. There are notable structural differences primarily due to the

additions to the final version. However, none of the changes fundamentally alter the characterization or plot of the original story.

15 In "Reading the Spaces of Age in Alice Munro's 'The Bear Came over the Mountain,'" Sara Jamieson argues that Munro's story also participates in "a gerontological turn that has been gaining momentum since the 1990s toward questioning the assumptions underlying the pervasive perception of the old age home as total institution" (4). As noted earlier, Munro's experience with her mother drove home the personal costs of caring for a family member at home (see Jamieson 14). In "Bear," Fiona chooses residential care and she is wealthy enough to pay the fees; by contrast, Marian has to take Aubrey out of Meadowlake or forfeit her home since she cannot afford to pay for both. As Jamieson astutely argues, by "writing against the idealization of home and community care ... Munro asks readers to recognize the need for residential care options" (14). When a person is ill, "home is not always the best place in which to grow old" (14).

16 For more information on Munro's reliance on comedy and jokes, see Redekop, *Mothers and Other Clowns* and Heble, *The Tumble of Reason*.

17 The description of the surreal flowers recalls the opening of Margaret Atwood's *Alias Grace* (1996), a novel that probes the hysteria diagnosis, and by extension the infamous reference to hysterics as sterile flowers.

18 The concern with being late recalls the implications associated with the lateness of the children from Green Hill in "Dance of the Happy Shades."

19 Nancy's difficulties also echo Antonin Artaud's agonized laments that he cannot "attain" his mind, that he has "lost" his understanding of words and "forgotten" the forms of thought (in Sontag, "Essay" xx).

20 As I note in my essay "Canadian Female Gothic on the Foreign Border: Margaret Atwood's Bodily Harm and Karen Connelly's Burmese Lessons":

In recognition of women writers' early and ongoing investment in the Gothic, Ellen Moers coined the term Female Gothic (1976). For Moers, the Female Gothic represents fears about women's entrapment within domestic spaces and anxieties about childbirth. Ultimately, Moers identifies the Female Gothic as "the mode par excellence that female writers have employed to give voice to women's deep-rooted fears about their own powerlessness and imprisonment within patriarchy" (5). In *The Madwoman in the Attic* (1979),

Sandra Gilbert and Susan Gubar develop the Female Gothic further, and specifically link the concept to female anxieties about authorship, "the split psyche produced by the woman writer's 'quest for self-definition'" (76) – a doubleness vividly illustrated by the Gothic doubling of Jane Eyre and her monstrous 'Other,' the imprisoned first wife Bertha Rochester. (230)

21   The hysteria diagnosis casts its shadow over "In Sight of the Lake" from the moment Nancy sees the flowers bursting from between the flagstones in the dream-like garden and extends to her final panicked realization that she is incarcerated in the nursing home, which triggers a classic example of the "hysterical fit." As the narrator explains, "She opens her mouth to yell but it seems that no yell is forthcoming. She is shaking all over and no matter how she tries she cannot get her breath down into her lungs. It is as if she has a blotter in her throat. Suffocation" (232). The references in this passage to the "blotter" in the throat and to "suffocation" explicitly gesture to the age-old hysteria diagnosis.

As medical historians observe, during the long turn between the nineteenth and twentieth centuries, women were viewed as inherently susceptible to hysteria; the term "hysteria" originates from the Greek word for uterus, "hystera," which derives from the Sanskrit word for stomach or belly. According to the ancient Egyptians, the cause of disturbances in adult women was the wandering movement of the uterus, which they believed to be "an autonomous, free-floating organism, upward from its normal pelvic position" (Micale 19). These ancient Egyptian beliefs, in turn, provided the foundation for classical Greek medical and philosophical accounts of hysteria. The Greeks adopted "the notion of the migratory uterus and embroidered upon the connection ... between hysteria and an unsatisfactory sexual life" (19). In *Timaeus*, Plato famously explains that "the womb is an animal which longs to generate children. When it remains barren too long after puberty, it is distressed and sorely disturbed, and straying about in the body and cutting off the passage of the breath, it impedes respiration and brings the sufferer into the extremist anguish and provokes all manner of diseases besides" (in ibid.). Owing to hysteria's association with choking and loss of air, in the 1600s, it was referred to as "the suffocation of the mother" (ibid. 47).

22   The quotations from Breton are derived from A.S. Kline's 2010 translation. I also cite the paragraph of the Richard Seaver and Helen Lane 1969 translation of *Manifestoes of Surrealism*.

23 This process is reminiscent of challenging the fanciful maps of early cartographers who famously wrote the phrases "Here be Monsters" over swaths of unknown territory.

24 See Kitwood, *Dementia Reconsidered*.

25 Nancy's preference for dreams recalls André Breton's confession about the relationship between his dreams and aging: "I am growing old," Breton confesses, "and more than that reality to which I believe I subject myself, it is perhaps the dream, the difference with which I treat the dream, which makes me grow old" (*Manifestoes* 14). Equally relevant are Sontag's cautionary words to readers approaching the work of Artaud – who was incarcerated in a host of asylums from his adolescence to the end of his life:

> The task of the reader … is not to react with the distance of Rivière [Artaud's psychiatrist] as if madness and sanity could communicate with each other only on sanity's own ground, in the language of reason. The values of sanity are not eternal or "natural," any more than there is a self-evident, common-sense meaning to the condition of being insane [and, I would add, "demented" or "feeble-minded"]. The perception that some people are crazy is part of the history of thought, and madness requires a historical definition. Madness means not making sense – means saying what doesn't have to be taken seriously. But this depends entirely on how a given culture defines sense and seriousness: the definitions have varied widely through history. ("Essay" liv)

CONCLUSION

1 My references to Benjamin in this chapter are drawn from my extensive research on the history of apocalyptic narratives, which culminated in my book *Rewriting Apocalypse in Canadian Fiction* (2005). I am grateful to the anonymous reviewer for pointing out that Mary Russo also refers to Walter Benjamin in her essay "Aging and the Scandal of Anachronism."

2 In light of my book's overarching concern with the shift from religious to medical consolation in the face of decline and death, it is notable that the first use of the word "placebo" dates back to 1225 AD where it referred to the Roman Catholic Church's Vespers for The Office of the Dead (OED). The word's contemporary association with "a drug, medicine, therapy, etc., prescribed more for the psychological benefit to the patient of being given treatment than for any direct

physiological effect" first arose in the Enlightenment period (1725). This shift represents a microcosmic example of the macrocosmic shift from a religious and elegiac tradition to the biomedical and Gothic approach to illness and death.

3 Please see Rankin "The Nocebo Effect."

4 Dr Samir Sinha spoke at the University of Toronto at Scarborough's International Health Film Series and Expo, 12 March 2015.

5 Please see Hebert et al. "Is the Risk of Developing Alzheimer's Disease Greater for Women than for Men?"; see also MacDonald "A Need for Change"; and Gullette "Our Frightened World."

6 I am very grateful to Katherine Schwetz for introducing me to Sedgwick's views on "paranoid reading."

7 See Donnelly "Psyche May Impact Risks for Dementia," A32.

8 As I noted earlier, Sara Jamieson reads Munro's "The Bear Came over the Mountain" biographically, in light of Munro's own family's efforts to care for her mother. According to Jamieson, Munro's story writes "against the idealization of home and community care," and argues for "residential care options" (14). Yet Munro's recent story "In Sight of the Lake" suggests that these facilities must also adopt a person-centred approach.

9 Black, "Understanding Alzheimer's Disease and Vascular Aging."

10 My thanks to Katherine Shwetz for alerting me to the shift to the language of terrorism in descriptions of illness post 9/11.

11 As Ingram explains: "The more goal setting you do and the more determination you have to achieve those goals, the more efficiency, organization, thoroughness, self-discipline and reliability you have, the more you demonstrate conscientiousness, an attribute easily determined by psychological tests. If you score in the ninetieth percentile on such tests, you have an 89 per cent reduced risk of Alzheimer's compared to those who score in the tenth percentile, at least according to an examination of nearly one thousand people over twelve years as part of the Religious Order Study" (146).

12 My thanks go to an anonymous reviewer of my manuscript – Reader A1 – for this eloquent summary of my perspective.

13 Yang, "Dementia."

14 See Beard and Neary, "Making Sense of Nonsense."

15 The basic pattern, however, is perhaps most powerfully articulated in historian Thomas Cole's story of a young Methodist preacher, Thomas Cartwright, publicly boasting about having pushed an 'old lady' down on the streets of Knox County, Kentucky, in the late nineteenth

century (84). Cartwright and his followers scorned the elderly because the former took the biblical metaphor of putting off "the old man" and putting on "the new man" (Eph. 4:22–4) literally. As Cartwright's fellow preacher and leader of the Second Great Awakening, Charles Finney proclaimed "the day of earth's redemption can never come, 'til the traditions of the elders are done away ... These traditions of the elders are the grand sources of most of the fatal errors of the present day" (in Cole 84). As this anecdote indicates, apocalyptic religious discourse was used by citizens of the newly independent United States to inscribe a particular relationship between generations, and to both identify and rid the nascent nation of what it deemed the source of its gravest errors.

16 The sign recalls my discussion of "The Peace of Utrecht" in chapter three. Both Helen's evocative use of the phrase "it was just time" and the references to time in Atwood's "Torching the Dusties" invite readers, as I suggested, "to consider *who* decides when and why the time is up" (134).

17 See my essay "'Their Dark Cells.'"

APPENDIX

Works on Dementia in Canada

Bauer, William. "What Is Interred with Their Bones." *Stories from Fiddlehead Greens: Stories from the Fiddlehead*. Edited by Roger Ploude and Michael Taylor. Ottawa: Oberon Press, 1979.

Hood, Hugh. "The Chess Match." *Stories from Fiddlehead Greens: Stories from the Fiddlehead*. Edited by Roger Ploude and Michael Taylor. Ottawa: Oberon Press, 1979.

Waltner-Toews, David. "A Sunny Day in Canada." *Stories from Fiddlehead Greens: Stories from the Fiddlehead*. Edited by Roger Ploude and Michael Taylor. Ottawa: Oberon Press, 1979.

Valgardson, W.D. "A Business Relationship." *Stories from Fiddlehead Greens: Stories from the Fiddlehead*. Edited by Roger Ploude and Michael Taylor. Ottawa: Oberon Press, 1979.

Elisabeth Vonarburg. *Le Silence de la Cité*. Paris: Denoël, 1981. Translated by Jane Brierley. *The Silent City*. Victoria, BC: Porcepic Books, 1988.

Alford, Edna. *A Sleep Full of Dreams*. Lantzville, BC: Oolichan Books, 1981.

Vanderhaeghe, Guy. "Dancing Bear." *Man Descending: Selected Stories*. Toronto: Macmillan of Canada, 1982.

Philips, Matthew O. "Matthew and Chauncy." *83: Best Canadian Stories*. Edited by David Helwig and Sandra Martin. Ottawa: Oberon Press, 1983.

Choyce, Lesley. "Dancing the Night Away." *Billy Botzweiler's Last Dance and Other Stories*. Toronto: blewointmentpress, 1984.

Gallant, Mavis. "Lena." *84: Best Canadian Stories*. Edited by David Helwig and Sandra Martin. Ottawa: Oberon Press, 1984.

Hailey, Arthur. *Strong Medicine*. Garden City, NY: Doubleday, 1984.

Itani, Frances. "Grandmother." *84: Best Canadian Stories*. Edited by David Helwig and Sandra Martin. Ottawa: Oberon Press, 1984.

Keeling, Nora. "Mine." *84: Best Canadian Stories*. Edited by David Helwig and Sandra Martin. Ottawa: Oberon Press, 1984.

Phillips, Edward O. *Where There's a Will*. Toronto: McClelland and Stewart, 1984.

Simmie, Lois. *Pictures*. Saskatoon: Fifth House, 1984.

Blaise, Clark. *Resident Alien*. Markham, ON: Penguin Books, 1986.

Hospital, Janette Turner. "After the Fall." *Dislocations*. Toronto: McClelland and Stewart, 1986.

Munro, Alice. "Fits." *The Progress of Love: Stories*. Toronto: McClelland and Stewart, 1986.

Thomas, Audrey. "Miss Foote." *Goodbye Harold, Good Luck*. Markham, ON: Viking/Penguin Books Canada, 1986.

Quarrington, Paul. *King Leary*. Toronto, ON: Doubleday Canada, 1987.

Maynard, Fredelle Bruser. *The Tree of Life*. Markham, ON: Viking, 1988.

Reaney, James. *Crazy to Kill: A Detective Opera*. Music by John Beckwith. Guelph, ON: Guelph Spring Festival, 1988.

Schein, Jonah. *Forget-Me-Not*. Toronto: Annick Press, 1988.

Dinniwell, Douglas. "Brunch." *89: Best Canadian Stories*. Edited by David Helwig and Maggie Helwig. Ottawa: Oberon Press, 1989.

Malyon, Carol. "Maude." *Vivid: Stories by 5 Women*. Edited by Beverley Daurio. Stratford, ON: Aya Press/The Mercury Press, 1989.

Rooke, Leon. "Saving the Province." *How I Saved the Province*. Lantzville, BC: Oolichan Press, 1989.

Shields, Carol. "Fuel for the Fire." *The Orange Fish*. Toronto: Random House, 1989.

Vanderhaeghe, Guy. *Homesick*. Toronto: McClelland & Stewart, 1989.

Wright, Richard B. *Sunset Manor*. Toronto: McClelland-Bantam, 1990.

Bushkowsky, Aaron. *Dancing Backwards: A New Two Act Play*. Toronto: Playwrights Canada, 1992.

Olson, Arthur. *The Dying of the Light: Living with Alzheimer's Disease*. Burnstown, ON: General Store Pub. House, 1992.

Carson, Anne. "The Anthology of Water." *Plainwater*. New York: A.A. Knopf, 1995.

Mootoo, Shani. *Cereus Blooms at Night*. Vancouver: Press Gang Publishers, 1996.

Gibson, Margaret. *Opium Dreams*. Toronto: McClelland & Stewart, 1997.

Closer and Closer Apart. Eugene Strickland. Dir. Bob White. Lunch Box Theatre Production, Calgary. October 1999. Performance.

Bruneau, Carol. *Purple for Sky*. Dunvegan, ON: Cormorant Books, 2000.

Sabatini, Sandra. *The One with the News*. Erin, ON: Porcupine's Quill, 2000.

Maclear, Kyo. *The Letter Opener*. Toronto: HarperCollins, 2006.

Barfoot, Joan. *Exit Lines*. Toronto: Alfred A. Knopf Canada, 2008.

Edwards, Caterina. *Finding Rosa: A Mother with Alzheimer's, a Daughter in Search of the Past*. Vancouver: Greystone, 2008.

Lemire, Jeff. *Essex County*. Atlanta: Top Shelf Productions, 2009.

Borrie, Cathie. *The Long Hello: The Other Side of Alzheimer's*. Vancouver: Nightwing Press, 2010.

Leavitt, Sarah. *Tangles: A Story About Alzheimer's, My Mother, and Me*. Calgary: Freehand Books, 2010.

O'Toole, Bet. *Lily's Song*. Toronto: Playwrights Canada, 2011.

DeBruin, Jennifer. *A Walk With Mary*. Renfrew, ON: General Store Pub. House, 2012.

Tremblay, Michel. *L'Oratorio de Noël: pièce en un acte*. Montréal: Leméac, 2012.

Cseke, Col. *Jim Forgetting*. Winnipeg: Scirocco Drama, 2013.

Hepburn, Janet. *Flee, Fly, Flown*. Toronto: Second Story Press, 2013.

Sobol, Julie Macfie, and Ken Sobol. *Love and Forgetting: A Husband and Wife's Journey Through Dementia*. Toronto: Second Story Press, 2013.

Pearson, Tom. *Please Don't Forget Me*. Toronto: Pegasus Books, 2014.

Hooper, Emma. *Etta and Otto and Russell and James*. Toronto: Penguin, 2015.

Remember. Dir. Atom Egoyan. Entertainment One, 2015. Film.

Tu te souviendras de moi. François Archambault. Dir. Fernand Rainville. Théâtre de la Manufacture, Québec City. November 2015. Performance.

Bibliography

Abou-Saleh, Mohammed T., C.L.E. Katona, and Anand Kumar, eds. *Principals and Practices of Geriatric Psychiatry*. 3rd ed. Chichester, West Sussex: Wiley, 2011.

Abrams, M.H. "Apocalypse: Theme and Romantic Variations." In *The Revelation of St John the Divine: Modern Critical Interpretations*, edited by Harold Bloom, 7–33. New York: Chelsea, 1998.

Achenbaum, W. Andrew. *Old Age in the New Land: The American Experience Since 1790*. Baltimore: John Hopkins University Press, 1978.

Ackerknecht, Erwin H. *A Short History of Medicine*. Rev. ed. Baltimore: Johns Hopkins University Press, 1982.

A.D.A.M. Education. "Alzheimer's Disease In-depth Report." *New York Times*, n.d. Accessed 12 December 2016. http://www.nytimes.com/health/guides/disease/alzheimers-disease/print.html.

Adderson, Caroline. *A History of Forgetting*. Toronto: Crean, 1999.

"The Advance of Old Age: The Physical Changes of Advancing Life. How to Attain a Green Old Age and Enjoy It." *St Louis Globe*. Reprinted in *Globe* [Toronto], 13 October 1888.

Agamben, Giorgio. *Homo Sacer: Sovereign Power and Bare Life*. Translated by Daniel Heller-Roazen. Stanford: Stanford University Press, 1998.

"ageism, n." *Oxford English Dictionary*. Oxford University Press. Last modified September 2012. Accessed 23 March 2016.

Alford, C. Fred. *What Evil Means to Us*. Ithaca: Cornell University Press, 1997.

Alzheimer, Alois. "A Characteristic Disease of the Cerebral Cortex." In *The Early Story of Alzheimer's Disease: Translation of the Historical Papers by Alois Alzheimer, Oskar Fischer, Francesco Bonfiglio, Emil Kraepelin,*

Gaetano Perusini, edited by Katherine Bick, Luigi Amaducci, and Giancarlo Pepeu, 1–4. Padova, Italy: Liviana Press, 1987.

"Alzheimer Disease." *Dorland's Illustrated Medical Dictionary*, edited by W.A. Newman Dorland. Philadelphia: Elsevier Health Sciences, 2011.

Alzheimer Society of Canada. "Alzheimer Society Milestones." *Alzheimer Society of Canada*. Last modified 1 August 2014. Accessed 12 December 2016. http://www.alzheimer.ca/en/About-us/Organization-history/Alzheimer-milestones.

– "Highlights of Our Work." *Alzheimer Society of Canada*. Last modified 5 August 2014. Accessed 12 December 2016. http://www.alzheimer.ca/en/About-us/Organization-history/Highlights-of-our-work.

– "Normal Aging vs Dementia." *Alzheimer Society of Canada*. Last modified 27 August 2015. Accessed 12 December 2016. http://www.alzheimer.ca/en/About-dementia/What-is-dementia/Normal-aging-vs-dementia.

– "Vision, Mission and Values." *Alzheimer Society of Canada*. Last modified 26 April 2016. Accessed 12 December 2016. http://www.alzheimer.ca/en/About-us/Vision-and-mission.

Alzheimer's Association. "Down Syndrome and Alzheimer's Disease." *Alzheimer's Association*. Accessed 12 December 2016. http://www.alz.org/dementia/down-syndrome-alzheimers-symptoms.asp.

– "Mild Cognitive Impairment." *Alzheimer's Association*. Accessed 12 December 2016. http://www.alz.org/dementia/mild-cognitive-impairment-mci.asp.

– "Parkinson's Disease Dementia." *Alzheimer's Association*. Accessed 12 December 2016. http://www.alz.org/dementia/parkinsons-disease-symptoms.asp.

"Alzheimer's Disease." In *Black's Medical Dictionary*, edited by Harvey Marcovitch. 42nd ed. London: A & C Black, 2010.

"Alzheimer's Disease." In *The Oxford Companion to the Mind*, edited by Richard L. Gregory. 2nd ed. Oxford: Oxford University Press, 2006.

"Alzheimer's Drugs May Harm People with Mild Memory Issues." *CBC News*. 16 September 2013. Accessed 12 December 2016. http://www.cbc.ca/news/health/alzheimer-s-drugs-may-harm-people-with-mild-memory-issues-1.1855890.

"Alzheimer's Generation." *Ottawa Citizen*, 14 June 2006.

"Alzheimer's: Should Prevention Rather than Cure Be the Focus?" *Vancouver Sun*, 24 November 2011.

"Alzheimer's Sidelines New Brunswick MP: Maurice Dionne Won't Seek Re-election." *Globe and Mail*, 15 May 1992.

"Alzheimer's: Silent Killer?" NBC News. One News Page Ltd. Accessed 12 December 2016. http://www.onenewspage.us/video/20140306/1661346/Alzheimer-Silent-killer.htm.

"Alzheimer's Sleuths Chase Clue Hidden in Protein." Hamilton Spectator, 13 January 1994.

Alzheimer's Society. "Rarer Causes of Dementia." Alzheimer's Society. Last modified March 2015. Accessed 12 December 2016. https://www.alzheimers.org.uk/site/scripts/documents_info.php?documentID=135Andrews, Jonathan. "Begging the Question of Idiocy: The Definition and Socio-Cultural Meaning of Idiocy in Early Modern Britain: Part I." History of Psychiatry 9, no. 33 (1998): 65–95.

Atwood, Margaret. Alias Grace. Toronto: McClelland and Stewart, 1996.

– The Edible Woman. Toronto: McClelland and Stewart, 1969.

– Surfacing. Toronto: McClelland and Stewart, 1972.

– "Torching the Dusties." In Stone Mattress: Nine Tales, 225–68. Toronto: McClelland, 2014.

"Baby-Boom Generation Could Be the Alzheimer's Generation" Guardian [Charlottetown, PEI], 16 June 2006.

Ballenger, Jesse. Self, Senility, and Alzheimer's Disease in Modern America: A History. Baltimore: Johns Hopkins University Press, 2006.

– "Medical Journalism in the War on Alzheimer's." To Conquer Confusion. Last modified 15 June, 2012. Accessed 12 December 2016. https://conquerconfusion.wordpress.com/2012/06/15/medical-journalism-in-the-war-on-alzheimers/.

Ballstadt, Carl, Elizabeth Hopkins, and Michael A. Peterman, eds. I Bless You in My Heart: Selected Correspondence of Catharine Parr Traill. Toronto: University of Toronto Press, 1996.

Barfoot, Joan. Exit Lines. Toronto: Alfred A. Knopf Canada, 2008.

Bartlett, Peter, and David Wright, eds. Outside the Walls of the Asylum: The History of Care in the Community 1750–2000. London: Athlone, 1999.

Barton, Adriana. "Anxiety May Speed Slide into Alzheimer's." Globe and Mail, 14 November 2014.

Basting, Anne Davis. Forget Memory: Creating Better Lives for People with Dementia. Baltimore: Johns Hopkins University Press, 2009.

– "Looking Back from Loss: Views of the Self in Alzheimer's Disease." Journal of Aging Studies 17 (2003): 87–99.

Bater, Ellen. "Alzheimer's: 'We Will Rage against the Hell of It.'" Kingston Whig [Kingston, ON], 17 November 2004.

Baucom, Ian. "The Human Shore: Postcolonial Studies in the Age of Natural Science." Keynote address presented at the annual meeting for the Canadian Association for Commonwealth Literature and Language Studies, University of New Brunswick, Fredericton, 28 May 2011.

Beach, Charles M. "Canada's Aging Workforce: Participation, Productivity, and Living Standards." In *A Festschrift in Honour of David Dodge's Contributions to Public Policy – A 2008 Conference*, 197–218. Ottawa: Bank of Canada, 2008.

Beard, Renée, and Tara M. Neary. "Making Sense of Nonsense: Experiences of Mild Cognitive Impairment." *Sociology of Health & Illness* 35, no. 1 (2013): 130–46.

Behuniak, Susan. "The Living Dead? The Construction of People with Alzheimer's Disease as Zombies." *Ageing and Society* 31, no. 1 (2011): 70–92.

Benjamin, Walter. "Theses on the Philosophy of History." In *Illuminations: Essays and Reflections*, 253–64. Translated by Harry Zohn. New York: Shocken, 1968.

Berrett, Trevor, and Betsy Pelz. "Alice Munro: 'Dance of the Happy Shades.'" *The Mookse and the Gripes*. Last modified 11 April 2013. Accessed 12 December 2016. http://mookseandgripes.com/reviews/2013/04/11/alice-munro-dance-of-the-happy-shades/.

Berrios, G.E. "Alzheimer's Disease: A Conceptual History." *International Journal of Geriatric Psychiatry* 5, no. 6 (1990): 355–65.

– "Dementia: A Historical Overview." In *Dementia*, edited by Alistair Burns, John O'Brien, and David Ames, 3rd ed. 5–17. London: Hodder Arnold, 2005.

– "Dementia: A Historical Overview." In *Dementia*, edited by David Ames, Alistair Burns, and John O'Brien, 5–17. 4th ed. London: Hodder Arnold, 2010.

– "Dementia during the Seventeenth and Eighteenth centuries: A Conceptual History." Psychological Medicine 17.4 (1987): 829–37.

– *History of Mental Symptoms: Descriptive Psychopathology Since the Nineteenth Century*. Cambridge: Cambridge University Press, 1996.

Bewell, Alan. *Wordsworth and the Enlightenment: Nature, Man, and Society in the Experimental Poetry*. New Haven: Yale University Press, 1989.

Bick, Katherine. "Foreword." In *The Early Story of Alzheimer's Disease: Translation of the Historical Papers by Alois Alzheimer, Oskar Fischer, Francesco Bonfiglio, Emil Kraepelin, Gaetano Perusini*, edited by Katherine Bick, Luigi Amaducci, and Giancarlo Pepeu, vii–viii. Padova, Italy: Liviana Press, 1987.

Bick, Katherine, Mary Luigi Amaducci, and Giancarlo Pepeu, eds. *The Early Story of Alzheimer's Disease: Translation of the Historic Papers by Alois Alzheimer, Oskar Fischer, Francesco Bonfiglio, Emil Kraepelin, Gaetano Perusini*. Padova, Italy: Liviana Press, 1987.

Black, Debra. "On the Trail of the Alzheimer's Gene." *Toronto Star*, 14 November 1992.

Black, Sandra. "Understanding Alzheimer's Disease and Vascular Aging: The Way Ahead." Keynote address presented at the New Frontiers Seminar Series, University of Toronto at Scarborough, 12 February 2015.

Blom, Joe Djuwe, and Sam Sussman. *Pioneers of Mental Health and Social Change, 1930–1989*. London: Third Eye, 1989.

Bonfiglio, Francesco. "Concerning Special Findings in a Case of Probably Cerebral Syphilis." In *The Early Story of Alzheimer's Disease: Translation of the Historical Papers by Alois Alzheimer, Oskar Fischer, Francesco Bonfiglio, Emil Kraepelin, Gaetano Perusini*, edited by Katherine Bick, Luigi Amaducci, and Giancarlo Pepeu, 19–31. Padova, Italy: Liviana Press, 1987.

Boswell, Arthur. "The Mayoralty Contest." *Daily Mail* [Toronto], 31 December 1885.

Botting, Fred. *Gothic*. London: Routledge, 1996.

Braak, Heiko, and Eva Braak. "Neurofibrillary Changes: The Hallmark of Alzheimer Disease." In *Concepts of Alzheimer Disease: Biological, Clinical, and Cultural Perspectives*, edited by Peter J. Whitehouse, Konrad Maurer, and Jesse J. Ballenger, 53–71. Baltimore: Johns Hopkins University Press, 2000.

Brave, Ralph, and Kathryn Slyva. "Exhibiting Eugenics: Response and Resistance to a Hidden History." *The Public Historian* 29, no. 3 (2007): 33–51.

Brayne, Carol. "The Relationship between Public Health, Population Perspectives, and the Concept of MCI." Keynote address presented at the Critical Intersections Conference at Trent University, Barrie, Ontario, 8 May 2015.

Brecht, Bertolt. *Brecht on Theatre: The Development of an Aesthetic*. Edited and translated by John Willet. London: Methuen, 1964.

Breton, André. "First Manifesto of Surrealism." Translated by A.S. Kline. *Poets of Modernity*. Accessed 12 December 2016. http://poetsofmodernity.xyz/POMBR/French/Manifesto.htm.

– *Manifestoes of Surrealism*. Translated by Richard Seaver and Helen R. Lane. Ann Arbor: University of Michigan Press, 1969.

Britton, Beth. "G8 Dementia Summit: The Real Work Begins Now." *Guardian*, 18 December 2013. Accessed 12 December 2016.

https://www.theguardian.com/social-care-network/2013/dec/18/
g8-dementia-summit-global-fight-back.

Brown, George. "Dr Ryerson's Last Pamphlet." *Globe* [Toronto], 7 January
1869.

Brown, Theodore M. "Mental Diseases." In *Companion Encyclopedia of
the History of Medicine*, edited by W.F. Bynam and R. Porter, 438–63.
New York: Routledge, 1983.

Bruneau, Carol. *Purple for Sky*. Dunvegan, ON: Cormorant Books, 2000.

Bundesen, Herman. "The Doctor Talks: Memory Loss and Fatigue Hit Old
Folk." *Globe and Mail* [Toronto], 6 March 1943.

– "Simple Living Habits Best Old Age Benefit: The Doctor Talks." *Globe
and Mail* [Toronto], 25 November 1940.

Butler, Judith. *Precarious Life: The Powers of Mourning and Violence*.
London: Verso, 2004.

Butler, Robert N. *The Longevity Revolution: The Benefits and Challenges
of Living a Long Life*. New York: PublicAffairs, 2008.

Butler, Robert N., Mia R. Oberlink, and Mal Schechter, eds. *The Promise
of Productive Aging: from Biology to Social Policy*. New York: Springer,
1990.

Cabajsky, Andrea. "Dementia in Early Canadian Writing." E-mail message
to the author, 8 November 2015.

Calasanti, Toni, and Neal King. "A Feminist Lens on the Third Age:
Refining the Framework." In *Gerontology in the Era of the Third Age:
Implications and Next Steps*, edited by Dawn C. Carr and Kathrin
Komp, 67–85. New York: Springer, 2011.

Calder, Patricia. "The Unexpected Gifts of Alzheimer's." *Globe and Mail*
[Toronto], 20 May 2011.

"Canadians Concerned." *Toronto Star*, 19 April 2011.

Carson, Anne. "The Anthropology of Water." In *Plainwater: Essays and
Poetry*, 119–235. New York: A.A. Knopf, 1995.

Carson, Jo. "The Elderly Deserve a Better Break from Doctors, Psychiatrist
Says." *Globe and Mail* [Toronto], 4 March 1975.

Chappell, Neena, Ellen Gee, Lynn McDonald, and Michael Stones. *Aging
in Contemporary Canada*. Toronto: Prentice Hall, 2003.

Chambers, Lori, and Edgar-André Montigny, eds. *Family Matters: Papers
in Post-Confederation Family History*. Toronto: Canadian Scholars'
Press, 1998.

Chang, Mary Ann. "Let Us Celebrate – ASMT'S 15th Anniversary!"
Alzheimer Alert 12, no. 3 (1996): 1–2.

Charcot, Jean-Martin. *Clinical Lectures on the Diseases of Old Age*.
Translated by L.H. Hunt. New York: Wood, 1881.

Chariandy, David. *Soucouyant*. Vancouver: Arsenal Pulp Press, 2007.

Charise, Andrea. "'Time's Feeble Children': Old Age and the Nineteenth-Century Longevity Narrative, 1793–1901." PhD diss., University of Toronto, 2013.

Cherry, Zena. "After a Fashion: Stress is the Salt of Life for Those Who Learn to Live with It." *Globe and Mail* [Toronto], 1 July 1966.

Chivers, Sally. "Barrier by Barrier: The Canadian Disability Movement and the Fight for Equal Rights." In *Group Politics and Social Movements in Canada*, edited by Miriam Smith, 307–28. Peterborough, ON: Broadview Press, 2008.

– *From Old Woman to Older Women: Contemporary Culture and Women's Narratives*. Columbus: Ohio State University Press, 2003.

– "The Show Must Go On: Aging, Care, and Musical Performance in *Quartet*." *Modern Drama* 59, no. 2 (Summer 2016): 213–30.

– *The Silvering Screen: Old Age and Disability in Cinema*. Toronto: University of Toronto Press, 2011.

Chivers, Sally, and Nicole Markotić, eds. *The Problem Body: Projecting Disability on Film*. Columbus: Ohio State University Press, 2010.

C.M.D. "Ministers of God on the Field of Politics." *Globe* [Toronto], 29 June 1861.

Chamberlain, Edward, and Sander L. Gilman, eds. *Degeneration: The Dark Side of Progress*. New York: Columbia University Press, 1985.

Cohen, Lawrence. "Introduction: Thinking about Dementia." In *Thinking about Dementia: Culture, Loss, and the Anthropology of Senility*, edited by Annette Leibing and Lawrence Cohen, 1–19. New Brunswick: Rutgers, 2006.

– *No Aging in India: Alzheimer's, the Bad Family, and Other Modern Things*. Berkeley: University of California Press, 1998.

Cole, Thomas. *The Journey of Life: A Cultural History of Aging in America*. New York: Cambridge University Press, 1992.

"Comet or Nurse." *Globe* [Toronto], 29 November 1886.

Cook, Eleanor. "'Powers' by Munro." E-mail message to the author, 11 February 2014.

Cook, Sharon Ann. "'A Quiet Place … to Die': Ottawa's First Protestant Old Age Homes for Women and Men." *Ontario History* 81 (1989): 25–40.

Comacchio, Cynthia R. *Nations Are Built of Babies: Saving Ontario's Mothers and Children, 1900–1940*. Montreal: McGill-Queen's University Press, 1993.

Corey, Paul. *Messiahs and Machiavellians: Depicting Evil in the Modern Theatre*. Notre Dame: University of Notre Dame Press, 2008.

"creep, v." *Oxford English Dictionary*. Oxford University Press. Last modified March 2016. Accessed 24 March 2016.

Cronk, Christine E. "Down Syndrome." In *The Cambridge Historical Dictionary of Disease*, edited by Kenneth F. Kiple. Cambridge: Cambridge University Press, 2003.

Cuddon, J.A., ed. *The Penguin Dictionary of Literary Terms and Literary Theory*. 3rd ed. London: Penguin, 1991.

Cumyn, Alan. *Losing It*. Toronto: McClelland, 2001.

D., J. "William Mitford, of Ottawa." *Christian Guardian* [Toronto], 20 January 1869.

Dalton, Arthur J., and Robyn A. Wallace. "What Can We Learn from Study of Alzheimer's Disease in Patients with Down Syndrome for Early-Onset Alzheimer's Disease in the General Population?" *Alzheimer's Research & Therapy* 3, no. 13 (2011). Accessed 12 December 2016. doi: 10.1186/alzrt72.

de Beauvoir, Simone. *Old Age*. Translated by Patrick O'Brian. Harmondsworth: Penguin, 1977.

Dean, Misao. "Dementia in Early Canadian Writing." E-mail message to the author, 9 September 2015.

"Death: Marion Poole." *Globe and Mail* [Toronto], 28 July 1977.

DeFalco, Amelia. "Caretakers/Caregivers: Economies of Affection in Alice Munro." *Twentieth Century Literature* 58, no. 3 (Fall 2012): 377–98.

– *Imagining Care: Responsibility, Dependency, and Canadian Literature*. Toronto: University of Toronto Press, 2016.

– *Uncanny Subjects: Aging in Contemporary Narrative*. Columbus: Ohio State University Press, 2010.

"degeneration, n." *Oxford English Dictionary*. Oxford University Press. Last modified March 2016. Accessed 23 March 2016.

Dessau, Lori. Personal interview, 8 July 2011.

Dillon, Lisa. "Parent-Child Co-residence among the Elderly in 1871 Canada and 1880 United States: A Comparative Study." In *Family Matters: Papers in Post-Confederation Canadian Family History*, edited by Lori Chambers and Edgar-André Montignym, 436–58. Toronto: Canadian Scholars' Press, 1998.

– *The Shady Side of Fifty: Age and Old Age in Late Victorian Canada and the United States*. Montreal: McGill-Queen's University Press, 2008.

Dillman, Rob. "Alzheimer Disease: Epistemological Lessons from History?" In *Concepts of Alzheimer Disease: Biological, Clinical, and*

Cultural Perspectives, edited by Peter J. Whitehouse, Konrad Maurer, and Jesse J. Ballenger, 129–57. Baltimore: Johns Hopkins University Press, 2000.

Donnelly, Laura. "Psyche May Impact Risks for Dementia; Women: Link between Anxiety, Alzheimer's." *The Province* [Vancouver, BC], 3 October 2014.

"Down's Syndrome." In *Black's Medical Dictionary*, edited by Harvey Marcovitch. 42nd ed. London: A & C Black, 2010.

"Dr Benjamin Rush." *Penn Medicine*. The Trustees of the University of Pennsylvania, 2016. Accessed 12 December 2016. http://www.uphs. upenn.edu/paharc/features/brush.html.

"Drapetomania." *Wikipedia*. Last modified 29 November 2016. Accessed 12 December 2016. https://en.wikipedia.org/wiki/Drapetomania.

Duffin, Jacalyn. *History of Medicine: A Scandalously Short Introduction.* Toronto: University of Toronto Press, 2000.

Dunn, Angela Fox. "Is There Any Need to Fear Old Age?" *Globe and Mail* [Toronto], 11 February 1982.

"Elder-Clowning." *Sheridan Centre for Elder Research*. Last modified 22 October 2014. Accessed 12 December 2016. https://serclab. wordpress.com/tag/elder-clowns/.

Ellenberger, Henri E. *The Discovery of the Unconscious: The History and Evolution of Dynamic Psychiatry*. London: Allen Lane, the Penguin Press, 1970.

Engstrom, Eric J. *Clinical Psychiatry in Imperial Germany: A History of Psychiatric Practice*. Ithaca: Cornell University Press, 2003.

– "Research Dementia in Imperial Germany: Alois Alzheimer and the Economies of Psychiatric Practice." *Cult Med Psychiatry* 31 (2007): 405–13.

Esman, Aaron, ed. and introd. *Essential Papers on Transference*. New York: New York University Press, 1990.

Estes, Carol. *The Aging Enterprise*. San Francisco: Jossey-Bass, 1979.

Evans, Robert G., Kimberlyn M. McGrail, Steven G. Morgan, Morris L. Barer, and Clyde Hertzman. "Apocalypse No: Population Aging and the Future of Health Care Systems." *Canadian Journal on Aging* 20, no. 1 (2001): 160–91.

Farrant, M.A.C. "Astounding Discovery, Marvellous Story, A Gift to Us All." Review of *Taking My Life*, by Jane Rule. *Globe and Mail*, 19 August 2011. Last modified 6 September 2012. Accessed 12 December 2016. http://www.theglobeandmail.com/arts/ books-and-media/taking-my-life-by-jane-rule/article592095/.

Faulkner, Joanne. "Negotiating Vulnerability through 'Animal' and 'Child': Agamben and Rancière at the Limit of Being Human." *Angelaki* 16, no. 4 (December 2011): 73–85.

Findley, Timothy. *Headhunter*. Toronto: HarperCollins, 1993.

– *The Last of the Crazy People*. New York: Meredith Press, 1967.

– *Pilgrim*. Toronto: HarperCollins, 1999.

– *The Wars*. Toronto: Clarke, Irwin, 1977.

Fox, Patrick. "The Role of the Concept of Alzheimer's Disease in the Development of the Alzheimer's Association in the United States." In *Concepts of Alzheimer Disease: Biological, Clinical, and Cultural Perspectives*, edited by Peter J. Whitehouse, Konrad Maurer, and Jesse J. Ballenger, 209–33. Baltimore: Johns Hopkins University Press, 2000.

Franzen, Jonathan. "My Father's Brain." *New Yorker*, 10 September 2001.

Freud, Sigmund. *Fragment of an Analysis of a Case of Hysteria ("Dora"). Case Histories I: "Dora" and "Little Hans."* Translated by Alix and James Strachey. London: Penguin, 1990.

– "Mourning and Melancholia." In *On the History of the Psycho-Analytic Movement and Other Works*, edited and translated by James Strachey, with Anna Freud, 237–58. London: Hogarth Press, 1961.

– "An Outline of Psychoanalysis." In *The Standard Edition of the Complete Psychological Works of Sigmund Freud, 1856–1939*. London: Hogarth Press, 1964–1974.

– *Studies in Hysteria*. New York: Nervous and Mental Disease Monographs, 1936.

Frye, Northrop. *The Anatomy of Criticism: Four Essays*. Princeton: Princeton University Press, 1957.

– *The Secular Scripture: A Study of the Structure of Romance*. Cambridge, MA: Harvard University Press, 1976.

Fuchs, Elinor. "Estragement: Toward an 'Age Theory' Theatre Criticism." *Performance Research* 19, no. 3 (2014): 69–77.

– "Rehearsing Age." Keynote address presented at the Playing Age Conference at the University of Toronto, Toronto, Ontario, 27–28 February 2015.

Funston, Mike. "Ticking Time Bomb; Canada Must Prepare Now for Inevitable Wave of Alzheimer's Patients, Experts Warn." *Toronto Star*, 16 January 2009.

"G8 Leaders Urge Governments to Band Together against Alzheimer's and Dementia." *CBS News*. Last modified 11 December 2013. Accessed 12 December 2016. http://www.cbsnews.com/news/g8-leaders-urge-governments-band-together-against-alzheimers-dementia/.

Garraty, John A., and Mark C. Carnes. "Dix, Dorothea Lynde." In *American National Biography*. New York: Oxford University Press, 1999.

Gee, Ellen M., and Gloria M. Gutman, eds. *The Overselling of Population Aging: Apocalyptic Demography, Intergenerational Challenges, and Social Policy*. Don Mills, ON: Oxford University Press, 2000.

Gerson, Carole. "Dementia in Early Canadian Writing." E-mail message to the author, 8 September 2015.

Gifford-Jones, W. "The Doctor Game: Charting Maze of Alzheimer's." *Globe and Mail* [Toronto], 2 February 1984.

Gilman, Charlotte Perkins. "The Yellow Wallpaper." In *The Charlotte Perkins Gilman Reader*, edited by Ann J. Lane, 3–20. London: University of Virginia Press, 1999.

Gilman, Sander L., Helen King, Roy Porter, G.S. Rousseau, and Elaine Showalter. *Hysteria Beyond Freud*. Berkeley: University of California Press, 1993.

Goddu, Teresa. *Gothic America: Narrative, History and the Nation*. New York: Columbia University Press, 1997.

Goffman, Erving. *Stigma: Notes on the Management of a Spoiled Identity*. Englewood Cliffs: Prentice-Hall, 1963.

Goldberg, Ann. *Sex, Religion, and the Making of Modern Madness: The Eberbach Asylum and German Society, 1815–1849*. New York: Oxford University Press, 1999.

Goldman, David L. "Dorothea Dix and Her Two Missions of Mercy in Nova Scotia." *The Canadian Journal of Psychiatry* 35, no. 2 (1990): 139–43.

Goldman, Marlene. "Canadian Female Gothic on the Foreign Border: Margaret Atwood's Bodily Harm and Karen Connelly's Burmese Lessons." *University of Toronto Quarterly* 82, no. 2 (2013): 225–41.

– *Dispossession: Haunting in Canadian Fiction*. Montreal and Kingston: McGill-Queen's University Press, 2012.

– "Purging the World of the Whore and the Horror: Gothic and Apocalyptic Portrayals of Dementia in Canadian Fiction." In *Popularizing Dementia: Public Expressions and Representations of Forgetfulness*, edited by Aagje Swinnen and Mark Schweda, 69–88. Bielefeld: Bielefeld University, 2015.

– *Rewriting Apocalypse in Canadian Fiction*. Montreal and Kingston: McGill-Queen's University Press, 2005.

– "'Their Dark Cells': Transference, Memory, and Postmemory in John Mighton's *Half Life*." In *Canadian Literature and Cultural Memory*, edited by Cynthia Sugars and Elinor Ty, 118–33. Toronto: Oxford University Press, 2014.

Goodey, C.F. "John Locke's Idiots in the Natural History of Mind." *History of Psychiatry* 5 (1994): 215–50.

Greenberg, Michael. "Just Remember This." Review of *Can't Remember What I Forgot: The Good News from the Front Lines of Memory Research*, by Sue Halpern. *New York Review of Books*, 4 December 2008. Accessed 12 December 2016. http://www.nybooks.com/articles/2008/12/04/just-remember-this/.

Groopman, Jerome. "Before Night Falls: A New Direction in Alzheimer's Research." *New Yorker*, 24 June 2013.

"Growing Senile? Suggest Sleep As Elixir." *Globe and Mail* [Toronto], 20 May 1957.

Gubrium, Jaber. "Narrative Practice and the Inner Worlds of Alzheimer Disease Experience." In *Concepts of Alzheimer Disease: Biological, Clinical, and Cultural Perspectives*, edited by Peter J. Whitehouse, Konrad Maurer, and Jesse J. Ballenger, 181–204. Baltimore: Johns Hopkins University Press, 2000.

Gullette, Margaret Morganroth. *Aged by Culture*. Chicago: University of Chicago Press, 2004.

– *Agewise: Fighting the New Ageism in America*. Chicago and London: University of Chicago Press, 2011.

– "Our Frightened World: Caregiving Fantasies in the Era of the New Longevity: Suicide and Euthanasia." Keynote Address presented at the Playing Age Conference at the University of Toronto, Toronto, Ontario, 27–28 February 2015.

– (Gullette, Margaret.) "Politics, Pathology, Suicide and Social Fates: Tony Kushner's *The Intelligent Homosexual's Guide to Capitalism and Socialism with a Key to the Scriptures*." *Modern Drama* 59, no. 2 (Summer 2016): 231–48.

– "Why I Hesitated about 'An Act Relative to Death with Dignity' and Then Voted for It." *Feminism & Psychology* 25, no. 1 (2015): 118–23.

Hachinski, Vladimir. "Shifts in Thinking about Dementia." *JAMA* 300, no. 18 (12 Nov. 2008): 2172–3.

Hacking, Ian. "Memory Sciences, Memory Politics." In *Tense Past: Cultural Essays in Trauma and Memory*, edited by P. Antze and M. Lambek, 67–87. London: Routledge, 1996.

"half-life, n." *Oxford English Dictionary*. Oxford University Press. Last modified March 2016. Accessed 24 March 2016.

Harris, Ruth. *Murders and Madness: Medicine, Law, and Society in the Fin de Siècle*. New York: Oxford University Press, 1989.

Hazam, Haim. *From First Principles: An Experiment in Ageing*. Westport, CT: Bergin & Garvey, 1996.

Hebert, Liesi E., Paul A. Scherr, Judith J. McCann, Laurel A. Beckett, and Denis A. Evans. "Is the Risk of Developing Alzheimer's Disease Greater for Women than for Men?" *American Journal of Epidemiology* 153, no. 2 (2001): 132–6.

"He Has No Policy." *Globe* [Toronto], 3 September 1886.

Heble, Ajay. *The Tumble of Reason: Alice Munro's Discourse of Absence*. Toronto: University of Toronto Press, 1994.

Heinik, Jeremia. "VA Kral, the Montreal Hebrew Old People's Home, and Benign Senescent Forgetfulness." *History of Psychiatry* 17, no. 3 (2006): 313–32.

Henderson, Jennifer. "Dementia in Early Canadian Writing." E-mail message to the author, 9 September 2015.

Higgs, Paul, and Chris Gilleard. "Aging, Abjection and Embodiment in the Fourth Age." *JAS* 25 (2011): 135–42.

– "Aging without Agency: Theorizing the Fourth Age." *Aging and Mental Health* 14, no. 2 (2010): 121–8.

– "Frailty, Abjection and the 'Othering' of the Fourth Age." *Health Studies Review* 23, no. 1 (2014): 10–19.

– "Frailty, Disability and Old Age: A Re-appraisal." *Health* 15, no. 5 (2011): 475–90.

– *Rethinking Old Age: Theorising the Fourth Age*. London: Palgrave, 2015.

Hinz, E.J., and J.J. Teunissen. "Milton, Whitman, Wolfe and Laurence: *The Stone Angel* as Elegy." *Dalhousie Review* 65, no. 4 (1985–86): 474–91.

Hirsch, Marianne. "The Generation of Postmemory." *Poetics Today* 29, no. 1 (2008): 103–28.

Hogle, Jerrold E. *The Cambridge Companion to Gothic Fiction*. Cambridge: Cambridge University Press, 2002.

– "Elegy and the Gothic: The Common Grounds." In *The Oxford Handbook of the Elegy*, edited by Karen Wiesman, 565–84. Oxford: Oxford University Press, 2010.

Hollander, John. *Vision and Resonance: Two Senses of Poetic Form*. New York: Oxford University Press, 1975.

Hollobon, Joan. "Can Be Treated: Depression in Aged Mistaken for Senility, Psychiatrists Told." *Globe and Mail* [Toronto], 9 November 1963.

– "Is the Boat Being Missed on Alzheimer's Disease?" *Globe and Mail* [Toronto], 19 February 1983.

Holstein, Martha. "Aging, Culture and the Framing of Alzheimer Disease." In *Concepts of Alzheimer Disease: Biological, Clinical, and Cultural Perspectives*, edited by Peter J. Whitehouse, Konrad Maurer, and Jesse J. Ballenger, 158–80. Baltimore: Johns Hopkins University Press, 2000.

"The Homemaker: 'Live Long and Like It' Proves Worth As Aim." *Globe and Mail* [Toronto], 12 September 1946.

Hopson, Debbie. "Every Moment of Absent-Mindedness Terrifies Me." *Globe and Mail*. Last modified 2 February 2015. Accessed 12 December 2016. http://www.theglobeandmail.com/life/facts-and-arguments/every-moment-of-absent-mindedness-terrifies-me/article22748764/.

Houston, R.A. "'Not Simple Boarding': Care of the Mentally Incapacitated in Scotland During the Long Eighteenth Century." In *Outside the Walls of the Asylum: The History of Care in the Community 1750–2000*, edited by Peter Bartlett and David Wright, 19–44. London: Athlone, 1999.

Howells, Coral Ann. *Contemporary Canadian Women's Fiction*. New York: Palgrave Macmillan, 2003.

Hughes, Sue. "G8 Dementia Summit Agrees on Steps against a 'Great Killer'" *Medscape*. Last Modified 13 December 2013. Accessed 12 December 2016. http://www.medscape.com/viewarticle/817789.

Hutcheon, Linda. *Irony's Edge: The Theory and Politics of Irony*. London: Routledge, 1994.

– *A Theory of Adaptation*. New York: Routledge, 2006.

Ignatieff, Andrew. Personal interview, 25 January 2011.

– Personal interview, 25 June 2014.

– "Thank You." E-mail message to the author, 26 January 2011.

– "My Follow Up." E-mail message to the author, 17 July 2014.

– "Finally." E-mail message to the author, 22 July 2014.

Ignatieff, Michael. "August in My Father's House." *Granta* 14 (August 1984): 38–50.

– "Deficits." *Granta Magazine* 27, no. 7 (July 1989): 78–90.

– *Scar Tissue*. Toronto: Viking, 1993.

"Improvement in Diet Will Delay Senility." *Globe* [Toronto], 28 July 1927.

Ingram, Jay. *The End of Memory: A Natural History of Aging and Alzheimer's*. Toronto: HarperCollins, 2014.

"Insanity in Britain." *Globe* [Toronto], 16 September 1907.

Irigaray, Luce. *This Sex Which Is Not One*. Translated by Catherine Porter and Carolyn Burke. Ithaca: Cornell University Press, 1985.

Jacklin, Kristin, Jessica E. Pace, and Wayne Warry. "Informal Dementia Caregiving among Indigenous Communities in Ontario, Canada." *Care Management Journals* 16, no. 2 (2015): 106–20.

Jacklin, Kristin, Jennifer D. Walker, and Marjory Shawande. "The Emergence of Dementia as a Health Concern among First Nations Populations in Canada." *The Canadian Journal of Public Health* 104, no. 1 (2013): e39–44.

Jacklin, Kristin, and Wayne Warry. "Forgetting and Forgotten: Dementia in Aboriginal Seniors." *Anthropology and Aging Quarterly* 33, no. 1 (2012): 13–21.

Jackson, Mark. *The Borderland of Imbecility: Medicine, Society and the Fabrication of the Feeble Mind in Late Victorian and Edwardian England.* Manchester: Manchester University Press, 2000.

James, Henry. *The Turn of the Screw.* Edited by Peter G. Beidler. Boston: Bedford Books of St Martin's Press, 1995.

Jamieson, Sara. "Reading the Spaces of Age in Alice Munro's 'The Bear Came over the Mountain.'" *Mosaic* 47, no. 3 (2014): 1–17.

Jewson, N.D. "The Disappearance of the Sick-Man from Medical Cosmology, 1770–1870." *Sociology* 10 (May 1976): 225–44.

Kaellis, Eugene, and Rhoda Kaellis. "Odds of Alzheimer's Disease Striking Increase with Age." *Vancouver Sun*, 6 March 1990.

Katz, Stephen. "Alarmist Demography: Power, Knowledge and the Elderly Population," *Journal of Aging Studies* 6, no. 3 (1992): 203–25.

– *Cultural Aging: Life Course, Lifestyle, and Senior Worlds.* Toronto: University of Toronto Press, 2009.

– "What is Age Studies?" *Age, Culture, Humanities: An Interdisciplinary Journal* 1 (Spring 2014): n.p. Accessed 12 December 2016. http://ageculturehumanities.org/WP/what-is-age-studies/.

Katz, Stephen, Paul Higgs, and Simon Williams. "Neuroculture, Active Ageing and the 'Older Brain': Problems, Promises and Prospects." *Sociology of Health and Illness* (2012): 1–15.

Katzman, Robert. "The Prevalence and Malignancy of Alzheimer [sic] Disease: A Major Killer." *Archives of Neurology* 33, no. 4 (1976): 217–18.

Katzman, Robert, and Katherine Bick. *Alzheimer's Disease: The Changing View.* San Diego: Academic, 2000.

Kay, Dennis. *Melodious Tears: The English Funeral Elegy from Spenser to Milton.* New York: Oxford University Press, 1990.

Kennedy, David. *Elegy.* London: Routledge, 2007.

Khatchaturian, Zaven. "Plundered Memories." *Sciences* 37, no. 4 (1997): 20–5.

Kilgour, Maggie. *The Rise of the Gothic Novel*. New York: Routledge, 1995.

Kirkwood, Leone. "Drug an Aid to Elderly Patients Who Were Vegetables, MD Says." *Globe and Mail* [Toronto], 7 January 1971.

Kitamura, Makiko. "Mid-life Stress Linked to Alzheimer's." *Star-Phoenix* [Saskatoon, SK], 5 October 2013.

Kitwood, Thomas. *Dementia Reconsidered: The Person Comes First*. Buckingham, UK: Open University Press, 1997.

Kleinman, Arthur. *The Illness Narratives: Suffering, Healing, and the Human Condition*. New York: Basic, 1988.

Kobayashi, Karen M., and André Smith. "Making Sense of Alzheimer's Disease in an Intergenerational Context: The Case of a Japanese Canadian Nisei (Second-Generation)-Headed Family." *Dementia* 1, no. 2 (June 2002): 213–25.

Kontos, Pia. "Embodied Selfhood: An Ethnographic Exploration of Alzheimer's Disease." In *Thinking About Dementia: Culture, Loss, and the Anthropology of Senility*, edited by Annette Leibing and Lawrence Cohen, 195–217. New Brunswick: Rutgers University Press, 2006.

Kontos, Pia, Karen-Lee Miller, Gail Joyce Mitchell, and Jan Stirling-Twist. "Presence Redefined: The Reciprocal Nature of Engagement between Elder-Clowns and Persons with Dementia." *Dementia: The International Journal of Social Research and Practice*. Accessed 12 December 2016. doi: 10.1177/1471301215580895.

Kotulak, Ronald. "Education Cuts Alzheimer's Risk, Studies Show." *Ottawa Citizen*, 6 May 1993.

Kraepelin, Emil. "Senile and Pre-senile Dementias." In *The Early Story of Alzheimer's Disease: Translation of the Historical Papers by Alois Alzheimer, Oskar Fischer, Francesco Bonfiglio, Emil Kraepelin, Gaetano Perusini*, edited by Katherine Bick, Luigi Amaducci, and Giancarlo Pepeu, 32–81. Padova, Italy: Liviana Press, 1987.

Kriebernegg, Ulla. "Defeating the Nursing Home Specter? Celebrations of Life in the Canadian Short Film 'Rhonda's Party.'" In *Crossroads in American Studies: Transnational and Biocultural Encounters*, edited by Frederike Offizier, Marc Priewe, and Ariane Schröder, 489–506. Heidelberg: Universitätsverlag Winter, 2016.

– "Putting Age in its Place: John Mighton's *Half Life* and Joan Barfoot's *Exit Lines*." *Age, Culture, Humanities: An Interdisciplinary Journal* 2 (2015): n.p. Accessed 12 December 2016. http://ageculturehumanities. org/WP/putting-age-into-place-john-mightons-half-life-and-joan-barfoots-exit-lines/.

Kral, V.A. *Selected Papers of V.A. Kral*. Edited by Harold Mersky. London: Department of Psychiatry, University of Western Ontario, 1989.

Kramer, Reinhold. *Mordecai Richler: Leaving St Urbain*. Montreal: McGill-Queen's University Press, 2008.

Kristeva, Julia. "On the Melancholic Imaginary." Translated by Louise Burchill. In *Discourse in Psychoanalysis and Literature*, edited by Shlomith Rimmon-Kenan, 104–23. New York: Methuen, 1987.

– *Powers of Horror: An Essay on Abjection*. Translated by Leon S. Roudiez. New York: Columbia University Press, 1982.

Krivel, Peter. "U of T Scientist Honoured for Alzheimer's Work." *Toronto Star*, 7 January 1997.

Kroetsch, Robert. "Unhiding the Hidden: Recent Canadian Fiction." *Journal of Canadian Fiction* 3, no. 3 (197): 43–5.

Kühl, Stefan. *The Nazi Connection: Eugenics, American Racism, and German National Socialism*. New York: Oxford University Press, 1994.

Kwentus, Joseph A. "Alzheimer's Disease." In *The Cambridge Historical Dictionary of Disease*, edited by Kenneth F. Kiple. Cambridge: Cambridge University Press, 2003.

L'Arche Canada. "Our History." *L'Arche Canada*. Accessed 13 December 2016. http://www.larche.ca:8080/en_CA/about-larche/our-history.

L.N. Geller, and H. Potter. "Chromosome Missegregation and Trisomy 21 Mosaicism in Alzheimer's Disease." *Neurobiology of Disease* 6, no. 3 (1999): 167–79.

Lacan, Jacques. "The Presence of the Analyst." In *Essential Papers on Transference*, edited by Aaron Esman, 480–91. New York: New York University Press, 1990.

Lage, José Manuel Martinez. "100 Years of Alzheimer's Disease." In *Alzheimer's Disease: A Century of Scientific and Clinical Research*, edited by George Perry, Jesus Avila, June Kinoshita, and Mark A. Smith, 15–26. Amsterdam: 10S, 2006.

Laing, R.D. *The Divided Self: An Existential Study in Sanity and Madness*. London: Tavistock Publishing, 1969.

Lambek, Michael. "Introduction." In *Irony and Illness: On the Ambiguity of Suffering in Culture*, edited by Michael Lambek and Paul Antze, 1–19. New York: Berghahn, 2004.

– "Introduction." In *Ordinary Ethics*, 1–36. New York: Fordham University Press, 2010.

Laplanche, Jean, and J.-B. Pontalis. *The Language of Psycho-Analysis*. Translated by D. Nicholson-Smith. New York: Norton, 1989.

Laslett, Peter. *A Fresh Map of Life: The Emergence of the Third Age*. London: Harvard University Press, 1989.

Laurence, Margaret. *The Stone Angel*. Toronto: McClelland, 1964.

Leacock, Stephen. *Sunshine Sketches of a Little Town*. Toronto: McClelland, 1994.

Learner, Barron H. "Rita Hayworth's Misdiagnosed Struggle." *Los Angeles Times*, 20 November 2006. Accessed 12 December 2016. http://articles.latimes.com/2006/nov/20/health/he-myturn20.

Leavitt, Sarah. *Tangles*. Calgary: Freehand, 2010.

Leckie, Robin. "The Unexpected Gifts of Alzheimer's." *Globe and Mail* [Toronto], 5 April 2012.

Lederman, Marsha. "A New Life for Ignatieff's Powerful Alzheimer's Novel." *Globe and Mail*. Last modified 24 October 2013. Accessed 12 December 2016. http://www.theglobeandmail.com/arts/theatre-and-performance/a-new-life-for-ignatieffs-powerful-alzheimers-novel/article4099682/.

Leibing, Annette, and Lawrence Cohen, eds. *Thinking about Dementia: Culture, Loss, and the Anthropology of Senility*. New Brunswick: Rutgers University Press, 2006.

Leighton, Alexander. *Caring for Mentally Ill People*. London: Cambridge University Press, 1982.

Lemire, Geoff. *Essex County*. Marietta: Top Shelf, 2009.

Leys, Ruth. *Trauma: A Genealogy*. Chicago: Chicago University Press, 2000.

The Liberal Conservative Students of Victoria. "To the Right Hon. Sir John Macdonald." *Daily Mail* [Toronto], 6 December 1886.

"Life Expectancy Rising: Maladies of Elderly Said Major Problem." *Globe and Mail* [Toronto], 29 September 1959.

Life, Patricia. "Long-Term Caring: Canadian Literary Narratives of Personal Agency and Identity in Late Life." PhD diss., University of Ottawa, 2014.

Lipovenko, Dorothy. "Alzheimer Group Counsels Families with Senile Member." *Globe and Mail* [Toronto], 17 January 1981.

– "Alzheimer's a Risk for Down's Adults." *Globe and Mail* [Toronto], 19 July 1995.

Lloyd-Smith, Alan. *American Gothic Fiction: An Introduction*. New York: Continuum, 2004.

Lock, Margaret. *The Alzheimer Conundrum: Entanglements of Dementia and Aging*. Princeton: Princeton University Press, 2013.

Locke, John. *An Essay Concerning Human Understanding*. Edited by Roger Woolhouse. New York and London: Penguin, 1997.

Loewald, H.W. "The Therapeutic Action of Psychoanalysis." In *Papers on Psychoanalysis*, 221–56. New Haven: Yale University Press, 1960.

Lowman, Josephine. "Why Grow Old? Medical Aid Holds Back Age Onset." *Globe and Mail* [Toronto], 16 August 1943.

Lyman, Karen A. "Bringing the Social Back In: A Critique of the Biomedicalization of Dementia." In *Aging and Everyday Life*, edited by Jaber F. Gubrium and James A. Holstein, 340–56. Malden, MA: Wiley-Blackwell, 2000.

Lynch, Gerald. "Stephen Leacock." *The Canadian Encyclopedia*. Last modified 4 March, 2015. Accessed 12 December 2016. http://www. thecanadianencyclopedia.ca/en/article/stephen-leacock/.

MacDonald, Bruce. "Will Senility Kill Canada's Senate?" *Globe and Mail* [Toronto], 29 April 1961.

MacDonald, Gayle. "A Need for Change in the Unbalanced Approach to Alzheimer's." *Globe and Mail*. Last modified 4 February 2015. Accessed 12 December 2016. http://www.theglobeandmail.com/ life/health-and-fitness/health/a-need-for-change-in-the-unbalanced-approach-to-alzheimers/article22786347/.

Maclear, Kyo. *The Letter Opener*. Toronto: HarperCollins, 2007.

Maddox, Brenda. *Freud's Wizard: Ernest Jones and the Transformation of Psychoanalysis*. Cambridge: Da Capo, 2007.

"The Man of Fifty." *Globe* [Toronto], 22 April 1930.

Marchione, Marilynn. "U.S. Alzheimer's Rate Seems to Be Dropping." *Tyler Morning Telegraph* [Tyler, TX], 15 July 2014. Accessed 12 December 2016. http://www.tylerpaper.com/TP-News+Health/ 202469/video-us-alzheimers-rate-seems-to-be-dropping-study-shows.

Marshall, Leni. "Ageility Studies: The Interplay of Critical Approaches in Age Studies and Disability Studies." In *Alive and Kicking at All Ages*, edited by Ulla Kriebernegg, Roberta Maierhofer, and Barbara Ratenbock, 21–40. Bielefeld: Transcript Verlag.

Mason, Jody. "Dementia in Early Canadian Writing." E-mail message to the author, 7 September 2015.

Matthews, Fiona E., Antony Arthur, Linda E. Barnes, John Bond, Carol Jagger, Louise Robinson, and Carol Brayne. "A Two-Decade Comparison of Prevalence of Dementia in Individuals Aged 65 Years and Older from Three Geographical Areas of England: Results of the Cognitive Function and Ageing Study I and II." *The Lancet* 382 (26 October 2013): 1405–12. Accessed 12 December 2016. doi: 10.1016/S0140-6736(13)61570-6.

Maurer, Konrad, and Ulrike Maurer. *Alois Alzheimer: His Life and Work*. Marburg: Prepress Print Production Services, 2002.

Maurer, Konrad, Stephan Volk, and Hector Gerbaldo. "The History of Alois Alzheimer's First Case." In *Concepts of Alzheimer Disease: Biological, Clinical, and Cultural Perspectives*, edited by Peter J. Whitehouse, Konrad Maurer, and Jesse J. Ballenger, 5–29. Baltimore: Johns Hopkins University Press, 2000.

McAree, J.V. "Asylums of Canada Disgrace to Nation." *Globe and Mail* [Toronto], 11 March 1947.

– "Mentally Deficient Still Multiplying." *Globe* [Toronto], 30 November 1939.

McLaren, Angus. *Our Own Master Race: Eugenics in Canada, 1885–1945*. Toronto: McClelland, 1990.

Micale, Mark. *Approaching Hysteria: Disease and Its Interpretations*. Princeton: Princeton University Press, 1995.

Mighton, John. *Half Life*. Toronto: Playwrights Canada, 2005.

Miller, Edgar. "Idiocy in the Nineteenth Century." *History of Psychiatry* 7 (1996): 361–73.

Milton, John. "Lycidas." *Representative Poetry Online*. Accessed 12 December 2016. https://rpo.library.utoronto.ca/poems/lycidas.

– *Paradise Lost: Book I. Representative Poetry Online*. Accessed 12 December 2016. https://rpo.library.utoronto.ca/poems/paradise-lost-book-i.

Mitchinson, Wendy. *Body Failure: Medical Views of Women, 1900–1950*. Toronto: University of Toronto Press, 2013.

Möller, Hans-Jürgen, and Manuel B. Graeber. "Johann F.: The Historical Relevance of the Case of the Concept of Alzheimer Disease." In *Concepts of Alzheimer Disease: Biological, Clinical, and Cultural Perspectives*, edited by Peter J. Whitehouse, Konrad Maurer, and Jesse J. Ballenger, 30–46. Baltimore: Johns Hopkins University Press, 2000.

Montigny, Edgar-André. "The Economic Role of the Elderly within the Family: Evidence from Turn-of-the-Century Ontario." In *Family Matters: Papers in Post-Confederation Canadian Family History*, edited by Lori Chambers and Edgar-André Montigny, 459–74. Toronto: Canadian Scholars' Press, 1998.

– *Foisted on the Government*. Montreal: McGill-Queen's University Press, 1997.

– "'Foisted upon the Government': Institutions and the Impact of Public Policy upon the Aged. The Elderly Patients at Rockwood Asylum, 1866–1906." *Journal of Social History* 28, no. 4 (1995): 819–36.

Moore, Jeffrey. *The Memory Artists*. Toronto: Viking, 2004.

Moorhouse, Aynsley. "An Artist's Statement, The Sounds of Forgetting: An Aural Exploration of Memory and Perception." *Occasion: Interdisciplinary Studies in the Humanities* 4 (14 June 2012). Accessed 12 December 2016. http://arcade.stanford.edu/occasion/artist%E2%80%99s-statement-sounds-forgetting-aural-exploration-memory-and-perception.

Mulan, Phil. *The Imaginary Time Bomb: Why an Ageing Population Is Not a Social Problem*. London: I.B. Tauris Publishers, 2000.

Munro, Alice. "The Bear Came over the Mountain." *New Yorker*, 27 December 1999.

– *The Beggar Maid: Stories of Rose and Flo*. New York: Knopf, 1979.

– "Dance of the Happy Shades." In *Dance of the Happy Shades*, 211–24. Toronto: McGraw-Hill Ryerson, 1968.

– *Lives of Girls and Women*. Toronto: McGraw-Hill Ryerson, 1971.

– "An Ounce of Cure." In *Dance of the Happy Shades*, 75–88. Toronto: McGraw-Hill Ryerson, 1968.

– "The Peace of Utrecht." In *Dance of the Happy Shades*, 190–210. Toronto: McGraw-Hill Ryerson, 1968.

– "Powers." In *Runaway*, 270–335. Toronto: McClelland, 2004.

– "In Sight of the Lake." In *Dear Life*, 217–32. Toronto: McClelland, 2012.

– "Walking on Water." In *Something I've Been Meaning to Tell You: Thirteen Stories*, 54–74. Toronto: McGraw-Hill Ryerson, 1974.

– *Who Do You Think You Are?: Stories*. Toronto: MacMillan of Canada, 1978.

Nascher, Ignatz Leo. *Geriatrics, the Diseases of Old Age and Their Treatment, Including Physiological Old Age, Home and Institutional Care, and Medico-Legal Relations*. London: Paul, 1914.

Nash, J. Madeleine. "The New Science of Alzheimer's." *Time*, 17 July 2000. Accessed 12 December 2016. http://content.time.com/time/world/article/0,8599,2047536,00.html.

National Academy on an Aging Society. *Demography is Not Destiny*. Washington, DC: National Academy on an Aging Society, 1999.

Neergaard, Lauran. "Report Sounds Alarm for Worldwide Alzheimer's 'Emergency.'" *Toronto Star*, 21 September 2009.

Neuberger, Julia. *Not Dead Yet: A Manifesto for Old Age*. London: HarperCollins, 2009.

Neufeldt, Aldred. "Growth and Evolution of Disability Advocacy in Canada." In *Making Equality: History of Advocacy and Persons with*

Disabilities in Canada, edited by Deborah Stienstra and Aileen Wight-Felske, 11–32. Toronto: Captus Press, 2003.

"nocebo, n." *Oxford English Dictionary*. Oxford University Press. Last modified September 2013. Accessed 24 March 2016.

Ondaatje, Michael. *Coming through Slaughter*. Toronto: Anansi, 1976.

"Oxygen Boost for Old Described as Quackery." *Globe and Mail* [Toronto], 10 October 1977.

"Parkinson's Disease." In *Mosby's Dictionary of Medicine, Nursing & Health Professions*, edited by Mosby, Inc. Philadelphia: Elsevier Health Sciences, 2012.

Paton, Maureen. "RD Laing: Was the Counterculture's Favourite Psychiatrist a Dangerous Renegade or a True Visionary?" *Independent* [London], 30 November 2015. Accessed 12 December 2016. http://www.independent.co.uk/life-style/health-and-families/rd-laing-was-the-countercultures-favourite-psychiatrist-a-dangerous-renegade-or-a-true-visionary-a6755021.html.

"Penfield Says Retired Should Not Go to Pot." *Globe and Mail* [Toronto], 8 June 1960.

"People with 10 Years of Education Less Likely to Get Alzheimer's: Report" *Gazette* [Montreal], 12 November 1994.

Perl, D. "Neuropathology of Alzheimer's Disease." *Mount Sinai Journal of Medicine* (2010): 32–42.

Perusini, Gaetano. "Histology and Clinical Findings of Some Psychiatric Disease of Older People." In *The Early Story of Alzheimer's Disease: Translation of the Historical Papers by Alois Alzheimer, Oskar Fischer, Francesco Bonfiglio, Emil Kraepelin, Gaetano Perusini*, edited by Katherine Bick, Luigi Amaducci, and Giancarlo Pepeu, 82–128. Padova, Italy: Liviana Press, 1987.

– "The Nosographic Value of Some Characteristic Histopathological Findings in Senility." In *The Early Story of Alzheimer's Disease: Translation of the Historical Papers by Alois Alzheimer, Oskar Fischer, Francesco Bonfiglio, Emil Kraepelin, Gaetano Perusini*, edited by Katherine Bick, Luigi Amaducci, and Giancarlo Pepeu, 129–47. Padova, Italy: Liviana Press, 1987.

Peters, Kevin R., and Stephen Katz. "Interview with Dr Ronald Petersen, 7 February 2013." *Dementia* 14, no. 3 (2015): 298–306.

– "Voices from the Field: Expert Reflections on Mild Cognitive Impairment." *Dementia* 14, no. 3 (2015): 285–97.

Picard, André. "'Alarming' Rise in Dementia Comes with a Crippling Price Tag." *Globe and Mail* [Toronto], 21 September 2010.

- "Developing Alzheimer's Linked to Lifestyle More than Genetics." *Globe and Mail* [Toronto], 22 July 2004.
- "New Research Indicates Seven Health Risks That Are Contributing to Alzheimer's." *Globe and Mail* [Toronto], 20 July 2011.

Pinel, Philippe. *Traité médico-philosophique sur l'aliénation mentale; ou la manie.* 2nd ed. Paris: Caille et Ravier, 1809.

"placebo, n." *Oxford English Dictionary.* Oxford University Press. Last modified March 2016. Accessed 24 March 2016.

Post, Stephen. "The Concept of Alzheimer's Disease in a Hypercognitive Society." In *Concepts of Alzheimer Disease: Biological, Clinical, and Cultural Perspectives,* edited by Peter J. Whitehouse, Konrad Maurer, and Jesse J. Ballenger, 245–56. Baltimore: Johns Hopkins University Press, 2000.

Powell, Sarah. "'I Can't Be Sure': Illness and Selfhood in Sarah Polley's *Away From Her.*" Graduate seminar paper, University of Toronto, 2014.

"The Premier and His Colleagues at Orillia." *Daily Mail* [Toronto], 1 December 1886.

Rae-Grant, Quentin, ed. *Images in Psychiatry: Canada.* Washington: American Psychiatric, 1996.

- *Psychiatry in Canada: 50 Years.* Ottawa: CPA, 2001.

Raluca Burlea, Suzana. "Encountering the Suffering Other in Illness Narratives: Between the Memory of Suffering and the Suffering Memory." PhD diss., Université de Montréal, 2010.

Rankin, Lissa. "The Nocebo Effect: Negative Thoughts Can Harm Your Health." *Psychology Today,* 6 August 2013. Accessed 12 December 2016. https://www.psychologytoday.com/blog/owning-pink/201308/the-nocebo-effect-negative-thoughts-can-harm-your-health.

Reaume, Geoffrey. *Remembrance of Patients Past: Patient Life at the Toronto Hospital For the Insane, 1870–1940.* Toronto: University of Toronto Press, 2009.

Redekop, Magdalene. *Mothers and Other Clowns: The Stories of Alice Munro.* London: Routledge, 1992.

Redhill, Michael. *Goodness.* Toronto: Coach House, 2005.

Revie, Nancy. "A Boomer is a Zoomer If They Want to Be." *Guelph Mercury,* 26 June 2014. Accessed 12 December 2016. http://www.guelphmercury.com/opinion-story/4598347-a-boomer-is-a-zoomer-if-they-want-to-be/.

Rex, Kathleen. "Grade 1 is Not Too Early to Find Out about Drugs, Psychiatrist Believes." *Globe and Mail* [Toronto], 21 September 1979.

Richler, Mordecai. *Barney's Version.* Toronto: Knopf, 1997.

– "The Summer My Grandmother Was Supposed to Die." In *An Anthology of Canadian Literature in English*, rev. and abbrev. ed., edited by Russell Brown, Donna Bennett, and Nathalie Cooke, 327–36. Toronto: Oxford University Press, 1991.

Riegel, Christian. *Writing Grief: Margaret Laurence and the Work of Mourning*. Winnipeg: University of Manitoba Press, 2003.

Riley II, Charles, A. *Disability in the Media: Prescriptions for Change*. Hanover, NH: University Press of New England, 2005.

"Rita Hayworth Dies at 68; 'Love Goddess' of '40s a Victim of Alzheimer's." *Gazette* [Montreal], 16 May 1987.

Robertson, J. Ross. "Commentary." *Toronto Telegram*, 31 December 1885.

– "The Contest on Monday." *Toronto Telegram*, 2 January 1886.

– "Editorial." *Toronto Telegram*, 26 December 1883.

Ross, Catherine Sheldrick. *Alice Munro: A Double Life*. Toronto: ECW Press, 1992.

Rothschild, David, and M.L. Sharp. "The Origin of Senile Psychoses: Neuropathologic Factors and Factors of a More Personal Nature." *Diseases of the Nervous System* 2 (1941): 49–54.

Rothschild, David, and Sidney L. Sands. "Sociopsychiatric Foundations for a Theory of the Reactions to Aging." *The Journal of Nervous and Mental Disease* 116, no. 3 (1952): 233–41.

Rotstein, Gary. "Alzheimer's Treatment Research Disappoints" *The Times and Transcript* [Moncton, NB], 1 December 2012.

Roy, Wendy. "The Word is Colander: Language, Loss, and Narrative Voice in Fictional Canadian Alzheimer's Narratives." *Canadian Literature* (Winter 2009): 41–61.

Rudy, Lisa Jo. "What Does It Mean to Be Neurotypical?" *Very Well*. Last modified 13 June 2016. Accessed 12 December 2016. https://www.verywell.com/what-does-it-mean-to-be-neurotypical-260047.

Rule, Jane. *Memory Board*. Toronto: Macmillan, 1987.

Russo, Mary. "Aging and the Scandal of Anachronism." In *Figuring Age: Women, Bodies, Generations*, edited by Kathleen Woodward, 20–33. Bloomington and Indianapolis: Indiana University Press, 1996.

Sabatini, Sandra. *The One with the News*. Erin: Porcupine's Quill, 2000.

Sacks, Peter M. *The English Elegy: Studies in the Genre from Spenser to Yeats*. Baltimore: Johns Hopkins University Press, 1985.

Salter, Jodie Lynne. "Intergenerational Storytelling and Transhistorical Trauma: Old Women in Contemporary Canadian Fiction." PhD diss., University of Guelph, 2012.

"A Sad Ruin." *Globe* [Toronto], 5 May 1886.

Savoy, Eric. "The Face of the Tenant: A Theory of American Gothic." In *American Gothic: New Interventions in a National Narrative*, edited by Robert K. Martin and Eric Savoy, 3–19. Iowa City: University of Iowa Press, 1998.

Scharf, Thomas. "Too Tight to Mention: Unequal Income in Her Old Age." In *Unequal Ageing: The Untold Story of Exclusion in Old Age*, edited by Paul Cann and Malcolm Dean, 25–52. Bristol: Policy Press, 2009.

Sedgwick, Eve Kosofsky. *The Coherence of Gothic Conventions*. New York: Arno, 1980.

– *Touching Feeling: Affect, Pedagogy, Performativity*. Durham: Duke University Press, 2003.

Selye, Hans. *The Stress of Life*. New York: McGraw-Hill, 1956.

"Senility Label Criticized." *Globe and Mail* [Toronto], 17 May 1963.

Shakespeare, William. *The Tempest*. Edited by Herbert E. Greene. New York: McMillan, 1913.

Shelley, Mary. *Frankenstein or The Modern Prometheus*. 1818. London: Oxford University Press, 1969.

Shenk, David. *The Forgetting: Alzheimer's Portrait of an Epidemic*. New York: Doubleday, 2001.

Sherman, David. "Dementia – A Fight We Can't Afford to Lose: U.S.-Born Scientist Hoping to Turn Toronto into One of Continent's Leading Research Centres for Alzheimer's, Related Conditions." *Toronto Star*, 12 August 2013.

– "Dementia Researcher Barry Greenberg Leading Canada's Efforts Against Growing Scourge." *Thestar.com*, 12 August 2013. Accessed 12 December 2016. https://www.thestar.com/life/health_wellness/2013/08/12/dementia_researcher_barry_greenberg_leading_canadas_efforts_against_growing_scourge.html.

Shorter, Edward. *A Historical Dictionary of Psychiatry*. New York: Oxford University Press, 2005.

– *A History of Psychiatry: From the Era of the Asylum to the Age of Prozac*. Toronto: John Wiley & Sons, 1997.

Showalter, Elaine. "Hysteria, Feminism, and Gender." In *Hysteria Beyond Freud*, 286–344. Berkeley: University of California Press, 1993.

– *Hystories: Hysterical Epidemics and Modern Culture*. New York: Columbia University Press, 1997.

Simmons, Harvey G. *Unbalanced: Mental Health Policy in Ontario, 1930–1989*. Toronto: Wall, 1990.

Sinha, Samir. "Introductory Remarks to the Film *You're Looking at Me Like I Live Here, But I Don't*." Introductory remarks presented at the University of Toronto at Scarborough's International Health Film Series and Expo, Toronto, Ontario, 12 March 2015.

"Sir John Indisposed." *Daily Mail* [Toronto], 3 December 1886.

Smith, Andrew. *Gothic Literature*. Edinburgh: Edinburgh University Press, 2007.

Smythe, Karen E. *Figuring Grief. Gallant, Munro, and the Poetics of Elegy*. Montreal: McGill-Queen's University Press, 1992.

Snell, James. "The Family and the Working-Class Elderly in the First Half of the Twentieth Century." In *Family Matters: Papers in Post-Confederation Canadian Family History*, edited by Lori Chambers and Edgar-André Montigny, 499–510. Toronto: Canadian Scholars' Press, 1998.

Sommer, Doris. "Attitude, Its Rhetoric." In *The Turn to Ethics*, edited by Marjorie Garber, Beatrice Hanssen, and Rebecca Walkowitz, 201–20. New York: Routledge, 2000.

Sontag, Susan. *AIDS and its Metaphors*. New York: Farrar, Strauss, and Giroux, 1989.

– "An Essay by Susan Sontag." In *Antonin Artaud: Selected Writings*, xvii–lix. New York: Farrar, 1976.

– *Illness as Metaphor*. New York: Farrar, 1978.

Sparshott, F. *The Theory of the Arts*. Princeton: Princeton University Press, 1982.

Spencer, J. "An Unusual Exchange." *Christian Guardian* [Toronto], 31 July 1861.

Spurgeon, David. "How Many Years Does It Take to Reach Old Age?" *Globe and Mail* [Toronto], 25 October 1962.

Sterling, Joe, and Ben Brumfield. "Canada's Alice Munro, 'Master' of Short Stories, Wins Nobel Prize in Literature." *CNN*, 10 October 2013. Accessed 12 December 2016. http://www.cnn.com/2013/10/10/living/nobel-prize-literature/.

Stewart, Graeme, ed. *Concrete Toronto*. Toronto: Coach House, 2007.

Stewart, Stormie. "The Elderly Poor in Rural Ontario: Inmates of the Wellington Country House of Industry, 1877–1907." In *Family Matters: Papers in Post-Confederation Canadian Family History*, edited by Lori Chambers and Edgar-André Montigny, 417–36. Toronto: Canadian Scholars' Press, 1998.

Stiles, Anne. "The Rest Cure, 1873–1925." In BRANCH: *Britain, Representation and Nineteenth-Century History*, edited by Dino Franco Felluga. *Romanticism and Victorianism on the*

Net. Accessed 12 December 2016. http://www.branchcollective.org/?ps_articles=anne-stiles-the-rest-cure-1873-1925.

Stoker, Bram. *Dracula*. Edited by Roger Luckhurst. Oxford: Oxford University Press, 2011.

Stoner, L.G. "Home Forum: The Question of Old Age." *Globe and Mail* [Toronto], 7 July 1944.

Strachey, Lytton. *Eminent Victorians: The Illustrated Edition*. New York: Weidenfeld & Nicolson, 1988.

"Stresses Need to Study Health of Elderly Folk." *Globe and Mail* [Toronto], 26 January 1951.

Sugars, Cynthia. "Canadian Gothic." In *A New Companion to the Gothic*, edited by David Punter, 409–27. West Sussex: Wiley-Blackwell, 2012.

Symons, Thomas H.B. "Ryerson, William." In *Dictionary of Canadian Biography*, vol. 10. University of Toronto/Université Laval, 1972. Accessed 12 December 2016. http://www.biographi.ca/en/bio/ryerson_william_10E.html.

Szabo, Sandor, Yvette Tache, and Arpad Somogyi. "The Legacy of Hans Selye and the Origins of Stress Research: A Retrospective 75 Years after His Landmark Brief 'Letter' to the Editor of *Nature*." *Stress* 15, no. 5 (Jan. 2012): 472–8.

Taylor, Paul. "On the Trail of the Mind Killer." *Globe and Mail* [Toronto], 21 January, 1993.

Thane, Pat. *Old Age in English History: Past Experience, Present Issues*. Oxford: Oxford University Press, 2000.

Thomas, Audrey. *Mrs Blood*. Vancouver: Talonbooks, 1970.

Townsend, Sally. "How Never to Grow Old." *Globe and Mail* [Toronto], 23 December 1944.

"trauma, n." *Oxford English Dictionary*. Oxford University Press. Last modified March 2016. Accessed 23 March 2016.

Turcotte, Martin, and Grant Schellenberg. *A Portrait of Seniors in Canada*. Ottawa: Statistics Canada, 2006.

Turner, B.S. *Can We Live Forever?* London: Anthem, 2009.

Tyhurst, J.S., F.C.R. Chalke, F.S. Lawson, B.H. McNeel, C.A. Roberts, G.C. Taylor, R.J. Weil, and J.D. Griffin. *More for the Mind: A Study of Psychiatric Services in Canada*. Toronto: Canadian Mental Health Association, 1963.

"Unetanneh Tokef." *Wikipedia*. Last modified 8 December 2016. Accessed 12 December 2016. https://en.wikipedia.org/wiki/Unetanneh_Tokef.

Valpy, Michael. "Being Michael Ignatieff." *Globe and Mail*. Last modified 22 August 2012. Accessed 12 December 2016. http://

www.theglobeandmail.com/news/politics/being-michael-ignatieff/
  article4325078/?page=all.
van der Kolk, Bessel A. "The Body Keeps the Score: Memory and the
  Evolving Psychobiology of Posttraumatic Stress." *Harvard Review of
  Psychiatry* 1, no. 5 (1994): 253–65.
Ventura, Héliane. "The Skald and the Goddess: Reading 'The Bear Came
  Over the Mountain' by Alice Munro." *Journal of the Short Story in
  English* 55 (Autumn 2010). Accessed 12 December 2016. https://jsse.
  revues.org/1121.
Vidal, F. "Brainhood, Anthropological Figure of Modernity." *History of the
  Human Sciences* 22, no. 1 (2009): 5–36.
Vickery, John. *The Prose Elegy: An Exploration of Modern American
  and British Fiction*. Baton Rouge: Louisiana State University Press,
  2009.
Volker, Roelcke, Paul Weindling, and Louise Westwood, eds. *International
  Relations in Psychiatry: Britain, Germany, and the United States to
  World War II*. New York: University of Rochester Press, 2010.
Warsh, Cheryl Krasnick. *Moments of Unreason: The Practice of Canadian
  Psychiatry and the Homewood Retreat, 1883–1923*. Montreal: McGill-
  Queen's University Press, 1989.
Watson, Sheila. *The Double Hook*. Toronto: McClelland and Stewart,
  1959.
– *Five Stories*. Toronto: Coach House, 1984.
Watts, Isaac. *The Psalms of David, imitated in the language of the New
  Testament, and applied to the Christian state and worship*. London:
  T. Longman, 1753.
Weiner, Myron F., and Anne M. Lipton, eds. *The American Psychiatric
  Textbook of Alzheimer Disease and Other Dementias*. Washington, D C
  and London: American Psychiatric Pub., 2009.
Whitehead, Ann. *Memory*. London: Routledge, 2009.
Whitehouse, Peter J. "History and the Future of Alzheimer Disease."
  In *Concepts of Alzheimer Disease: Biological, Clinical, and Cultural
  Perspectives*, edited by Peter J. Whitehouse, Konrad Maurer, and Jesse J.
  Ballenger, 291–306. Baltimore: Johns Hopkins University Press, 2000.
Whitehouse, Peter J. and Daniel George. *The Myth of Alzheimer's: What
  You Aren't Being Told about Today's Most Dreaded Diagnosis*. Detroit:
  Gale Cengage Learning, 2009.
– "The War (on Terror) on Alzheimer's." *Dementia* 13, no. 1 (January
  2014): 120–30.

Whitehouse, Peter J., Konrad Maurer, and Jesse Ballenger, eds. *Concepts of Alzheimer's Disease: Biological, Clinical, and Cultural Perspectives.* Baltimore: Johns Hopkins University Press, 2000.

Whitman, Walt. "When Lilacs Last in the Dooryard Bloom'd." 1865. *Poetry Foundation.* Accessed 12 December 2016. https://www.poetry-foundation.org/poems-and-poets/poems/detail/45480.

Wilde, Oscar. *The Picture of Dorian Gray.* Edited by Andrew Elfenbein. New York: Pearson Longman, 2007.

Wilson, Ethel. *The Innocent Traveller.* Toronto: MacMillan, 1949.

Wolfe, Thomas. *Look Homeward, Angel.* New York: Grossett & Dunlap, 1929.

Woodward, Kathleen. "Introduction." In *Figuring Age: Women, Bodies, Generations,* edited by Kathleen Woodward, ix–xxix. Bloomington and Indianapolis: Indiana University Press, 1999.

– "Inventing Generational Models: Psychoanalysis, Feminism, Literature." In *Figuring Age: Women, Bodies, Generations,* edited by Kathleen Woodward, 149–70. Bloomington and Indianapolis: Indiana University Press, 1999.

– *Statistical Panic: Cultural Politics and Poetics of Emotions.* Durham: Duke University Press, 2009.

Woolf, Virginia. *Diary.* Vol. 3. Edited by Anne Oliver Bell. London: Penguin/Hogarth, 1982.

Wordsworth, William. "The World is Too Much with Us." *Representative Poetry Online.* Accessed 12 December 2016. http://rpo.library.utoronto.ca/poems/world-too-much-us.

Wright, David. *Downs: The History of a Disability.* New York: Oxford University Press, 2011.

Wright, David, James Moran, and Sean Gouglas. "The Confinement of the Insane in Victorian Canada: The Hamilton and Toronto Asylums, c. 1861–1891." In *The Confinement of the Insane: International Perspectives 1800–1965,* edited by Roy Porter and David Wright, 100–28. Cambridge: Cambridge University Press, 2013.

Yang, Jennifer. "Dementia: A Private Tragedy Looms as a Public Catastrophe Worldwide." *Thestar.com,* 22 March 2015. Accessed 12 December 2016. https://www.thestar.com/news/world/2015/03/22/dementia-a-private-tragedy-looms-as-a-public-catastrophe-worldwide.html.

Yeats, William Butler. "Sailing to Byzantium." In *W.B. Yeats: Selected Poetry,* edited by A. Norman Jeffares, 104–5. London: Macmillan, 1968.

Young, Alan. *The Harmony of Illusions: Inventing Post-Traumatic Stress Disorder*. Princeton: Princeton University Press, 1995.

Zeiger, Melissa. *Beyond Consolation: Death, Sexuality, and the Changing Shapes of Elegy*. Ithaca: Cornell University Press, 1997.

Zeilig, Hannah. "Dementia As a Cultural Metaphor." *The Gerontologist* 52, no. 4 (2014): 258–67.

Index

abjection: and Alzheimer's disease, 32; and animality, 241; and dementia in literature, 131, 143, 146–8, 236, 265; inversion of elegy, 192; Kristeva and, 32, 123, 236; literary figures of, 261–2, 270, 326, 374n32; and old age, 272. *See also* Kristeva, Julia

Adderson, Caroline, 44; *A History of Forgetting*, 237, 238–45, 247–53, 262, 265–8, 273, 276–7, 282, 320

ageism, 117–18, 159–60, 242, 321–3, 349n58, 367n14

age studies, 7, 11, 39; and critical paranoia, 320; and disability studies, 344n10; and literary studies, 8, 10–12, 345n14. *See also* aging; Basting, Anne Davis; Fuchs, Elinor; Gullette, Margaret Morganroth; old age

aging, 8, 10–11, 21, 50, 84–5, 95, 120, 152, 270–2, 350n68; and Alzheimer's disease, 11, 17, 18, 73, 205, 306; and decline, 121, 128, 133, 136–7, 256, 313, 336; and disease, 49, 66, 68, 95–6,

167–8, 357n4, 366n12; fear of, 41, 83–4; Gothic forms of, 34, 79, 91, 95; and institutionalization, 50, 94, 96, 105–6; in the media, 81, 84, 114–16, 124–5, 148, 159; medicalization of, 40, 91–2, 119–20, 149, 224; and memory loss, 13, 123–4, 164; "menace" of, 78–9, 88, 90, 172; and modernization, 96, 112–13, 128, 365n6; religious views of, 91–2, 114, 119, 129; socio-psychiatric theory of, 155, 158; stress and, 42, 155, 165–6, 379n11; and waste, 111–12, 114, 119, 121, 128, 140; women and, 49, 50, 66, 68, 76, 237. *See also* apocalyptic demography; decline; degeneration; Kraepelin, Emil; old age

Aging, National Institute on, 193

AIDS, 3–4, 15, 22, 149–50, 270, 320–2, 343n4

Alias Grace (Atwood), 389

Alzheimer, Alois, 52–9, 59–61, 308, 354–5n17; discovery of Alzheimer's, 37, 39, 49–50